SMOKING AND HEALTH RESEARCH FRONTIERS

SMOKING AND HEALTH RESEARCH FRONTIERS

CALVIN B. FONG
EDITOR

Nova Science Publishers, Inc.
New York

For permission to use material from this book please contact us:
Telephone 631-231-7269; Fax 631-231-8175
Web Site: http://www.novapublishers.com

LIBRARY OF CONGRESS CATALOGING-IN-PUBLICATION DATA

Smoking and health research frontiers / Calvin B. Fong (editor)
p.; cm.
Includes bibliographical references and index.
ISBN 1-60021-480-0
1. Smoking—Health aspects. 2. Passive smoking. 3. Smoking cessation. I. Fong, Calvin B.
[DNLM: 1. Smoking—adverse effects. 2. Maternal Exposure --adverse effects. 3. Tobacco Smoke Pollution—adverse effects.
QV 137 S6662 2006]
RA1242. T6S5884 2006
362.29'6--c22
2006032297

Published by Nova Science Publishers, Inc. ✦ New York

CONTENTS

PREFACE

Smoking is a greater cause of death and disability than any single disease, says the World Health Organisation. According to their figures, it is responsible for approximately five million deaths worldwide every year. Tobacco smoking is a known or probable cause of approximately 25 diseases including cancer, heart attacks and strokes. The WHO says that its impact on world health is still not fully assessed. This new book offers leading edge research from around the globe with a focus on smoking cessation and the effects of passive smoking on health.

Chapter 1 - Collaborations among various disciplines concerned with smoking cessation and prevention are gaining in currency. Such collaborations are predicated, in part, on recognizing both the implicit assumptions in different fields and the consequences of these assumptions. These issues, however, are usually not considered in transdisciplinary research. In this article, we demonstrate how indices, such as the risk ratio, attributable fraction, or R-squared, have different implications for causal inference and interventions, depending on study setting and research goals.

Chapter 2 - Second-hand smoke (SHS) is also referred as passive smoke, involuntary smoke, environmental tobacco smoke, and environmental cigarette smoke. The sources of SHS include exposure from relatives at home, work place, and in public. Experimental and epidemiologic studies have observed the intake and metabolism of SHS (National Research Council (U.S.).

Part of the importance of SHS stems from the fact that the levels of some carcinogens, e.g., polycyclic aromatic hydrocarbon (PAH), benzo(a)pyrene (BP) and 4-aminobiphenyl (4-ABP, an arylamine), are actually higher in undiluted SHS than in mainstream smoke (i.e., active smoke) (National Research Council 1986). In addition, the size of the particles in SHS is smaller than those in mainstream smoke and, therefore, these particles are more likely to be deposited in the lung (Dockery and Trichopoulos 1997; Hecht 1999). The association between SHS and lung cancer or childhood asthma has been studied extensively. While it is well-recognized that 80-90% of all lung cancer is attributable to cigarette smoking, only 15% of all smokers develop this disease and about 10% of all diagnosed lung cancers are never smokers (Hammond and Seidman 1980).

In summary, for different health effects, significant associations have been observed in genetic markers, including risk modification by germline polymorphisms, gene expression changes, and somatic alterations.

Some gaps in our knowledge of SHS health effects remain. The associations between sequence variants of genes involved in phase I and II metabolism and cell cycle pathways and the risk of lung cancer have been widely explored for SHS exposure and conclusive findings are not yet available.

Chapter 3 - Although tobacco smoking is a widely recognized health hazard and a major cause of preventable mortality, smoking remains prevalent in our society. Approximately 30% of women and 35% of men of reproductive age smoke. But more importantly, the incidence of smoking is increasing among adolescents and specifically teenage girls. Environmental tobacco smoke (ETS), or passive smoke, is a significant source of exposure to a large number of substances known to be hazardous to human health. Recently, substantial harmful effects of cigarette smoke on the ability to become pregnant have become apparent. The deleterious effect of passive smoke exposure is similar to active smoking with respect to fertility. Women who smoke take longer to achieve a natural pregnancy, require more hormonal stimulation during IVF treatment with reduced success, and reach menopause earlier than their non-smoking counterparts. Toxicants found in passive smoke have been isolated at higher levels in the serum and follicular fluid of women exposed to ETS compared to non-smokers implying that cigarette smoke may act as an ovarian toxicant as one mechanism to disrupt fertility. However, the male contribution to infertility cannot be excluded. The paternal effect on infertility is largely dependant on sperm function. The effect of cotinine, for example, has been shown to alter sperm function, and may be an underlying mechanism of impaired fertility. Paternal smoking is associated with sperm with a higher incidence of DNA abnormalities that may account for higher implantation failures and miscarriage rates. Both the female and male gamete are sensitive to toxic exposure(s) and slight alterations to either the sperm or oocyte may be lethal at the peri-implantation stage of embryo development leading to sub-fertility. Passive smoke exposure may induce toxic effects and compromise fertility through several direct or indirect mechanisms.

Chapter 4 - Multiple sources of evidence have linked secondhand smoke to cardiovascular disease (CVD) in adults. While the prevalence of this exposure has decreased in the past 20 years, a substantial proportion of the population (43%) still remains exposed. The relative risk of CVD in passive smokers is approximately 1.25 when controlled for confounding variables. Potential mechanisms appear to be oxidant gas exposure, which leads to endothelial dysfunction, resulting in multiple abnormalities of the vascular system (arterial thickening, and the pro-inflammatory, pro-thrombotic, and pro-atherogenic state). Additional mechanisms accounting for the causal relationship between secondhand smoke exposure and CVD include mitochondrial damage leading to energy perturbations and alterations in autonomic function, leading to decreased heart rate variability, a risk factor for higher mortality rates in patients with chronic heart failure. Children are at high risk due to home exposure, but there is has been limited research in this area, with most research on the effects of tobacco smoke exposure in childhood focusing on the respiratory system. Non-invasive diagnostic research tools will be useful in determining the effects of tobacco smoke exposure during childhood on the developing cardiovascular system.

Chapter 5 - The influence of passive smoking on human health has been studied for several decades. Currently a wide range of damaging effects due to chronical involuntary exposure of nosmokers to secondhand smoke is commonly accepted. Infants and children are the most vulnerable target population. A specific interest is focused on the antenatal exposure of fetuses. As smoking is associated with many other social, behavioral and habitual factors, the national studies involving different populations are needed for better understanding of the passive smoking and health problem.

The European Longitudinal Study of Pregnancy and Childhood (ELSPAC) includes

6 countries with the total cohort of 40.000 children and their parents. In the Czech Republic, all women in the urban city of Brno and the rural district Znojmo who were pregnant in the period between 1990/91 (cca 6.000 persons) were asked to participate in this study.

The data about parents life style, family history, education, social and living conditions, stress events and health are repeatedly collected from the second trimester (first time at 18th month of women pregnancy) through the rest of pregnancy and delivery. The follow-up measurements of newborns, infants and children include the data about many conditions influencing the child´s physical, psychical and behavioral development, skills and health. The sources of data are parents, physicians, later on teachers and children themselves as well. Within the Czech cohort, about 40% of women reported the smoking history in their life, 25% of them smoked during 9 months before pregnancy. Relatively high rate of quitting could be seen and the prevalence of those who smoked during the whole pregnancy was 8%. Unfortunately, within the 6 months after delivery, all former smokers started to smoke again.

The Czech cohort of ELSPAC confirms the previously published results:

antenatal exposure to cigarette smoke is associated with fetal growth retardation

maternal smoking during pregnancy and after delivery is associated with shorter period of breast feeding

breast feeding had the significant protective effect on infants health

postnatal exposure to maternal smoking is associated with significantly increased incidence of infants respiratory and gastrointestinal diseases, as well as with higher level of medical care including hospitalization

mothers smoking is the main factor influencing the children´ exposure to ETS, also in families where with the smoking mother other smokers are living

although older children are more exposed to ETS, the relations between the exposure and their health decreased, with an exception of wheezing

only weak association both of antenatal and postnatal exposure to passive smoking to children´alergy were seen

the disadvantageous antenatal developmental conditions manifested in the low birthweight are in significant relations to conduct disorders seen at the 3rd and 6th year of age.

Pregnancy is a great opportunity to smoking cessation. Nonsmoking parents behavior must be kept also after delivery and – best of all – forever. The role of physicians and other health professionals in motivating smokers to smoking cessation and in treatment of those who are dependent is crucial and essential.

Chapter 6 - Tobacco smoking is an unhealthy lifestyle linked with infertility and fetal abnormalities. Both first- and second-hand tobacco smoke can result in ill effects on female reproductive integrity and disturbances in the maternal-embryo/feto-placental functional unit. Numerous harmful substances from tobacco smoke can pass the placental barrier or accumulate in placental structures. Cigarette smoke contains several thousands of chemicals and approximately 30 metal ions, including cadmium, arsenic, lead, nickel, chromium, aluminum, antimony, copper, iron, and radioactive elements. Many metals are highly reactive and contribute to the production of oxidative stress, a starting point of toxic and carcinogenic effects of tobacco smoke. In the general population, cigarette smoke is the chief environmental source of cadmium, a confirmed human carcinogen.

By affecting woman's health and the internal environment of her descendant(s), toxic metals may cause immediate and delayed ill effects on virtually all organ systems. Women of childbearing age and growing infants are prone to deficiencies of essential elements (iron, zinc, copper, calcium) and thus are especially sensitive to toxic-essential metal interactions. During pregnancy, toxic metals can compromise fetal health directly *in utero*, by passing the placental barrier, and indirectly, by accumulation in the placenta and inhibition of nutrient transfer to the fetus.

Toxic metals can interfere with principal placental functions, maintenance of pregnancy and fetal viability, by affecting the production of placental hormones. Their accumulation in the placenta may compromise prevention of placental-fetal rejection by maternal immune system and fetal response to antigen exposure *in utero*.

Only a few studies so far have validated the concept of placental steroid disruption due to metal exposure. Cadmium ions accumulate in human placental (trophoblast) cells where they suppress progesterone release without apparent inhibition of syncytial development. Increase in placental cadmium is commensurate with a decrease in placental progesterone concentrations in women exposed to cigarette smoke during pregnancy. Animal studies support the findings of cadmium-induced ovarian and placental steroid disruption during pregnancy. A concomitant low iron diet has an additive effect on cadmium-induced placental steroid disruption.

Human placenta can be used as a 'dual purpose specimen' for monitoring harmful substances in both the maternal and internal fetal environment when epidemiological variables for evaluation of exposure conditions are considered. Assessment of placental function by steroid disruption as an indicator of fetal distress *in utero* may serve as a useful noninvasive test for evaluation of risk for infant health in relation to prenatal exposure to common pollutants in environmental tobacco smoke.

Chapter 7 - Free radicals levels in a healthy organism are strictly controlled by enzymatic and non-enzymatic antioxidants. In smokers, exogenous free radicals contained both in the mainstream smoke as well as in the sidestream smoke, may affect the control mechanisms involved in the oxidative balance regulation and therefore contribute to the oxidative stress, and may initiate the development of pathological changes. These processes can be followed and observed by measurements of non-enzymatic antioxidants levels. Vitamin E, being a fat-soluble antioxidant in biological membranes and plasma lipoprotein capsules, belongs to the most important non-enzymatic antioxidants. The evaluation of the actual vitamin E status in the body is very important for the estimation of vitamin E supplementation in persons showing its deficiency.

The literature review indicates that the alpha-tocopherol (the main form of vitamin E) level in plasma is in active smokers on average by 5% lower, however the data are discrepant (from –28.7% to +5.0%). Similar discrepancies are observed among reports on gamma-tocopherol metabolism. The differences in plasma levels between smokers and nonsmokers range from –3.0% to +20%. Diversity of plasma alpha- and gamma-tocopherol levels values in nonsmokers and persons exposed to environmental tobacco smoke (passive smokers) is similar to those observed among active smokers but the number of reports is minute.

Studies performed with use of deuter-labeled tocopherols unequivocally indicate a significantly faster diminishing of plasma tocopherols in smokers in comparison with nonsmokers, but this results are not confirmed in meta-analysis indicating that smoking is moderately, and frequently insignificantly associated with changes in plasma tocopherol levels. This is probably caused by physiological factors (absorption, transport, distribution) affecting vitamin E biokinetics in smokers and nonsmokers. This may also be caused by the body increased antioxidative mobilization in response to oxidative stress evoked by tobacco smoke.

This article discusses the effects of tobacco smoke on plasma alpha- and gamma-tocopherol levels in smokers and the possible causes of markedly divergent data.

Chapter 8 - The impact of smoking on general health has been widely studied and is directly related to several important medical problems including cancer, low birth weight, and pulmonary and cardiovascular disease. Such a great interest is encouraged by the number of smokers in the world; more than 1,300 billion (WHO, 2005). In the past 25 years, there has also been an increasing awareness of the role of cigarette consumption in oral health problems such as periodontal disease and dental implant failures. In the field of periodontics, it has been reported that smokers have a 2.7 times greater probability of presenting periodontal disease than non-smokers, independent of age, sex and plaque index; furthermore, the disease is more severe in smokers than in former and non-smokers.

In addition, it has been reported that chronic smoking compromises periodontal health, demonstrated by an increased number of periodontally diseased sites with loss of periodontal bone height. In the field of implantology, a greater incidence of early and late implant failures has been observed for smokers when compared to non-smokers. In order to further evaluate the effect of cigarette smoke on the tissues around the tooth and dental implants, our group has been using a cigarette smoke exposure chamber and an animal model. By exposing the animals to this model of passive smoking, we have learned that ligature-induced periodontitis and the bone around titanium implants may be affected by cigarette smoke inhalation.

This chapter will then attempt to discuss recent available evidences on the impact of smoking on the periodontal and peri-implant tissues, and provide the reader with an overview of the data we have collected on the effect of cigarette smoke inhalation and its cessation on both tissues.

Chapter 9 - ETS may deteriorate oral health as that has been demonstrated regarding with general health. The effects of ETS on oral health may be first noticed by practitioners who routinely see objective symptoms in oral cavity. Alternative pathway is epidemiological study where data-bases including information in large-scale survey on exposure to ETS and oral health are analyzed. Causal relationships must be discussed, further, based on evidences which could explain biological mechanisms. The authors address the possible effect of passive smoking on gingival pigmentation and dental diseases, pediatric caries and periodontal disease, in this chapter.

Oral symptoms could be addressed by both smokers and practitioners more easily relative to those of general diseases since the oral cavity is visible. Gingival pigmentation is strongly associated with active smoking. A dose-response relationship was exhibited in several epidemiological studies. Melanin pigmentation in the gingiva is common phenomena globally, however, current smokers are more likely exhibiting melanin pigmentation in the gingiva than non-smokers. Melanocytes were identified at the basal layer of the gingival epithelium. Tobacco smoking could stimulate production of melanin. Prevalence of pigmentation decreased in relation to the number of years following smoking cessation. These findings indicate a causal association.

An epidemiological study conducted in two workplace locations separately exhibited the association of active smoking with gingival pigmentation. Another finding of the study was a distinct difference in the prevalence of gingival pigmentation between groups of non-smokers in the workplaces, factory and office. We guess that smoking may have been prohibited in the factory and allowed in the office. This finding is indicative of the effect of passive smoking on gingival pigmentation. A dentist who works in the northern part of Japan suggested the effect of passive smoking on gingival pigmentation in children. The authors gathered digital images of gingiva in children and smoking status of their parents who visited a dental clinic where the weather is relatively cold. The investigation demonstrated an association of gingival pigmentation of children with parents who smoke. A possible mechanism are discussed based on findings of the effect of active smoking on gingival pigmentation.

The authors review several studies on pediatric caries and a few studies on periodontal disease in terms of the effects of passive smoking. They discuss strength of evidence and the possible mechanisms.

In: Smoking and Health Research Frontiers
Editor: Calvin B. Fong, pp. 1-8
ISBN 1-60021-480-0

Chapter I

Smoking Cessation and Prevention: Implications of Study Design, Research Setting, and Goals

Edmond D. Shenassa[1,] and Constantine Daskalakis[2]*
[1]Brown Medical School, Department of Community Health; Division of Epidemiology;
[2]Thomas Jefferson University, Department of Medicine, Division of Clinical Pharmacology, Section of Biostatistics.

Abstract

Collaborations among various disciplines concerned with smoking cessation and prevention are gaining in currency. Such collaborations are predicated, in part, on recognizing both the implicit assumptions in different fields and the consequences of these assumptions. These issues, however, are usually not considered in transdisciplinary research. In this article, we demonstrate how indices, such as the risk ratio, attributable fraction, or R-squared, have different implications for causal inference and interventions, depending on study setting and research goals.

Introduction

Collaborations among various disciplines concerned with smoking cessation and prevention are gaining in currency. Such efforts, including those promoted by the National Cancer Institute, the Tobacco Etiology Research Network, and others, are propelled in part by our developing understanding that smoking is best understood from a transdisciplinary

* Correspondence concerning this article should be addressed to Dr. Edmond D. Shenassa, Sc.D., Assistant Professor, Brown Medical School, 121 S. Main St. Providence, RI 02912. Phone: 401-863-6361; Fax: 401-863-1889; E-mail: edmond_shenassa@brown.edu.

perspective (Shenassa, et al., 2003). Gaining a transdisicplinary perspective is predicated, in part, on accurate communication between disciplines (Klein, 1996; Shenassa & Earls, 2001; Nash, et al., 2003). An important step in facilitating such communication is recognizing both the implicit assumptions in different fields and the consequences of these assumptions.

In this chapter, we examine the implications of study design, specifically the prevalence of an independent variable of interest (i.e., exposure or risk factor), with respect to the context of interpretation and applicability of study findings. The prevalence of an independent variable in a study often reflects the sampling scheme that is most commonly used in a particular field. In balanced designs, the prevalence is usually 50% by design, since this tends to maximize efficiency. Such designs are particularly common in experimental or quasi-experimental studies. On the other hand, unbalanced designs, where the prevalence is typically much lower or much higher than 50%, are more common in observational studies, particularly population-based ones. These differences in the prevalence of exposure, implied by the study design, can have important implications regarding the interpretation of associations between variables of interest and application of findings from one setting to another. This is particularly true when the aim is to apply research findings to intervention programs.

Below, we first demonstrate that, although the magnitude of the association between the two variables may not vary across different study designs, the potential prevention or intervention yield depends on the prevalence of the exposed individuals in the study population, which is implicitly influenced by the study design. Next, we use a published study to demonstrate how a few simple calculations can provide additional information with important public health implications.

Association Versus Intervention Yield: A Hypothetical Example

A number of studies have reported an independent positive association between maternal smoking during pregnancy and various adverse health outcomes among the offspring (e.g., Buka et al., 2003; Wackshlag et al., 2002; Shenassa & Brown, 2004; Grant, 2005). Therefore, let us consider a hypothetical clinic-based longitudinal study that recruits and follows women who smoke during a pregnancy and women who do not (as well as their offspring) in equal numbers, with the goal of assessing future nicotine dependence among the offspring. Such a balanced design is highly efficient in detecting outcome differences between groups. The hypothetical results of this study are presented in Table 1.

In this example, a child's estimated risk of nicotine dependence is two and a half times higher if the mother smoked during pregnancy than if she did not (Table 1). The estimated *risk ratio* (RR) is 2.5, with a 95% confidence interval (95% CI) of 1.25 to 5.00 and an associated chi-squared p-value of 0.005. We would conclude that the increase in risk associated with *in utero* exposure to tobacco smoke is both clinically (magnitude of the risk ratio) and statistically (p-value) significant. If this association reflects a truly causal mechanism, preventing maternal smoking during pregnancy might reduce the subsequent risk of nicotine dependence among adult offspring. In fact, if the association is entirely causal, by preventing all 40 women smokers in the study sample from smoking, we would expect 8 rather than 20 of their offspring to eventually become nicotine dependent (i.e., the same proportion that was observed among women who did not smoke during pregnancy). In other words, about 12 of the 28 observed cases of nicotine dependence would be prevented, a 43% yield. This "yield" of preventable cases from removal of exposure is often called the *population attributable fraction* (AF). In the context of intervention programs, population attributable fraction corresponds to the proportion of smokers who would quit smoking when a particular risk factor is successfully removed or rendered neutral.

Table 1. Mother's smoking during pregnancy and child's subsequent nicotine dependence: hypothetical data for a balanced prospective study.

		Child nicotine dependent?		
		yes	no	
Mother smoked during pregnancy?	yes	20	20	40
	no	8	32	40
		28	52	80

Let us now consider the broader implications of such a research finding. What would be the results of an actual program aimed at women in the general community who smoke during their pregnancies? The answer depends on the prevalence of exposure in the community. Although the prevalence in the study sample was artificially set to 50% by design, it will naturally be much lower in the general population. Depending on various characteristics of the community members, the prevalence of women who smoke during pregnancy is likely to be close to 15%. Therefore, let us consider a hypothetical community where the target population consists of 80,000 pregnant women (and their offspring), 15% of whom smoke during pregnancy. Assuming that the hypothetical study results shown in Table 1 were unbiased with respect to a child's risks of nicotine dependence, the expected outcomes for the 80,000 offspring in the target population are shown in Table 2.

Table 2. Mother's smoking during pregnancy and child's subsequent nicotine dependence: hypothetical data for a community population.

		Child nicotine dependent?		
		yes	no	
Mother smoked during pregnancy?	yes	6,000	6,000	12,000
	no	13,600	54,400	68,000
		19,600	60,400	80,000

In this community population, the child's risk of nicotine dependence is 50% if the mother smokes and 20% if she doesn't (RR = 2.5), identical to the findings from the clinic-based study sample. However, even if we were to prevent all 12,000 pregnant women from smoking during their pregnancy, we would still expect to see 2,400 of their children develop nicotine dependence (i.e., 20%, the same proportion as when the mother does not smoke during pregnancy). So, at best, we can prevent 3,600 cases of nicotine dependence out of a total of 19,600 observed in the community, a population attributable fraction of 18%. The much lower yield in the community setting relative to the clinic setting (18% vs. 43%) is entirely due to the different prevalence of the exposure in the two settings. Of course, these two different yields have considerably different public health implications (Shenassa & Earls, 2001; Shenassa, 2002).

For a particular association, as reflected in the risk ratio, the yield increases as the prevalence of the exposure increases (Figure 1). This may be an intuitive conclusion, but it is too often not consiered in communicating and applying findings across disciplines. Consequently, consideration of this measure [consideration of prevalence of exposure?] can broaden the interdisciplinary reach of studies, and strengthen the authors' argument that their findings have public health implications, particularly when they suggest that their findings have implications for prevention and/or intervention programs.

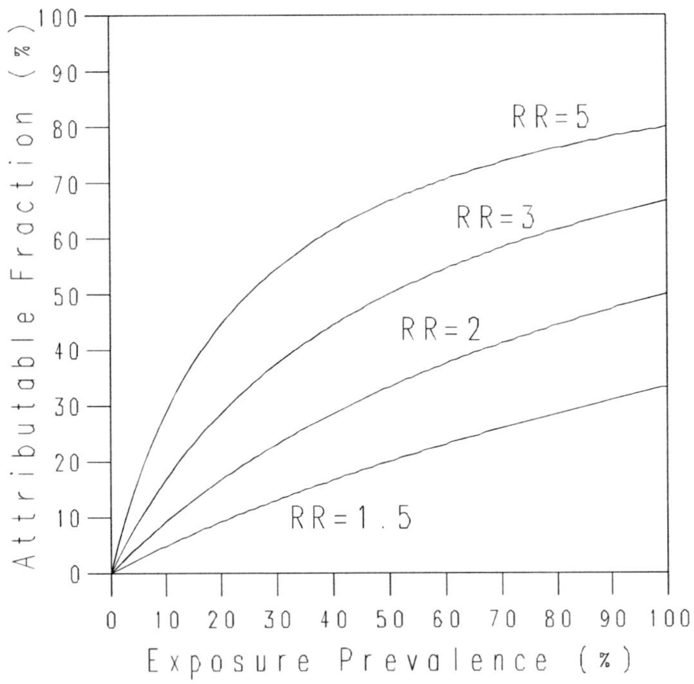

Figure 1. The population attributable fraction (AF) corresponding to various risk ratios (RR), as a function of exposure prevalence.

A similar point applies to the R-squared (R^2) as a measure of explained variability.* In the study sample, the R^2 equals 0.078. Although very low, this value of the R^2 might still be considered quite satisfactory, given that it is due to a single predictor of the child's nicotine dependence and would certainly increase if other predictors were to be accounted for.

* Here, we are actually referring to a pseudo-R-squared for dichotomous outcomes, since the usual R-squared is only appropriate for continuous outcomes. The pseudo-R-squared is computed differently from the usual R-squared, but has a similar interpretation (i.e., the proportion of the outcome's variability that can be attributed to the independent predictor).

However, the R^2 in the community population would be 0.049. This difference is entirely due to the difference in the prevalence of smoking among pregnant women in the study sample and in the community.

ASSOCIATION VERSUS INTERVENTION YIELD: AN ACTUAL EXAMPLE

To illustrate the points raised above, we now turn to an actual study of risk factors for smokeless tobacco use among 808 male high school athletes in West Virginia (Goebel et al., 2000). We chose this work because of its excellent execution, exposition, and particularly clear and detailed presentation of the data. Table 3 is based on results presented in that paper's Table 1. In their paper, the authors accurately concluded that, among other factors, "playing football, smoking cigarettes and having parents who would permit use at home are correlated with the decision to use smokeless tobacco" (p. 324).

Table 3. Smokeless tobacco use, by risk factor, in a West Virginia study (abstracted from Goebel et al., 2000).

		N	Tobacco user n (%)	OR	RR	AF
Plays football	yes	290	69 (23.8)	1.47	1.35	11%
	no	518	91 (17.6)			
Has tried cigarettes	yes	405	137 (33.8)	9.03	5.93	71%
	no	403	23 (5.7)			
Has family permitting use	yes	124	77 (62.1)	12.50	5.12	39%
	no	684	83 (12.1)			

OR: odds ratio; RR: risk ratio; AF: population attributable fraction.

The authors then suggested that "[in] addition to student refusal assertion training, education to counteract advertising, and education on physical consequences of tobacco beginning in elementary school, researchers designing prevention programs in West Virginia should consider interventions to consider the permissive attitude of Appalachia adults. Furthermore, targeting sports participants for prevention programs, especially football players, may be beneficial in our state" (Goebel et al., 2000, p. 324). Although it would be ideal to have such a multidimensional approach to intervention, public health interventions often require some guidance as how to prioritize and focus scarce resources. Having information on the yield (i.e., population attributable fraction), along with other relevant data such as cost of various programs, would facilitate informed decisions (Shenassa, 2002).

In the case of the West Virginia study, the authors did not provide such guidance. From reading the paper's results, it might seem that efforts should best be directed towards the strongest risk factors (e.g., teens who have tried cigarettes and homes with permissive family), but that is not necessarily the case. The intervention yield also depends on the prevalence of each risk factor in the target population. Assuming that the study sample reflected the state's target population (which seems reasonable, given information presented in the paper), simple computation of the population attributable fraction (for details, see Appendix) shows that an intervention with teens who have permissive homes would have a yield of 39%, while an intervention with football players would have a yield of only 11%. These potential benefits must be balanced against the potential costs of needing to target the approximately 15% (124/808) of homes with permissive families or the 36% (290/808) of all male high school students who play football.

Discussion

For simplicity, our discussion ignored potential confounding factors. Obviously, any health outcome is influenced by numerous factors, and such factors may differ between the groups that are compared. Therefore, in realistic situations, we would attempt to control for such (measured) covariates, and estimate adjusted measures of association. The computational details and relationships between the various measures (i.e., risk ratio, R-squared, and attributable fraction) are beyond the scope of this paper, but the points raised here are equally applicable to that more complicated context as well.

In conclusion, research studies often conclude that factors that exhibit a high risk ratio or explain a substantial proportion of variability of the outcome maybe useful for targetting intervention programs. In this paper, we have argued that such an association between a risk factor and a health outcome does not necessarily imply that an intervention targeting that risk factor will be efficient or desirable. A high RR may correspond to a high yield and/or R^2 in one setting but not in another. This point is of particular importance when communicating findings across disciplines or when applying research findings to intervention programs. Different fields of inquiry have distinct perspectives and goals (e.g., description, causal inference, public health intervention or prevention, etc.). Therefore, it is not surprising that they often rely on different statistical tools in the course of research. Since there is no single "best" tool for all goals and settings, recognizing the implicit assumptions and inter-relations of these tools is a crucial step in effectively communicating across disciplines.

Appendix

The attributable fraction in the population (AF_{pop}) is the proportion of cases seen in the entire population that are due to the risk factor of interest (e.g., proportion of cases of nicotine dependence among offspring due to the mother's smoking during pregnancy). It can be computed as (Levin, 1953; Miettinen, 1974)

$$AF_{pop} = \frac{p_e(RR-1)}{p_e(RR-1)+1} = \frac{p_e(r_1-r_0)}{p_e(r_1-r_0)+r_0},$$

where p_e is the prevalence of exposure (i.e., proportion of pregnant women who smoke);

r_1 and r_0 represent the child's risk of later developing nicotine dependence if the mother smoked and didn't smoke during pregnancy, respectively; and

$RR = r_1/r_0$ is the relative risk for mother's smoking during pregnancy.

In the case of adjusted analyses (either via stratification or logistic regression), the simple formula above is not valid. Applicable formulas are given in Miettinen (1974), Walter (1976), and Greenland (1984).

The pseudo-R-squared (R^2) can be roughly interpreted as the proportion of the outcome's variability (here, offspring's nicotine dependence) that can be attributed to the predictor of interest (here, mother's smoking during pregnancy). It is a likelihood ratio measure, computed as

$$R^2 = 1 - \frac{\ell_1}{\ell_0}$$

with

$$\begin{aligned}\ell_1 &= p_e r_1 \ln(r_1) + p_e(1-r_1)\ln(1-r_1) + \\ &\quad (1-p_e) r_0 \ln(r_0) + (1-p_e)(1-r_0)\ln(1-r_0) \\ \ell_0 &= [p_e r_1 + (1-p_e) r_0]\ln[p_e r_1 + (1-p_e)\ r_0] + \\ &\quad [p_e(1-r_1) + (1-p_e)(1-r_0)]\ln[p_e(1-r_1) + (1-p_e)(1-r_0)]\end{aligned}$$

and notation as above.

REFERENCES

Buka SL, Shenassa ED, Niaura R. Elevated risk of tobacco dependence among offspring of mothers who smoked during pregnancy: a 30-year prospective study. *Am J Psychiatry.* Nov 2003;160(11):1978-1984.

Goebel, L.J., Crespo, R.D., Abraham, R.T., Masho, S.W. & Clover, E.D. (2000). Correlates of youth smokeless tobacco use. *Nicotine & Tobacco Research 2*, 319-325.

Grant, S., *Qualitatively and quantitatively similar effects of active and passive maternal tobacco smoke exposure on in utero mutagenesis at the HPRT locus. BMC Pediatr*, 2005. 29(5): p. 20.

Greenland, S. (1984). Bias in methods for deriving standardized morbidity ratios and attributable fraction estimates. *Statistics in Medicine 3*:131-141.

Klein, J.T., (1996). *Crossing Boundaries: Knowledge, Disciplinarities, and Interdisciplinarities*. Charlottesville: University Press of Virginia.

Levin, M.L. (1953). The occurrence of lung cancer in man. *Acta Unio Internationalis Contra Cancrum 19*: 531-541.

Miettinen, O.S. (1974). Proportion of disease caused or prevented by a given exposure, trait, or intervention. *American Journal of Epidemiology 99*: 325-332.

Nash, J., Collins, B., Loughlin, S., et al. Training the transdisciplinary scientist to address tobacco use behavior. *Nicotine & Tobacco Research.* Dec 2003;5 Suppl 1:S41-53.

Shenassa, E. (2002). Delivering the goods: The relevance of classification accuracy to the design of community intervention and prevention programs. *Journal of Community Psychology 30*:197-210.

Shenassa ED, Brown MJ. Maternal smoking and infantile gastrointestinal dysregulation: the case of colic. *Pediatrics.* Oct 2004;114(4):e497-506.

Shenassa, ED., & Earls, F. (2001). On the application of psychology to public health: Identification versus explanation. *Journal of Community Psychology 29*: 83-85.

Shenassa ED, McCaffery JM, Swan GE, et al. Intergenerational transmission of tobacco use and dependence: a transdisciplinary perspective. *Nicotine Tob Res.* Dec 2003;5 Suppl 1:S55-69.

Wakschlag, L.S., Pickett, K.E., Cook, E., Jr, Benowitz, N.L, Leventhal, B.L. (2002) Maternal smoking during pregnancy and severe antisocial behavior in offspring: a review. *American Journal of Public Health 92(6)*:966-74.

Walter, S.D. (1976). The estimation and interpretation of attributable risk in health research. *Biometrics 32*:829-849.

In: Smoking and Health Research Frontiers
Editor: Calvin B. Fong, pp. 9-61

ISBN 1-60021-480-0

Chapter II

GENETIC SUSCEPTIBILITY TO SECOND-HAND SMOKE

***Yen-Ching Chen*[1,3], *Jen-Hau Chen*[2] *and David C. Christiani*[3,4]**

[1]Channing Laboratory, Department of Medicine, Brigham and Women's Hospital, Harvard Medical School, Boston, MA, USA;

[2]Department of Internal Medicine, National Taiwan University Hospital, Taipei, Taiwan;

[3]Occupational Health Program, Department of Environmental Health, Harvard School of Public Health, Boston, MA, USA;

[4]Pulmonary and Critical Care Unit, Department of Medicine, Massachusetts General Hospital, Harvard Medical School, Boston, MA, USA.

ABSTRACT

Second-hand smoke (SHS) is also referred as passive smoke, involuntary smoke, environmental tobacco smoke, and environmental cigarette smoke. The sources of SHS include exposure from relatives at home, work place, and in public. Experimental and epidemiologic studies have observed the intake and metabolism of SHS (National Research Council (U.S.).

Part of the importance of SHS stems from the fact that the levels of some carcinogens, e.g., polycyclic aromatic hydrocarbon (PAH), benzo(a)pyrene (BP) and 4-aminobiphenyl (4-ABP, an arylamine), are actually higher in undiluted SHS than in mainstream smoke (i.e., active smoke) (National Research Council 1986). In addition, the size of the particles in SHS is smaller than those in mainstream smoke and, therefore, these particles are more likely to be deposited in the lung (Dockery and Trichopoulos 1997; Hecht 1999). The association between SHS and lung cancer or childhood asthma has been studied extensively. While it is well-recognized that 80-90% of all lung cancer is attributable to cigarette smoking, only 15% of all smokers develop this disease and about 10% of all diagnosed lung cancers are never smokers (Hammond and Seidman 1980).

In summary, for different health effects, significant associations have been observed in genetic markers, including risk modification by germline polymorphisms, gene expression changes, and somatic alterations.

Some gaps in our knowledge of SHS health effects remain. The associations between sequence variants of genes involved in phase I and II metabolism and cell cycle pathways and the risk of lung cancer have been widely explored for SHS exposure and conclusive findings are not yet available.

Keywords: Second-hand smoke, genetic susceptibility, biomarkers.

INTRODUCTION

Second-hand smoke (SHS) is also referred as passive smoke, involuntary smoke, environmental tobacco smoke, and environmental cigarette smoke. The sources of SHS include exposure from relatives at home, work place, and in public. Experimental and epidemiologic studies have observed the intake and metabolism of SHS (National Research Council (U.S.). Committee on Passive Smoking. 1986; Hecht, Carmella et al. 1993; Hackshaw, Law et al. 1997; Parsons, Carmella et al. 1998; Repace, Jinot et al. 1998). Part of the importance of SHS stems from the fact that the levels of some carcinogens, e.g., polycyclic aromatic hydrocarbon (PAH), benzo(a)pyrene (BP) and 4-aminobiphenyl (4-ABP, an arylamine), are actually higher in undiluted SHS than in mainstream smoke (i.e., active smoke) (National Research Council 1986). In addition, the size of the particles in SHS is smaller than those in mainstream smoke and, therefore, these particles are more likely to be deposited in the lung (Dockery and Trichopoulos 1997; Hecht 1999). The association between SHS and lung cancer or childhood asthma has been studied extensively. While it is well-recognized that 80-90% of all lung cancer is attributable to cigarette smoking, only 15% of all smokers develop this disease and about 10% of all diagnosed lung cancers are never smokers (Hammond and Seidman 1980) (Figure 1A). Epidemiological investigations have found 1.6- and 1.2-fold increased risk of lung cancer among non-smokers exposed to SHS based on data from the USA and Europe, respectively (1992; Boffetta, Agudo et al. 1998), and a risk of 1.3 was reported by the Surgeon General and National academy of Sciences (1986; 1986). Since the completion of Human Genome Project in the early 2000s, abundant genome data allow us to explore the association between SHS exposure and human health effects at the genetic level. Unlike phenotypic markers, genetic markers are stable over time and are easy to measure. Therefore, it is possible to assess variations in genes involved in xenobiotic detoxification, metabolism, DNA repairs, apoptosis, cell cycle control, angiogenesis, tumor suppressor, and other cellular responses related to SHS exposure.

Some polymorphisms (see Table 1-3, later in text), sequence variants of *GSTP1, GSTM1, CYP1A 1, CYP1B1, p53, NAT2, NAD(P)H:quinone oxidoredictase 1 (NQO1), O6-alkylguanine DNA alkyltransferase (AGT), alpha1-antitrypsin (α1-AT)*, expression of *K-ras, Bax,* or *Nrf2*-dependent antioxidant and cytoprotective genes, and hypermethylation of *MGMT*, have been related to exposure to SHS. However, previous studies have been restricted to Caucasians. Studies that compare different ethnic groups are important for a more complete understanding of variations of genetic profiles and risk related to SHS. Moreover, it is important to consider other environmental or occupational exposures, e.g. arsenic, asbestos (Amos, Xu et al. 1999; Nelson, Christiani et al. 1999), chromium (VI) (Hu,

Feng et al. 2004), nickel and vinyl chloride (Williams and Sandler 2001), cadmium (Yang, Julan et al. 2006), UV radiation, and dietary aflatoxin (Dogliotti, Hainaut et al. 1998), smoked meat, cheese, and fish (Whyatt, Garte et al. 1995), which may interact with SHS and lead to more severe or complicated health effects. Large regions of the human genome have not been explored for SHS-related health effects. Besides association studies, linkage analyses and microarray studies are useful approaches to narrow and identify the susceptibility genes related to SHS exposure. Once susceptibility genes are identified, genes involved in the same molecular or biological pathway could be analyzed together to comprehensively assess the effect of SHS. This article includes a review of existing literature addressing genetic susceptibility to SHS and presents perspectives for future studies in this field.

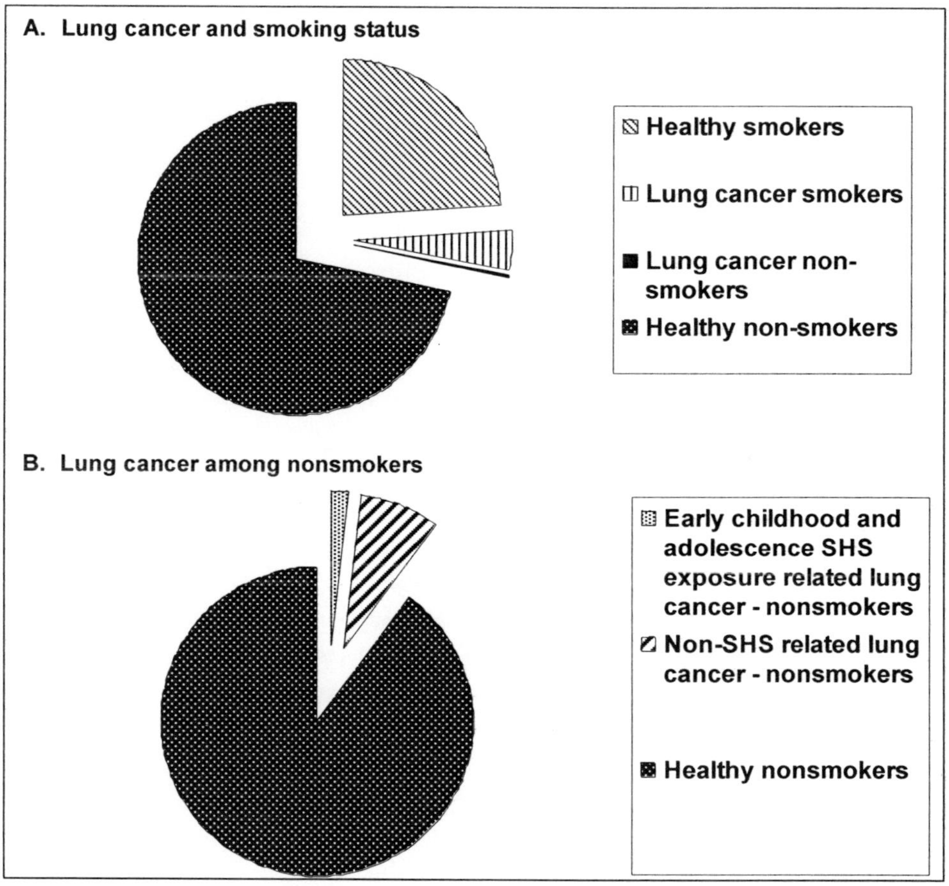

Figure 1: Second-hand smoke, active smoke and lung cancer (Hammond and Seidman 1980; Janerich, Thompson et al. 1990; Weiss 1997; Samet, Brenner et al. 1998).

Carcinogens in Second-Hand Smoke

SHS contains over 4,000 compounds (2005), 69 of which are known carcinogens and could be divided into: PAH, heterocyclic compounds, nitrosamines, aromatic amines, N-heterocyclic amines, aldehydes, volatile hydrocarbons, miscellaneous organic compounds, and inorganic compounds (Hoffmann and Hoffmann 2001). Some are more commonly reported, including PAH, 4-ABP (Schonberger and Van Schayck 1998; Faraglia, Chen et al. 2003), BP (Merlo, Andreassen et al. 1998; London, Smart et al. 2000; De Flora, Balansky et al. 2003; Wolf, Kutz et al. 2005), BP diol-epoxide (BPDE) (Stierum, Hageman et al. 1997; Song, Lippman et al. 2005), benzene, 4-(methylnitrosoamino)-1-(3-pyridyl)-butanone (NNK) (National Research Council 1986; Abdel-Rahman and El-Zein 2000; De Flora, Balansky et al. 2003), 7H-dibenzo[c,g]carbazole (DBC) (Mitchell and Warshawsky 1999), acetaldehyde (Matsuda, Kawanishi et al. 1998), 1,3-butadiene (Norppa 2004), styrene (Norppa 2004), acrolein (Borchers, Carty et al. 1999; Borchers, Wesselkamper et al. 1999), cadmium (Yang, Julan et al. 2006), and arsenic (Chen, Su et al. 2005), etc. In addition, the ratio of levels of BP in SHS to the mainstream has been used as a good surrogate of BP exposure and has been reported to be 2.5-3.5 (Hecht 1999). The details of 69 carcinogens in cigarette smoke is available in Monograph 13: Risks associated with smoking cigarettes with low machine-measured yields of tar and nicotine, National Cancer Institute (Hoffmann and Hoffmann 2001) on the website (http://cancercontrol.cancer.gov/tcrb/monographs/13/). Among these carcinogens, 11, 8 and 47 are confirmed, probably, and possibly human carcinogens.

Health Effects Related to Second-Hand Smoke

Several health effects have been linked to SHS and can be divided into (1) respiratory health effects: lung cancer (Malats, Camus-Radon et al. 2000; Hou, Falt et al. 2002; Hung, Boffetta et al. 2003), asthma (Colilla, Nicolae et al. 2003; Raherison, Taytard et al. 2003; Kurz and Ober 2004; Choudhry, Avila et al. 2005; Meyers, Postma et al. 2005), chronic obstructive pulmonary disease (COPD) (Silverman and Speizer 1996; Borchers, Wert et al. 1998; Walter, Gottlieb et al. 2000; Mayer and Newman 2001; Girod and King 2005), mucus hypersecretion, inflammation, airway hyperreactivity (Borchers, Wert et al. 1998; Borchers, Wesselkamper et al. 1999), and lung function changes (von Ehrenstein, von Mutius et al. 2002), (2) reproductive and developmental effects: oral cleft (Little, Cardy et al. 2004) and low birth weight (Martin and Bracken 1986), (3) cardiovascular effects: atherosclerosis (Heeschen, Jang et al. 2001), cardiovascular disease (myocardial infarction, cerebral stoke, and sudden cardiac death) and cardiovascular function (e.g., blood pressure and heart rate) (Humble, Croft et al. 1990; Stoney, Lentino et al. 1998; Dautzenberg 2004), (4) other cancers: cancers of nasal sinus, cervix, breast, bladder, and ovary (1999; IARC 2004; Reynolds, Hurley et al. 2004; 2005; Chen, Su et al. 2005; Baker, Odunuga et al. 2006), and (5) eye and nose irritation (1999), angiogenesis (Heeschen, Jang et al. 2001; Zhu, Heeschen et al. 2003), worsening of cystic fibrosis (1999), and diabetes (Houston, Houston et al. 2006). Other diseases like Parkinson's disease, chronic pancreatitis, pancreatic cancer, cancers of liver, kidney, oral and nasal cavities, esophagus, larynx, pharynx, stomach, urinary tract, and cervix (Talamini, Bassi et al. 1999; Phillips 2002; Parain, Hapdey et al. 2003; Dautzenberg 2004) have been explored among smokers. However, the association between SHS exposure and these health effects are unclear.

Females are more commonly affected. Most women are non-smokers and thus more likely to expose to SHS containing higher levels of some carcinogens than those in the mainstream smoke. The number of lung cancer cases among non-smokers is increasing, and a large proportion of them are female adenocarcinoma (Harris, Zang et al. 1993; Kabat 1996; Chen, Chen et al. 2004). In the USA, adenocarcinoma is the most common subtype of lung cancer, accounting for 40% and 50-80% of lung cancer in smokers and never-smokers, respectively (Pulling, Divine et al. 2003). Besides adenocarcinoma, ovarian damage (Matikainen, Perez et al. 2001), complicated pregnancy (e.g., placenta praevia, placental abnormalities) (Martin and Bracken 1986; Kukla, Hruba et al. 2001), and spontaneous abortion (1999) are also related to SHS exposure among women. The high smoking rate among males makes it difficult to assess the health effects resulting from SHS exposure among men. Therefore, the female populations have been frequently selected as the group among which to assess the relationship between genetic susceptibility and SHS exposure to reach statistical power (Schonberger and Van Schayck 1998; Gealy, Zhang et al. 1999; Vahakangas, Bennett et al. 2001; Kiyohara, Wakai et al. 2003; Ng, Tan et al. 2005; Yang and Pyo 2005). For example, the overall smoking prevalence in Chinese women in Singapore has been 3% since the 1980s (1993), but the incidence of lung cancer in the 1980s was comparable with that among women in Canada and the UK, where smoking prevalence was much higher (Parkin, Muir et al. 1992; Burns 1994). Lung cancer incidence for female smokers was 2.3 in a meta-analysis including 8 studies in China (Liu 1992). Because of the significant difference in smoking rates between Chinese females and women in the West (MacLennan, Da Costa et al. 1977; Koo and Ho 1990), further studies are needed to elaborate the ethnic and geographic differences.

Children are another subpopulation susceptible to SHS because they have higher chance of SHS exposure, immature metabolic system, and higher levels of cell division and growth (Perera 1997; Krajinovic, Sinnett et al. 2002). About 17% of lung cancers among nonsmokers are attributable to high levels of SHS exposure during early childhood and adolescence (Janerich, Thompson et al. 1990; National Research Council 1993; Perera 1997) (Figure 1B). Exposure *in utero* to active maternal cigarette smoking and passive maternal cigarette exposure are two routes by which a fetus can be exposed to SHS (Byrd and Howard 1995). According to the Third National Health and Nutrition Examination Survey, 43% of children (age 4-11) were exposed to SHS at home (Pirkle, Flegal et al. 1996). About 10% of current smokers had a child at home, and the state-specific prevalence ranged from 12.3% in California to 34.2% in Kentucky (1997) for children (age<18) exposed to SHS. The perinatal and childhood health effects related to maternal SHS exposure include (1) fetal growth: behavior problems, decreased intellectual achievement (Martin and Bracken 1986; Olds, Henderson et al. 1994; Streissguth, Sampson et al. 1994), lower neonatal birth weight, small-for-gestational age, and premature delivery (Martin and Bracken 1986; Mainous and Hueston 1994; Dejin-Karlsson, Hanson et al. 1998; Hanke, Kalinka et al. 1999; Wu, Zhang et al. 2001; Hong, Lee et al. 2003; Yang, Julan et al. 2006), (2) congenital malformation: oral cleft palate (Little, Cardy et al. 2004), and (3) fetal loss: infant mortality (Kharrazi, DeLorenze et al. 2004) and sudden infant death (1999; Adgent 2006),(4) cancer: hematopoietic malignancies (e.g., acute lymphoblastic leukemia) (Shu, Ross et al. 1996; Ji, Shu et al. 1997; Sorahan, Prior et al. 1997; Finettc, O'Neill et al. 1998; Canalle, Burim et al. 2004) and brain tumor (Baldwin and Preston-Martin 2004), and (5) allergic and respiratory effects: asthma (Casimir 1996; Lorente, Romo et al. 1998; Bjorksten 1999; de Blic 1999; Ronmark, Jonsson et al. 1999; Chan-Yeung, Manfreda et al. 2000; Gilliland, Li et al. 2002; Peden 2002; Kurz and Ober 2004; Arruda, Sole et al. 2005; Bener, Janahi et al. 2005; Wenten, Berhane et al. 2005; Li, Romieu et al. 2006), wheezing, cough, phlegm, chronic bronchitis, pneumonia, middle ear infection (General 1986; National Research Council 1986; 1992; 1997; Cook and Strachan 1997; 1998; Chen, Rennie et al. 1998; Gergen, Fowler et al. 1998; Strachan and Cook 1998; 1999; Gilliland, Li et al. 2002; Arshad, Kurukulaaratchy et al. 2005), and atopic eczema (Kramer, Lemmen et al. 2004). However, some studies suggested that children whose mothers smoked during their pregnancy were not at an increased risk of cancer (Pershagen, Ericson et al. 1992; Klebanoff, Clemens et al. 1996; Sorahan, Prior et al. 1997). It is more difficult to recruit children than adults, but it is important to do research on them, because early SHS exposure figures greatly in predicting disease risk in later life.

Lung Cancer

Lung cancer is the most well-known disease related to SHS and is the 1st and 2nd cause of death in the USA for men and women, respectively (Parkin, Pisani et al. 1999; 2003). The American Cancer Society reported the incidence rate of cancer of the lung and bronchus (Jemal, Siegel et al. 2006) in males as 77.8, 76.7, 113.9, 59.4, 42.6, and 44.6 per 100,000 and age-adjusted to the 2000 US standard population for all races, whites, African Americans, Asian Americans/Pacific Islanders, American Indians/Alaska Natives, and Hispanic Latinos, respectively. For females, the incidence rates were 48.9, 51.1, 55.2, 28.3, 23.6, and 23.3 per 100,000 for the same standard population and ethnic groups above. In the USA, tobacco use increased from 1915 (Sellers, Potter et al. 1992) and lung cancer risk from SHS increased approximately 1.6-fold (1992; Fontham, Correa et al. 1994; Cardenas, Thun et al. 1997; Boffetta, Agudo et al. 1998). A meta-analysis of 37 studies reported the excess risk of lung cancer increased 24% among nonsmokers live with smokers (Hackshaw, Law et al. 1997). A large case-control study (Boffetta, Agudo et al. 1998) including 7 European countries found that a 1.16- and 1.15-fold increased, but not significant, risk of lung cancer among individuals exposed to SHS from the spouse and at the workplace, respectively. The cessation of exposure from both sources decreases the excess risk (Boffetta, Agudo et al. 1998). Active smoking accounted for 90% of lung cancer deaths, and lung cancer in lifelong never smokers accounted for 11,000 deaths in 1995 (Samet, Brenner et al. 1998). Among adult nonsmokers, SHS exposure lead to about 3,000 lung cancer death and 35,000 deaths from ischemic heart disease each year (2006).

Besides passive and active smoking, several other factors have been reported to modify the risk of lung cancer. These include diet (Fontham 1990; Alavanja, Brownson et al. 1992; Ko, Lee et al. 1997), occupational exposure (Boffetta 1993; Collier and Pritsos 2003), prior lung disease (Alavanja, Brownson et al. 1992; Gao 1996; Ko, Lee et al. 1997), and indoor air pollutants (e.g., fumes from cooking oils) (Gao 1996; Wang, Zhou et al. 1996; Ko, Lee et al. 1997), coal or wood combustion (Gao 1996; Ko, Lee et al. 1997), and family history of lung cancer (Wang, Zhou et al. 1996). Comprehensive inclusion of various risk factors could provide better prediction of lung cancer risk.

Asthma

Asthma has become an important public health problem. Recent studies suggest that maternal smoke exposure during pregnancy is an important risk factor for childhood asthma and wheezing (Martinez, Cline et al. 1992; Gilliland, Li et al. 2001; von Mutius 2002). However, this association was not found by others (1992; 1997; Cook and Strachan 1997; 1998; Strachan and Cook 1998; 1999; 2000). In addition, some studies have suggested that an interaction between family history of asthma or atopy and exposure to tobacco smoke in early childhood, but not *in utero,* influences the risk of asthma (Ronmark, Jonsson et al. 1999; Jaakkola, Nafstad et al. 2001; Larsson, Frisk et al. 2001; von Mutius 2002). Besides SHS exposure, factors like air pollution from traffic or industries, dust mite, pet allergens, cold air, respiratory infections, medication, and exercise can exacerbate asthma symptoms (1992; 1997; Cook and Strachan 1997; 1998; Strachan and Cook 1998; 1999; Barnes 1999; Jordaan, Ehrlich et al. 1999; Gold 2000; Ehrlich, Jordaan et al. 2001; Thorn, Brisman et al. 2001). The population-attributable risk for SHS exposure in children has been estimated to range from 9% for asthma prevalence to 25% for hospital admissions due to lower respiratory symptoms (Rushton, Courage et al. 2003).

Chronic Obstructive Pulmonary Disease (COPD)

Chronic obstructive pulmonary disease (COPD) is a disease with permanent narrowing of small bronchi, or destruction of acini (emphysema); chronic bronchitis and emphysema are related diseases. Some irritants in cigarette smoke (e.g., aluminum silicate and kaolinite) have been related to COPD (Girod and King 2005). Indians have a higher incidence rate of COPD than other ethnic groups: it has been diagnosed in 4.1% of subjects, with a male-to-female ratio of 1.56:1 and a smoker-to-nonsmoker ratio of 2.65: 1 (Jindal, Aggarwal et al. 2006). In this population, nonsmokers with SHS exposure had a 1.4-fold risk of COPD (95% CI=1.21-1.61) as compare to those without SHS exposure. Individuals with exposure to both SHS and solid fuel combustion had a higher risk of COPD than those with SHS exposure alone (Jindal, Aggarwal et al. 2006). The gender differences on COPD risk reflect that smoking is an important risk factor for men who have higher smoking rate. Like lung cancer, other environmental factors may lead to synergistic effects. This is possibly a result of combination of environmental exposure and genetic susceptibility.

Acute Lymphoblastic Leukemia (ALL)

Acute lymphoblastic leukemia (ALL) is the most common malignancy affecting children and accounts for 30% of all childhood cancers (Canalle, Burim et al. 2004). Accumulating evidence shows that either maternal exposure to SHS or a history of paternal, but not maternal, smoking was associated with an increase risk of leukemia and lymphoma in children under 5 years of age (Shu, Ross et al. 1996; Ji, Shu et al. 1997; Sorahan, Prior et al. 1997). However, very few studies have explored the association between SHS exposure and the risk of ALL.

Diabetes

Smoking has been linked to impaired response to glucose tolerance tests and insulin resistance (Janzon, Berntorp et al. 1983; Attvall, Fowelin et al. 1993) and increased incidence of diabetes (Rimm, Manson et al. 1993; Rimm, Chan et al. 1995; Kawakami, Takatsuka et al. 1997; Wannamethee, Shaper et al. 2001; Will, Galuska et al. 2001), but this result was not replicated in other studies (Wannamethee, Shaper et al. 2001). The role of SHS exposure to diabetes has not been explored until very recently (Houston, Houston et al. 2006). In a population composed of Caucasians and African Americans, the 15-year incidence of glucose intolerance was highest among smokers (21.8%), followed by never smokers with SHS exposure (17.2%), former smokers (14.4%), and lowest among never smokers without SHS exposure (11.5%) (Houston, Houston et al. 2006). Some studies have shown a dose-response association between smoking and incidence of diabetes (Rimm, Manson et al. 1993; Kawakami, Takatsuka et al. 1997).

Intermediate Biomarkers for Second-Hand Smoke Exposure

Intermediate biomarkers are very useful in predicting the internal dose of tobacco smoke exposure, the degree of metabolism and activation/deactivation of carcinogens, angiogenesis, cell cycle, and immune response. Examples include urinary tobacco-specific N-nitroso compounds (Hecht 2002), cytogenetic endpoints in pulmonary alveolar macrophages, bone marrow and peripheral blood erythrocytes, apoptosis and proliferating cell nuclear antigen, DNA adducts (e.g., 8-hydroxy-2-deoxyguanosine (8-OHdG), BPDE-DNA adducts, ^{32}P-postlabelled bulky adduct, oxidative damage to DNA) (Hong, Kim et al. 2001; Phillips 2002; Georgiadis, Demopoulos et al. 2004; IARC 2004), protein adducts formed by 4-ABP and PAH (Maclure, Katz et al. 1989; Hammond, Coghlin et al. 1993; Hecht 1998), sequence variants (detailed later in text), gene expression (e.g., *p53* and *K-ras*), thiobarbituric acid-reactive substances (index of lipid peroxidation and oxidative stress) (De Flora, Izzotti et al. 2005), aplasia of the chest wall muscles, ipsilateral anomalies of upper extremity due to maternal cigarette smoking (Slezak and Sasiadek 2000), deficiency of α1-antitrypsin (Silverman and Speizer 1996), cotinine (a metabolite of nicotine); vascular endothelial growth factor (VEGF), monocyte chemoattractant protein 1 (MCP-1) levels, and circulating endothelial progenitor cells (EPC) related to tumor angiogenesis (Zhu, Heeschen et al. 2003); sister chromatid exchanges (SCEs) (Vineis, Bartsch et al. 1994; Tang, Warburton et al. 1999); levels of oxidative stress measured by proinflammatory nuclear transcription factor-kappa B, activator protein-s (mouse brain) (Manna, Rangasamy et al. 2006); and activation of COX-2, mitogen activated protein kinase and c-Jun N-terminal kinase (Manna, Rangasamy et al. 2006).

Some biomarkers can indicate the site where carcinogens were ingested into body. For example, BP and NNK accumulated in the central and peripheral lung, respectively, which is due to different lipid solubilities (Gerde, Muggenburg et al. 1997; Gerde, Muggenburg et al. 1998; Pulling, Divine et al. 2003). The half-life of the cytogenetic markers differ greatly and can therefore reflect various lengths of SHS exposure. Cotinine has a plasma half-life of 21 to 48 hour in nonsmokers (Sepkovic, Haley et al. 1986; Ahijevych, Tyndale et al. 2002). PAH-albumin has a half-life of 21 days (Tang, Warburton et al. 1999). SCEs in lymphocytes can reflect SHS exposure in previous years (Tang, Warburton et al. 1999).

Biomarkers related to active smoking may not be useful for SHS exposure and related health effects. For example, single-strand DNA breaks were increased among smokers but not among SHS-exposed nonsmokers (Holz, Meissner et al. 1993). Some DNA adducts, e.g., BPDE-DNA, bulky DNA and 8-OHdG, were significantly associated with SHS exposure in some studies (Mooney, Santella et al. 1995; Zenzes, Puy et al. 1998; Georgiadis, Topinka et al. 2001) but not in others (Holz, Meissner et al. 1993; Daube, Scherer et al. 1997; Petruzzelli, Celi et al. 1998; Besaratinia, Maas et al. 2002). In addition, elevation of SCEs is not common in passive smokers (Sorsa, Husgafvel-Pursiainen et al. 1989; Sardas, Karahalil et al. 1995). On the contrary, hemoglobin adducts of 4-ABP and adducts of 3-ABP found in nonsmokers exposed to SHS were similar to adducts found in smokers, but the levels were significantly higher among individuals heavily exposed than those with undetectable SHS exposure (Maclure, Katz et al. 1989; Hammond, Coghlin et al. 1993; Hecht 1998). Elevated levels of some adducts have been observed in SHS-exposed non-smoking women and children compared to unexposed ones, e.g., PAH-DNA, PAH-albumin, and 4-ABP-hemoglobin adducts (Crawford, Mayer et al. 1994; Whyatt, Santella et al. 1998; Tang, Warburton et al. 1999). Therefore, key features of ideal biomarkers for SHS exposure would be (1) changes in the markers are significantly different between smokers and SHS-exposed nonsmokers, (2) the markers are sensitive to SHS exposure, and (3) the markers can be easily detected among SHS-exposed individuals. In addition, there is also ethnic differences among children. A US study found that African–American children had higher levels of cotinine and PAG-albumin than Hispanic children after controlling for SHS exposure (Tang, Warburton et al. 1999).

Biomarkers of Biologically Effective Dose/Early Effect

Several markers (e.g., carcinogen metabolites and DNA and protein adducts) were used to estimate the biological effective dose. Findings from association studies using this type of biomarker were summarized in Table 1.

Table 1. Association studies use biomarkers of biologically effective does/early effect.

Gene	Genotype	Study population	Outcome	Findings	Reference
1-OHP					
CYP1A1 *GSTT1* *GSTM1*	*MspI* *Null* *Null*	Italian nonsmokers	Urinary 1-hydroxyperene	NS	(Merlo, Andreassen et al. 1998)
DNA adduct					
CYP1A1	*CYP1A1*4 (C2453A)* *CYP1A1*2A (MspI)* *CYP1A1*2B (A2455G)*	Greek nonsmokers	DNA adducts	NS NS NS	(Georgiadis, Topinka et al. 2005)
	MspI *MspI+GSTM1 null* *MspI +GSTP1 (Ile/Val)* *MspI +EPHX slow*	Greek with significant SHS exposure	DNA adducts	S S S S	(Georgiadis, Demopoulos et al. 2004)
	MspI *Ile462Val*	Korean women and their newborns	Neonatal 8-hydroxy-deoxyguanosine and malondialdehyde	NS NS	(Hong, Kim et al. 2001)
CYP1B1	*Leu432Val*	Workers in a Hungarian alumina plant	DNA adducts	S	(Schoket, Papp et al. 2001)
	Arg48Gly + *Ala119Ser* *Leu432Val* *Asn453Ser*	Greek with negligible SHS exposure	DNA adducts	S S S	(Georgiadis, Demopoulos et al. 2004)
CYP2E1	*Maternal PstI (G-1259C)*	Korean women and their newborns	Neonatal 8-hydroxy-deoxyguanosine and malondialdehyde	NS	(Hong, Kim et al. 2001)
EPHX	*His139Arg* *Tyr113His*	Greek nonsmokers	DNA adducts	S S	(Georgiadis, Demopoulos et al. 2004)
GSTT1	*Null* *Null+CYP1A1 MspI*	Greek nonsmokers	DNA adducts	NS	(Georgiadis, Demopoulos et al. 2004)
	Null	Korean women and their newborns	Neonatal 8-hydroxy-deoxyguanosine and malondialdehyde	NS	(Hong, Kim et al. 2001)
GSTM1	*Null+CYP1A1 MspI*	Greek nonsmokers	DNA adducts	S	(Georgiadis, Demopoulos et al. 2004)
	Null *Null+GSTP1 AG orGG*	Polish nonsmokers	PAH-DNA adducts in human mononuclear white blood cells	NS	(Butkiewicz, Grzybowska et al. 2000)
	Null	Korean women and their newborns	Neonatal 8-hydroxy-deoxyguanosine and malondialdehyde	S (8-OHdG) NS(MDA)	(Hong, Kim et al. 2001)
GSTP1	*Ile/Val* *Ile/Val + GSTM1 null*	Polish nonsmokers	PAH-DNA adducts in human mononuclear white blood cells	NS	(Butkiewicz, Grzybowska et al. 2000)
	Ile/Val +CYP1A1 MspI	Greek nonsmokers	DNA adducts	S	(Georgiadis, Demopoulos et al. 2004)
EPHX	*Tyr113His* *His139Arg*	Greek	DNA adducts	NS	(Georgiadis, Demopoulos et al. 2004)
NAT2	*Slow acetylator*	Males with low or null nicotine-cotinine levels	DNA adducts (4-ABP)	S	(Vineis, Bartsch et al. 1994)

Table 1. Association studies use biomarkers of biologically effective does/early effect. (Continued)

Gene	Genotype	Study population	Outcome	Findings	Reference
XPD	*Exon 10* *Exon 23* *Exon 10* *AA+exon23GG*	Swedish nonsmoking populaton	DNA adducts	S S S	(Hou, Falt et al. 2002)
IgE					
CD14	*+1437* *-159 TT*	Latinos (Puertp Ricans, Mexicans, and African Americans)	IgE levels	S	(Choudhry, Avila et al. 2005)

Carcinogen Metabolites

Cotinine is a metabolite of nicotine, which is highly specific for tobacco smoke, and its level can be measured in the blood, saliva, or urine (2006). In the USA, cotinine could be detected in 70% to 43% of population from 1988-91 to 2002 (2006). About 20% of children have been exposed to SHS at home and their cotinine levels are 2-fold higher than those in adults (2006). In a study composed of African-American and Hispanic children, cotinine level was significantly elevated among the SHS exposed children ($P<0.05$) (Tang, Warburton et al. 1999). However, no studies have evaluated how genetic changes affect the association between these markers and SHS-related health effects.

Urinary 1-hydroxyperene (1-OHP) is the metabolite of pyrene. *CYP1A1* MspI, *GSTM1, or GSTT1* null genotypes were not associated with urinary 1-OHP levels among Italian police officers exposed to PAHs (Merlo, Andreassen et al. 1998). The level of hair nicotine, which is one of the main components in tobacco smoke, from people working in the bars or restaurants (Al-Delaimy, Fraser et al. 2001); urinary 4-Methylnitrosamino-1-(3-pyridyl)-1-butanol (NNAL), which is a metabolite of tobacco-specific carcinogen 4-(methylnitrosamino)-1-(3-pyridyl)-1-butanone (NNK) from infants to estimate SHS exposure from their family members (Hecht, Carmella et al. 2006).

DNA Adducts

Several studies have investigated how genetic polymorphisms modify the association between SHS exposure and the levels of DNA adducts. Below are detailed by genes.

CYPs

Cytochrome P450 (CYPs) are drug-metabolizing enzymes involved in phase I activation. Because of their role in activation of toxicants taken into the human body, genes encoding these enzymes have been more widely explored for SHS exposure than genes involved in other pathways. *CYP1A1* MspI, C2453A, and A2455G variant carriers showed a higher, but not significant, level of PAH-DNA adducts and aberrant chromosome after SHS exposure (Georgiadis, Topinka et al. 2005). Significantly higher level of DNA adducts was observed for *CYP1A1* MspI (Georgiadis, Topinka et al. 2005), combination of *CYP1A1* MspI/*GSTM1* null, *CYP1A1* MspI /*GSTP1* (Ile/Val), and *CYP1A1* MspI /*EPHX* slow polymorphism but not for *CYP1A1**4 (C2453A) (Georgiadis, Demopoulos et al. 2004). As a whole, the levels of DNA adducts were not modified by *CYP1A1* genotypes and SHS exposure. On the contrary, the genetic polymorphism of *CYP1B1,* Leu432Val, was related to elevated levels of DNA adducts in white blood cells of workers in a Hungarian aluminum plant who were exposed to PAH (Schoket, Papp et al. 2001). In addition, among Greek nonsmokers, *CYP1B1* variant carriers (Arg486Gly+Ala119Ser, Leu432Val, or Asn453Ser) with significant SHS exposure had significantly higher PAH-DNA adduct levels and aberrant chromosomes (Georgiadis, Demopoulos et al. 2004).

GSTs

Glutathione S-transferase (GSTs) are phase II detoxification enzymes encoded by four classes of polymorphic genes: alpha, mu, pi, and theta (Daniel 1993; Awasthi, Sharma et al. 1994; Wilce and Parker 1994). Alteration in the mu and theta class genes have been linked to tobacco-associated lung cancer (Bennett, Alavanja et al. 1999). Enzyme activity reach saturation with high-level carcinogen exposure among individuals who had either high or low GST activity, but this phenomenon was not observed with low-level exposure (Kiyohara, Wakai et al. 2003). Therefore, genetic polymorphisms of these genes may be ideal to assess the effects of low-level tobacco exposure, SHS.

In a Greek nonsmoking population, the DNA adduct level was highest among individuals carrying *GSTM1* null and *CYP1A1* MspI variant (1.27 ± 1.15 adducts per 108 nucleotides), and lowest among individuals with the *CYP1A1* and *GSTM1* wild type (0.83±1.08 adducts per 108 nucleotides) (P = 0.006) (Georgiadis, Demopoulos et al. 2004). However, DNA adduct levels were not significantly elevated among nonsmokers carrying *GSTM1* null or the combination of *GSTM1* null/*CYP1A1* MspI and *GSTP1* (Ile/Val)/*GSTM1* null (Georgiadis, Demopoulos et al. 2004). In a Polish nonsmoking population, the levels of PAH-DNA adducts in white blood cells were not modified by *GSTM1* null, *GSTP1* Val, the combination of *GSTM1* null and *GSTP1* AG or GG genotypes, or the combination of genotypes of *GSTM1* and *GSTP1,* but the adduct levels were significantly higher in summer among smokers carrying *GSTP1* AG or GG genotype (Butkiewicz, Grzybowska et al. 2000).

NAT2

NAT2 (N-acetyltransferase 2) is expressed in the liver and in the mucus of colon and bladder (Hein 1988; Hayes, Bi et al. 1993; Frederickson, Messing et al. 1994). NAT2 activates and deactivates hydrazine drugs, carcinogens, and arylamine, which widely exist in industry, cooked food and environmental contaminants (Hein 1988; Hein, Doll et al. 1993; Vatsis, Weber et al. 1995). Its polymorphisms can be categorized into three phenotypes: rapid, intermediate, and slow acetylator, which were determined by mutations at positions 481 (NAT2*5A), 590 (NAT2*6A) and 857 (NAT2*7A), respectively (Blum, Demierre et al. 1991). The cutpoint to differentiate slow and rapid acetylator is 0.6 for the ratio of 5-acetylamino-6-formylamino-3-methyluracil to 1-methylxanthine (Bartsch, Caporaso et al. 1990; Butler, Lang et al. 1992; Cribb, Isbrucker et al. 1994). The 4-ABP adducts were significantly higher among *NAT2* slow acetylators than rapid acetylators at low or null nicotine-cotinine levels, and this phenomenon was not observed at higher nicotine-cotinine levels (Vineis, Bartsch et al. 1994).

EPHX

EPHX (Microsomal epoxide hydrolase) is an important phase I gene, because of its ability to hydrolate PAH epoxy metabolites to the carcinogenic form. The two polymorphic variants in exons 3 (Tyr113His) and 4 (His139Arg) were found to confer lower and higher activity, respectively (Hassett, Aicher et al. 1994). However, the association between genetic polymorphisms of *EPHX* and the risk of lung cancer has not been established. Nonsmokers with the *EPHX* "fast" phenotype (Arg139Arg) had lower DNA adduct levels than those with the "slow" phenotype (His139His), therefore sequence variants of *EPHX* also plays a role in phase II detoxification (Georgiadis, Demopoulos et al. 2004). Individuals carrying *CYP1A1* MspI variant and *EPHX* "slow" polymorphisms had significantly higher DNA adduct levels (Georgiadis, Demopoulos et al. 2004).

XPD

The XPD (Xeroderma pigmentosum complementation group D) protein is involved in transcription-coupled nucleotide excision repair (NER) and forms a complex with the basal transcription factor IIH polypeptide 2 (TFIIH) during transcription-coupled repair. NER consists of global genome repair and transcription-coupled repair pathways, both of which repair bulky DNA adducts and UV-induced DNA damage (Bohr, Smith et al. 1985; Hou, Falt et al. 2002). Mutations in *XPD* cause a severe depression of NER and some cancer-prone effects (de Boer and Hoeijmakers 2000). In a Swedish nonsmoking population, there was a significant trend of increasing adduct level when the number of *XPD* variant allele in exon 10 ($p=0.02$) or exon 23 increased ($p=0.001$). The trend increased further when individuals carry the combination of exon 10 AA and exon 23 GG genotype ($p=0.02$) (Hou, Falt et al. 2002).

MDA, 8-OHdG

In a Korean population, neonatal malondialdehyde (MDA, an index of lipid peroxidation) and 8-OHdG were not affected by maternal SHS exposure and genotypes of *CYP1A1 MspI* and Ile462Val, *CYP2E1 PstI,* and *GSTT1 null* (Hong, Kim et al. 2001). However, maternal *GSTM1* null genotype and SHS exposure was associated with an increasing neonatal oxidative damage (8-OHdG) ($P=0.007$) but not significant for MDA (Hong, Kim et al. 2001).

Besides the examples above, BPDE-DNA adducts, ^{32}P-postlabelled bulky adduct, urinary 5'-Hydroxymethyluracil, and 8-Oxo-7,8-dihydroguanine are also DNA adducts. Among them the last two markers are oxidative DNA damage and repair (Bianchini, Donato et al. 1998) and.

Protein Adducts

Protein adducts formed by 4-ABP and PAH (Maclure, Katz et al. 1989; Hammond, Coghlin et al. 1993; Hecht 1998) have been used for estimate exposure to tobacco smoke. In a study composed of African-American and Hispanic children, 4-ABP-hemoglobin adducts and PAH-albumin were significantly higher ($P < 0.05$) among SHS-exposed children as compare to those without exposure (Tang, Warburton et al. 1999). In a study composed of Caucasians and Asians, the 4-ABP adducts (DNA adducts in bladder cells) were significantly higher among *NAT2* slow acetylators than rapid acetylators at low or null nicotine-cotinine levels, and this phenomenon was not observed at higher nicotine-cotinine levels (Vineis, Bartsch et al. 1994).

IgE, Eosinophils

CD14 is involved in modulating plasma IgE levels (Holt, Sly et al. 1997; O'Donnell, Toelle et al. 2004) and is part of the receptor complex for endotoxin, which has been found in cigarette smoke particles (Hasday, Bascom et al. 1999; Larsson, Szponar et al. 2004; Vercelli 2004). Endotoxin has been reported as a risk factor of respiratory disease among smokers or SHS-exposed nonsmokers (Hasday, Bascom et al. 1999; Larsson, Szponar et al. 2004). Linkage studies showed that human chromosome 5q31, where *CD14* is located, is the region linked to asthma and its related phenotypes (e.g., atopy and airway hyperresponsiveness) (Hoffjan and Ober 2002; Hoffjan, Nicolae et al. 2003). In a Latino population, there was a significant interaction between plasma IgE levels, *CD14* -159 genotypes, and SHS exposure ($p= 0.0002$) (Choudhry, Avila et al. 2005). SHS-exposed individuals with *CD14* -159 TT genotype showed the lowest IgE levels regardless of ethnicity (Choudhry, Avila et al. 2005). In a Dutch population, elevated IgE+ cells and eosinophils were observed in the nasal mucosa for children exposed to SHS, but the levels were not elevated for Langerhans cells, T cells, B cells and granulocytes, macrophages, and mast cells, (Vinke, KleinJan et al. 1999),

VEGF, MCP-1, ECP

In a Lewis lung cancer model, SHS exposure significantly increased levels of vascular endothelial growth factor (VEGF), monocyte chemoattractant protein 1 (MCP-1), and circulating endothelial progenitor cells (EPC), which were related to tumor angiogenesis (Zhu, Heeschen et al. 2003). Though angiogenesis is considered an important process related to carcinogenesis, its role in SHS-related health effects is unclear.

Biomarkers of Second-Hand Smoke Genetic Effects

Biomarkers discussed in this section include change of gene expression, somatic alterations in tissue, post-translational changes (e.g., SCEs and CAs) and epigenetic modification (e.g., DNA methylation). These studies are mainly experimental or functional studies. The advantages of experimental and functional studies as compare to association studies include that (1) easy to adjust or change the experiment status, (2) studies performed in a well controlled environment and therefore less interferences, (3) small sample size, and

(4) easy to observe the physiological changes resulting from SHS exposure. Association study is an approach commonly used to explore the relationship between sequence variants of genes and SHS related health effects. This approach is important because (1) many factors could be included, but not necessary controlled, in the study, therefore the findings are close to the real world, (2) large sample size could reach enough statistical power, and (3) collection and determination of genetic polymorphic markers are relatively stable, easier, faster, and cheaper than performing experimental studies. Therefore, these markers could be widely applied in large studies. Because of the large number of experimental studies, Table 2 only listed the findings from human *in vivo* studies.

Table 2. Association studies use biomarkers of second-hand smoke genetic effects.

Gene	*Genotype/genetic changes*	Study population	Outcome	Findings	Reference
Gene expression					
CYP1A1		Polish	Placental mRNA expression levels	NS	(Whyatt, Garte et al. 1995)
CYP1B1		Taiwanese nonsmokers	Expression levels	S	(Wu, Wu et al. 2004)
AhR		Taiwanese nonsmokers	Expression levels in the peripheral leukocytes	NS	(Wu, Wu et al. 2004)
Somatic mutation					
p53	*G:C to A:T transitions (mutations in exons 4-8)*	European Caucasian nonsmokers without SHS exposure	Lung cancer tumors	S	(Husgafvel-Pursiainen, Boffetta et al. 2000)
	G:C to A:T transitions	Caucasian nonsmoking females with SHS exposure	Lung cancer tumors	S	(Vahakangas, Bennett et al. 2001)
	G:C to A:T transitions	American nonsmoking women	Carcinoid lung tumors	S	(Gealy, Zhang et al. 1999)
	G→T transversion (lung cancers) *G→A transition (non-lung cancer)*	European nonsmokers	Lung cancer tumors	S (smokers vs. nonsmokers) S (lung cancer vs. non-lung cancers)	(Hainaut and Pfeifer 2001)
Gene	*Genotype/genetic changes*	Study population	Outcome	Findings	Reference
K-ras	*Mutations on codon 12 or 13*	Caucasian ex- and nonsmoking females	Lung cancer tumors	NS	(Vahakangas, Bennett et al. 2001)
	Mutations in exon 1	American nonsmoking females	Carcinoid lung tumors	NS	(Gealy, Zhang et al. 1999)
	Mutation in codon 12 (transition vs. transversion)	Never smokers (99 Whites and 44 Hispanics)	Lung adenocarcinoma	NS	(Pulling, Divine et al. 2003)
HPRT	*Exon2-3 genomic HPRT deletions*	Maternal SHS exposure and their newborns	HPRT mutational spectrum in newborns	S (SHS exposed vs. non-exposed)	(Finette, O'Neill et al. 1998)

Table 2. Association studies use biomarkers of second-hand smoke genetic effects.

Gene	*Genotype/genetic changes*	Study population	Outcome	Findings	Reference
Chromosome aberrations					
CYP1B1	*Arg48Gly + Ala119Ser* *Leu432Val* *Asn453Ser*	Greek with negligible SHS exposure	Chromosome aberrations	NS NS NS	(Georgiadis, Demopoulos et al. 2004)
CYP1A1	*MspI* *MspI+GSTM1 null* *MspI +GSTP1 (Ile/Val)* *MspI +mEH*	Greek with significant SHS exposure	Chromosome aberrations	S NS NS NS	(Georgiadis, Demopoulos et al. 2004)
	*CYP1A1*4 (C2453A)* *CYP1A1*2A (MspI)* *CYP1A1*2B (A2455G)*	Greek nonsmokers	Chromosome aberrations	NS NS NS	(Georgiadis, Topinka et al. 2005)
GSTT1	*Null* *Null+CYP1A1 MspI*	Greek nonsmokers	Chromosome aberrations	NS	(Georgiadis, Demopoulos et al. 2004)
GSTM1	*Null+CYP1A1 MspI*	Greek nonsmokers	Chromosome aberrations	NS	(Georgiadis, Demopoulos et al. 2004)
GSTP1	*Ile/Val +CYP1A1 MspI*	Greek nonsmokers	Chromosome aberrations	NS	(Georgiadis, Demopoulos et al. 2004)
Post-translational changes					
Chromosomal aberrations		Caucasian-predominant population (71%)	Chromosomal aberrations in newborns umbilical cord blood	S (*in utero* exposure, yes vs. no)	(Pluth, Ramsey et al. 2000)
Epigenetic effects					
p16, DAPK, RASSF1A	*Promoter methylation*	Caucasians : 82% Others : 18%	*K-ras mutation spectrum*	NS (smokers vs. nonsmokers)	(Divine, Pulling et al. 2005)
MGMT/AGT	*Methylation*	Never smoker (99 Whites and 44 Hispanics)	*Methylation*	S (Never-smokers: 66% vs. smoker: 47%)	(Pulling, Divine et al. 2003)

Gene Expression

CYPs (Cytochrome P450)

In Sprague-Dawley rats, the *in utero* SHS exposure induces pulmonary *CYP1A1* in the first day of life, but not fetal *CYPs* genes (Lee, Royce et al. 2000). Compared to placentas from nonsmoking women, *CYP1A 1* mRNA levels were significantly increased in placentas from current smokers ($P < 0.001$) and ex-smokers ($P < 0.01$) but were marginal increased for placentas from those with SHS exposure (Whyatt, Garte et al. 1995). In a Polish population, the *CYP1A 1 MspI* RFLP was not a significant determinant of *CYP1A 1* mRNA levels among nonsmokers (Whyatt, Garte et al. 1995). In a Taiwanese population, expression levels of *CYP1B1,* but not *CYP1A1,* were significantly increased in peripheral leukocytes when non-smoking cases were compared to controls (Wu, Wu et al. 2004).

AhR (Aryl Hydrocarbon Receptor)

Aryl hydrocarbon receptor (AhR) regulates xenobiotic-metabolizing enzymes (e.g., CYPs) and its ligand includes various aromatic hydrocarbons (e.g., PAH). In C57BL/6N and DBA/2N mice study, compounds in SHS binds to the AhR and stimulates its transformation, nuclear localization, dioxin responsive element binding, and activation of *CYP1A1* gene transcription (Gebremichael, Tullis et al. 1996). In a Taiwanese population, there was no significant elevation of expression of *AhR* in the peripheral leukocytes when non-smoking lung cancer cases were compared to controls (Wu, Wu et al. 2004). No other association studies have been performed so far.

11β-HSD2 (11β-Hydroxysteroid Dehydrogenase Type 2)

The enzyme encoded by *11β-hydroxysteroid dehydrogenase type 2 (11β-HSD2)* plays a role in fetal development, especially fetal birth weight (Stewart, Rogerson et al. 1995; Murphy, Zakar et al. 2002). This gene may play a role in maternal SHS exposure and the fetal health effects. A human tophoblast cell model showed that exposure to cadmium, a component in tobacco smoke, led to decrease in levels of 11β-HSD2 protein and mRNA, *11β-HSD2* promoter activity, and repression of *11β-HSD2* transcription (Yang, Julan et al. 2006). This gene may play a role in the fetal health effects of maternal SHS exposure, but no association studies have been performed.

COX-2

COX-2, also called prostaglandin-endoperoxide synthase 2 (PTGS2) is expressed in a limited number of cell types and is responsible for the prostanoid biosynthesis involved in inflammation and mitogenesis. The expression of this gene is deregulated in epithelial tumors (Kurie and Dubois 2001). In a mice study, SHS exposure led to increased levels of reactive oxygen species, which lead to increase of nuclear transcription factor-kappa B (NF-kB) activation, higher levels of proinflammatory NF-kB and activator protein-1, activation of mitogen-activated protein kinase and c-Jun N-terminal kinase in different regions of the brain, and activation of COX-2 in all the regions of the brain (Manna, Rangasamy et al. 2006). Because COX-2 plays a role in the innate immune response, its genetic polymorphisms may be associated with SHS-related health effects.

CXCR1 (CXC Chemokine Receptors 1)

The protein encoded by CXC chemokine receptors 1 (*CXCR1),* a receptor for interleukin 8 (IL8), is a member of the G-protein-coupled receptor family. CXCR1 binds to IL8 with high affinity and transduces the signal through a G-protein activated second messenger system. CXCR1 and CXCR2 mediate neutrophil recruitment to inflammatory sites (Catusse, Liotard et al. 2003). Therefore, SHS exposure may regulate the chemokines (IL-8) and their receptors (CXCR1), and then the following tumorigenesis. An animal study indicated that chicken exposed to SHS differentially stimulated the CXCR1 isoform I in primary fibroblast (Li, Lu et al. 2000).

NK-1R (Neurokinin-1 Receptor)

Neurokinin-1 receptor (NK-1R) is a receptor for neurokinin substance P, which is released from sensory C-fiber terminals and immunoinflammatory cells (Wong, Sun et al. 2002). An *in situ* hybridization study found 2-fold increase of *NK-1R* expression among lung samples from nonsmokers as compare to those from smokers (Bai, Zhou et al. 1995). The different sensitivity of *NK-1R* expression makes it an ideal marker to differentiate SHS exposure. In C57BL/6 mice, SHS exposure was related to downregulation of NK-1R mRNA in heart tissue, upregulation in the liver and kidney, but the *NK-1R* expression was not significantly change in the lungs and spleen tissues (Wong, Sun et al. 2002). However, no association studies has been reported.

Muc2 and Muc5ac

Mucin glycoproteins are adhesive, viscous, and elastic, they could trap objects enter airway and remove them through mucociliary movement (Borchers, Wert et al. 1998). Rats and mice exposed to acrolein, a compound in photochemical smog and tobacco smoke, showed increasing mucus hypersecretion, as a result of elevation of expression of *MUC5ac* and levels of macrophages and neutrophils (Borchers, Wert et al. 1998). However, this phenomenon was not observed for *MUC2* gene (Borchers, Wert et al. 1998; Borchers, Wesselkamper et al. 1999). Therefore, chronic inflammation plays a role in mucus hypersecretion, a characteristic of COPD.

Ki-67, PCNA, p21, Cyclin D1, p53, Filaggrin, Loricin, and Cytokeratins 1 and 10

Cell cycle and cell differentiation have been known to play a role in carcinogenesis. Exposure of mice and rat oral keratinocytes to nicotine changed of the mRNA and protein levels of nicotinic acetylcholine receptors and the cell cycle and cell differentiation markers Ki-67, PCNA, p21, cyclin D1, p53, filaggrin, loricrin, and cytokeratins 1 and 10, which may lead to some pathobiologic effects of tobacco products in oral tissues (Arredondo, Nguyen et al. 2001).

Bax

The protein encoded by *BCL2-associated X protein (BAX)* belongs to the BCL2 protein family, members of which act as anti- or pro-apoptotic regulators in a wide variety of cellular activities. The expression of *BAX* is regulated by the tumor suppressor *p53* and has been shown to be involved in p53-mediated apoptosis. An animal study found that PAH exposed mice showed an induction of the expression of *Bax* in oocytes, followed by apoptosis (Matikainen, Perez et al. 2001). No association studies have been performed.

Antioxidant Enzymes

Tobacco smoke increases oxidative stress and thus slightly increased gene expression of protein disulfide isomerase (PDI) and catalase in a rat model as below. Administered high dose of ascorbic acid (vitamin C) to osteogenic disorder Shionogi (ODS) rat, which lacks ascorbic acid synthesis enzyme, significantly decreased of the expression of genes encode antioxidant enzymes (e.g., CuZn-superoxide dismutase (SOD), MnSOD, catalase and PDI) and xenobiotic metabolizing enzymes (e.g., CYP1A2) (Ueta, Tadokoro et al. 2003). The reduction of expression of plasma glutathione peroxidase was not significant (Ueta, Tadokoro et al. 2003). Therefore, vitamin C intake may reduce the oxidative stress resulting from cigarette smoking.

Ribosomal Protein L31 and Zis

Injection BP into male Sprague–Dawley rats, increasing growth and proliferation rate (athrogenic phenotype), suppression of mRNA level for *ribosomal protein L31* and *Zis* genes, overexpression of gas-5 and mitochondrial mRNAs were observed in the cultured vascular smooth muscle cells (Lu, Alejandro et al. 2002). In the same study, these findings were confirmed by in situ hybridization experiments *in vivo*.

Somatic Mutations

p53

p53 is a tumor suppressor gene involved in cell growth and proliferation. Some studies found that *p53* mutation occurs more frequently in smokers (26%) and former smokers (67%) than never-smokers exposed to spousal SHS (13%) and lifetime never-smokers (10-19%) (Husgafvel-Pursiainen, Boffetta et al. 2000; Vahakangas, Bennett et al. 2001). However, another study found that *p53* mutation frequency was similar between smokers and nonsmokers (Gealy, Zhang et al. 1999). These disparities may result from different *p53* mutations, study population, and small sample size used in the latter studies. The type and spectra of *p53* mutation were consistently and significantly different between smokers and nonsmokers (Gealy, Zhang et al. 1999). For example, G:C to T:A transversions and some mutational hotspots in codon 157-158, 179, 245-249, 273 and 282 (Cherpillod and Amstad 1995; Denissenko, Pao et al. 1996; Hernandez-Boussard and Hainaut 1998) were more frequently observed among smokers (19-31%) as compared to G:C to A:T transitions, which were more common among never smokers (22-57%) (Gealy, Zhang et al. 1999; Husgafvel-Pursiainen, Boffetta et al. 2000; Hainaut and Pfeifer 2001; Vahakangas, Bennett et al. 2001). In a European Caucasian population, G:C to T:A transversions were associated with elevated risk of lung cancer when compared ever-smokers to never smokers with SHS exposure (OR=2.9, 95% CI=1.2-7.2) or compared ever-smokers to never smokers without SHS exposure (OR=4.4, 95% CI=1.2-16.2) (Husgafvel-Pursiainen, Boffetta et al. 2000). In summary, G:C to A:T transitions in *p53* are markers observed among nonsmokers and thus may be useful markers for predicting SHS-related effects.

K-ras

Kirsten ras (K-ras) is an oncogene and encodes a protein belongs to small GTPas superfamily. It has two isoforms different in the C-terminal region as a result of alternative splicing. A mice study showed that *K-ras* mutation in exon 2 maybe a specific target for SHS (Witschi, Oreffo et al. 1995). For *p53* mutant mice, the *K-ras* mutation spectrum was similar in tumors from the different groups (group a: 5 months SHS exposure+4.5 months recover period, group b: 9.5 months continuative SHS exposure) (Yao, Wang et al. 2005). In one study, the mutations in *K-ras* codon 12 accounted for 30-40% of lung adenocarcinoma among smokers and former uranium miners; less than 11% of adenocarcinoma cases were found among nonsmokers (Vahakangas, Bennett et al. 2001). In a Caucasian female nonsmoking population, mutations on *K-ras* codon 12 and 13 were not associated with lung cancer risk (Vahakangas, Bennett et al. 2001). Similar findings were observed in an American nonsmoking female population for mutation in exon 1 for the risk of carcinoid lung tumors (Gealy, Zhang et al. 1999) and in another Caucasian-predominant population for mutations in codon 12 and the risk of lung adenocarcinoma (Pulling, Divine et al. 2003). The difference in frequencies of *K-ras* mutation between smokers and nonsmokers were not sufficient to make them ideal markers for SHS exposure. This may explain the null findings between smokers and nonsmokers in prior studies.

P16, DAPK, RASSF1A

P16, located in chromosome 9p21, is involved chromosomal inversions, translocations, heterozygous deletions, and homozygous deletions in malignant cell lines from various tumors (Liggett and Sidransky 1998). *Death-associated protein kinase 1 (DAPK1)* is a tumor suppressor gene and is a positive mediator of interferon induced programmed cell death (Lee, Rho et al. 2005). *Ras effector homolog 1 (RASSF1A)* is a tumor suppressor gene and encodes a protein similar to the RAS effector proteins. Loss or altered expression of *RASSF1A* has been associated with the pathogenesis of a variety of cancers (Byun, Lee et al. 2001). The inactivation of this gene was found to be correlated with the hypermethylation of its CpG-island promoter region (Liu, Yoon et al. 2002). SHS-related adenocarcinoma was partly induced through cell cycle control by *p16* (Jarmalaite, Kannio et al. 2003), signal transduction by *RASSF1A*, and apoptosis via *DAPK* and *RASSF1A* (Tang, Khuri et al. 2000; Dammann, Schagdarsurengin et al. 2003). In an animal study, an additive effect was observed in SHS-exposed mice with a mutant *p53* transgene and *p16* deletion (Wang, Zhang et al. 2005). Possible association between genetic polymorphisms of these genes and SHS-related health effects have not been assessed.

HPRT

Hypoxanthine–guanine phosphoriboslytransferase (HPRT) is involved in the purine salvage pathway, which phosphoribosylates purine analogs and leads to cytotoxicity (Finette, O'Neill et al. 1998). Among SHS-exposed newborns, a significant difference in *HPRT* mutational spectra, increasing genomic deletions mediated by V(D) recombinase, was observed in those exposed *in utero* to cigarette smoke (Finette, O'Neill et al. 1998). Therefore, the sequence variants in *HPRT* may serve as a good indicator for fetal SHS exposure.

Post-Translational Changes

Sister Chromatid Exchanges (SCEs)

Sister chromatid exchanges (SCE) is a marker reflect the genetic damages resulting from exposure to carcinogens (Tucker, Eastmond et al. 1997). SCEs were correlated with DNA adducts and somatic mutations (Carrano 1986) and were related to SHS-exposure previously

(Morimoto, Miura et al. 1984). Because of the long half-life, SCEs in lymphocytes can reflect SHS exposure in past years (Tang, Warburton et al. 1999). However, elevation of SCEs is not common in passive smokers (Sorsa, Husgafvel-Pursiainen et al. 1989; Sardas, Karahalil et al. 1995). In a population composed of Hispanic and African-American children, the SCE level was marginally increased when compared SHS-exposed children to those without exposure (P=0.076) (Tang, Warburton et al. 1999). The SCE level was higher among African-American children than the level among Hispanic children after controlling for SHS exposure (P=0.059).

Chromosomal Aberrations (CAs)

Chromosomal aberrations (CAs) are structural aberrations comprising chromosome-type and chromatid-type breaks and rearrangements (Norppa 2004). CAs can predict cancer risk among nonsmokers but not depend on the time between the chromosome analysis and cancer diagnosis (Bonassi, Hagmar et al. 2000), this could be explained by individual susceptibility (Norppa 2004). *CYP1A1* MspI, C2453A, and A2455G variant carriers showed a higher, but not significant, level of aberrant chromosome after SHS exposure (Georgiadis, Topinka et al. 2005). In a Caucasian-predominant population, a significant association between the newborn *CYP1A1 MspI* polymorphism and CA frequencies was observed in the newborns umbilical cord blood (heterozygotes vs. wild type: p=0.02), but not for other genes (*CYP2D6* and *CYP1A1,* and phase II genes: *NAT1, NAT2, GSTT1, GSTM1, GSTP1*, and *epoxide hydrolase*) (Pluth, Ramsey et al. 2000). Exposure to tobacco smoke *in utero* also appeared to increase fetal translocation frequencies (maternal smoking status, yes vs. no: p=0.045) (Pluth, Ramsey et al. 2000).

Epigenetic Effects

Promoter Methylation

In a Caucasian-predominant population, the prevalence of methylation of the *p16, DAPK,* and *RASSF1A* genes were similar between adenocarcinomas from smokers and nonsmoker and were also independent of *K-ras* mutation (Divine, Pulling et al. 2005). *O6-methylguanine-DNA methyltransferase (MGMT)* or *O6-alkylguanine DNA alkyltransferase (AGT)* encodes a DNA repair enzyme that removes the guanine at the O6 position and transfers the alkyl group to an internal cysteine acceptor site (Cohet, Borel et al. 2004) to protect carcinogenesis from alkylating agents (Pulling, Divine et al. 2003). For example, the adduct *O*6-alkylguanine, which is the metabolite of *N*-nitroso compounds (IARC 2004), can be inactivated by MGMT. When DNA repair by MGMT failed, transition mutation in *K-ras* may take place (Pulling, Divine et al. 2003). *MGMT* methylation was more frequent in tumors from never-smokers than from smokers (66 vs. 47%) (Pulling, Divine et al. 2003). Transcriptional silencing may occur when methylation of a CpG island in the *MGMT* promoter region is affected (Esteller, Hamilton et al. 1999; Esteller, Toyota et al. 2000). Because the methylation of *MGMT* was more frequent in tumors from never-smokers, it might be a good marker for SHS related health effects.

Biomarkers of Heritable Susceptibility to Second-Hand Smoke

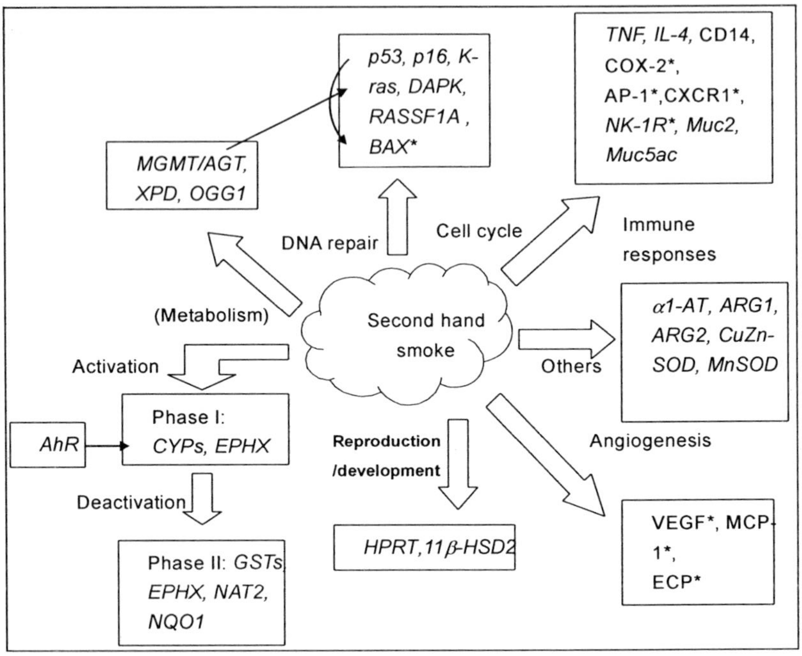

Figure 2: Genes and enzymes involved in pathways related to second-hand smoke exposure. *Association studies were not available.

There is abundant evidence of the association between active tobacco smoke and various ill effects on health. A great deal of genetic data have been generated since the completion of Human Genome Project. However, few studies have assessed genetic susceptibility and the risk of SHS-related health effects. To date, associations between genetic polymorphisms and the risk of some SHS-related health effects or intermediate status have been assessed for *GSTP1* (Miller, De Vivo et al. 2003; Canalle, Burim et al. 2004), *GSTT1* (Hong, Lee et al. 2003), *GSTM1* (Nyberg, Hou et al. 1998; Bennett, Alavanja et al. 1999; Kiyohara, Wakai et al. 2003; Wenzlaff, Cote et al. 2005), *NAT2* (Vineis, Bartsch et al. 1994; Nyberg, Hou et al. 1998; Schonberger and Van Schayck 1998), *CYP1A1* (Merlo, Andreassen et al. 1998; Hung, Boffetta et al. 2003; Georgiadis, Topinka et al. 2005; Ng, Tan et al. 2005), *CYP1B1* (Wenzlaff, Cote et al. 2005), *p53* (mice and human) (Gealy, Zhang et al. 1999; Husgafvel-Pursiainen, Boffetta et al. 2000; Vahakangas, Bennett et al. 2001; De Flora, Balansky et al. 2003; Yao, Wang et al. 2005), *NAD(P)H:quinone oxidoredictase 1 (NQO1)* (Bock, Wenzlaff et al. 2005), *O(6)-alkylguanine DNA alkyltransferase (AGT)* (Cohet, Borel et al. 2004), *xeroderma pigmentosium complementation group D (XPD)* (Hou, Falt et al. 2002), *tumor necrosis factor (TNF)* (Wenten, Berhane et al. 2005), *CD14* (Choudhry, Avila et al. 2005), *8-oxoguanine DNA glycosylase (OGG1)* (Sunaga, Kohno et al. 2002), *alpha1-antitrypsin (α1-AT)* (children) (von Ehrenstein, von Mutius et al. 2002), *Arginase II (ARG2)* (Li, Romieu et al. 2006), *epoxide hydrolase (EPHX1)* (Wu, Zhang et al. 2001), and *supF (E. coli)* (Matsuda, Kawanishi et al. 1998).

Based on the existing studies, the genetic markers listed above and discussed in earlier sections could be categorized into different biological pathways: (1) metabolism (activation/deactivation), (2) DNA repair, (3) cell cycle, (4) immune response, (5) reproduction/development, (6) angiogenesis, and (7) others (Figure 2). The findings regarding of genetic polymorphisms of individual genes or their joint effects are detailed below. Findings from association studies are summarized in Table 3.

Table 3. Association studies use biomarkers of heritable susceptibility to second-hand smoke.

Gene	*Genotype*	Study population	Outcome	Findings	Reference
Metabolism (Activation)					
CYP1A1	*Msp I (T6235C)*	Chinese nonsmokers	Lung cancer	S	(Song, Tan et al. 2001)
	Msp I *Ile462Val*	Japanese nonsmokers	Lung adenocarcinoma	NS NS	(Sunaga, Kohno et al. 2002)
	Msp I	Lifetime nonsmoking Japanese women	Lung cancer	NS	(Kiyohara, Wakai et al. 2003)
	Msp I *Ile462Val (A4889G)* *Msp I+GSTM1 null* *Msp I+GSTT1 null*	Lifetime Chinese female nonsmokers	Lung cancer	S S NS NS	(Ng, Tan et al. 2005)
	Ile462Val *Ile462Val + GSTM1 null*	Caucasians nonsmokers (pooled analysis)	Lung cancer	S S	(Hung, Boffetta et al. 2003)
	MspI *Ile462Val*	Never smokers (Caucasians: 82%, African Americans: 18%)	Lung cancer	NS NS	(Wenzlaff, Cote et al. 2005)
	Msp I	Caucasian-predominant population (68%)	Lung cancer	NS	(Vineis, Veglia et al. 2003)
	Ile462Val	Caucasian female never-smokers	Lung cancer	NS	(Bennett, Alavanja et al. 1999)
	MspI	Italian traffic police officers	Lung Cancer	NS	(Merlo, Andreassen et al. 1998)
	Msp I *C2453A* *A2455G*	Children with SHS exposure (Caucasians: 95%)	Childhood acute lymphoblastic leukemia	NS NS NS	(Infante-Rivard, Krajinovic et al. 2000)
CYP1B1	*Leu432Val* *Leu432Val + NQO1* *C609T* *Leu432Val + GSTM1null* *Leu432Val + GSTP1 Ile105Val*	Never smokers (Caucasians: 82%, African Americans: 18%)	Lung cancer	S S S S	(Wenzlaff, Cote et al. 2005)
Metabolism (Deactivation)					
GSTT1	*Null*	European nonsmoking Caucasians	Lung cancer	NS	(Malats, Camus-Radon et al. 2000)
	Null	Caucasian female never-smokers	Lung cancer	NS	(Bennett, Alavanja et al. 1999)
	Null	Nonsmokers (Caucasian: 95%)	Lung cancer (all, adenocarcinoma, non small cell lung cancer)	NS	(Nazar-Stewart, Vaughan et al. 2003)
	Null	Never smokers (Caucasians: 82%, African Americans: 18%)	Lung cancer	NS	(Wenzlaff, Cote et al. 2005)
	Null	Caucasians nonsmokers (pooled analysis)	Lung cancer	NS	(Hung, Boffetta et al. 2003)

Table 3. Association studies use biomarkers of heritable susceptibility to second-hand smoke. (Continued)

Gene	*Genotype*	Study population	Outcome	Findings	Reference
	Null	Japanese nonsmokers	Lung adenocarcinoma	NS	(Sunaga, Kohno et al. 2002)
	Null *Null+CYP1A1 Ile462Val*	Greek nonsmokers	Lung cancer	NS NS	(Georgiadis, Demopoulos et al. 2004)
	Null *Null+CYP1A1 MspI* *Null+CYP1A1 Ile462Val*	Chinese female lifetime nonsmokers	Lung cancer	NS S NS	(Ng, Tan et al. 2005)
GSTM1	*Null*	Caucasian female never-smokers	Lung cancer	S	(Bennett, Alavanja et al. 1999)
	Null	Japanese nonsmokers	Lung adenocarcinoma	S	(Sunaga, Kohno et al. 2002)
	Null	Lifetime non-smoking Japanese women	Lung Cancer	S	(Kiyohara, Wakai et al. 2003)
	Null *Null+ GSTP1 Val*	Never smokers (Caucasians: 82%, African Americans: 18%)	Lung cancer	S S	(Wenzlaff, Cote et al. 2005)
	Null *Null +CYP1A1 MspI* *Null +CYP1A1 Ile462Val*	Lifetime Chinese female non-smokers	Lung cancer	NS NS NS	(Ng, Tan et al. 2005)
	Null *Null + NAT2 slow acetylator*	Swedish never smokers	Lung cancer	NS S	(Nyberg, Hou et al. 1998)
	Null	European nonsmoking Caucasians	Lung cancer	NS	(Malats, Camus-Radon et al. 2000)
	Null	Nonsmokers (Caucasians: 62%)	Lung cancer	NS	(Tang, Rundle et al. 1998)
	Null	Nonsmokers (Caucasian: 95%)	Lung cancer (all types, adenocarcinoma, non small cell lung cancer)	NS	(Nazar-Stewart, Vaughan et al. 2003)
	Null+CYP1A1 Ile462Val	Caucasians non-smokers (pooled analysis)	Lung cancer	S	(Hung, Boffetta et al. 2003)
	Null	Caucasian: 61% Hispanics: 24.5% African Americans: 4% Asians: 5%	Asthma and wheezing in children (in utero SHS exposure)	S	(Gilliland, Li et al. 2002)
GSTP1	*Ile/Val (A→G)*	US Caucasians	Lung cancer	NS	(Miller, De Vivo et al. 2003)
	Ile/Val +GSTM1 Null	Never smokers (Caucasians: 82%, African Americans: 18%)	Lung cancer	S	(Wenzlaff, Cote et al. 2005)
NOQ1	*Ser187Pro (T allele)*	Nonsmokers (Caucasians, 77% African Americans, 23%)	Lung cancer	NS	(Bock, Wenzlaff et al. 2005)
	Ser187Pro *Pro/Pro + GSTT1 null*	Japanese nonsmokers	Lung adenocarcinoma	NS NS	(Sunaga, Kohno et al. 2002)
NAT2	*Slow acetylator*	Non-smoking Chinese females	Lung cancer	S	(Seow, Zhao et al. 1999)
	Slow acetylator *Slow acetylator + GSTM1 null*	Swedish never smokers	Lung cancer	NS S	(Nyberg, Hou et al. 1998)

Table 3. Association studies use biomarkers of heritable susceptibility to second-hand smoke. (Continued)

Gene	*Genotype*	Study population	Outcome	Findings	Reference
DNA repair					
MGMT/ AGT	*143Val + 178Arg*	Caucasians	Adenocarcinoma Small cell carcinoma Squamous cell carcinoma	S NS NS	(Cohet, Borel et al. 2004)
XPD	*Exon 10 and 23*	Swedish never smoker (<1 cigarette/day during a year)	Lung cancer	S	(Hou, Falt et al. 2002)
OGG1	*Ser326Cys*	Japanese nonsmokers	Lung adenocarcinoma	NS	(Sunaga, Kohno et al. 2002)
Immune response					
TNF	*TNF G-308*	Children Caucasian: 54% Hispanic: 32% Others: 14%	Respiratory illness-related school absences	S	(Wenten, Berhane et al. 2005)
IL-1	*IL-1A -889, IL-1B -511, IL-1A +3954*	German nonsmokers	Periodontal disease	NS	(Meisel, Schwahn et al. 2004)
CD14	*+1437* *-159* *-810*	Latinos (Puertp Ricans, Mexicans, and African Americans)	Asthma severity and lung functions	S (asthma severity, FEV1) S (asthma severity, IgE) S (IgE)	(Choudhry, Avila et al. 2005)
Others					
αl-AT	*PiMS*	German children with SHS exposure	Lung function	S	(von Ehrenstein, von Mutius et al. 2002)
ARG1 *ARG2*	*A/G, T/A, C/T, T/C* *G/C, T/C* *G/A, T/C*	Mexican children	Childhood asthma and atopy	NS S NS	(Li, Romieu et al. 2006)

Metabolism (Activation/Deactivation)

CYPs (Cytochrome P450)

CYP1A1

CYP1A1 MspI and Ile462Val are two SNPs commonly studied and are in high linkage disequilibirum with each other (Hayashi, Watanabe et al. 1991). However, both variant alleles are rare in Caucasians and African Americans (Kiyohara 2000; Georgiadis, Demopoulos et al. 2004). For *CYP1A1* MspI, significant elevated risk of lung cancer was observed among nonsmokers in a Chinese population (odds ratio (OR)=3.2, 95% confidence interval (CI)=1.5-6.7) (Song, Tan et al. 2001). An insignificant association was found in two Japanese nonsmoking populations (Sunaga, Kohno et al. 2002; Kiyohara, Wakai et al. 2003), a Chinese lifetime nonsmoking female population (Ng, Tan et al. 2005), two Caucasian nonsmoking populations (Hung, Boffetta et al. 2003; Wenzlaff, Cote et al. 2005), a pooled population composed of Caucasian and Asian non-smokers (Vineis, Veglia et al. 2003), and an Italian nonsmoking population (Merlo, Andreassen et al. 1998). For joint effects, Chinese female nonsmokers carrying MspI CC genotype showed a two-fold increased risk of lung cancer when they were also null for *GSTT1* (OR=2.7, 95 CI=1.1-6.9) as compare to other genotype combinations combined (Ng, Tan et al. 2005). But an increased lung cancer risk was found for the combination of MspI CC genotype and *GSTM1* null (Ng, Tan et al. 2005). The vast majority of prior studies showed null associations; therefore, the MspI polymorphism may not be an important risk factor for SHS-related lung cancer.

The sequence variant *CYP1A1* Ile462Val was significantly associated with lung cancer in a pooled Caucasian nonsmoking population including 14 case-control studies (all lung cancer: OR=2.99, 95% CI=1.51-5.91; adenocarcinoma: OR=4.85, 95% CI=2.03-11.6) (Hung, Boffetta et al. 2003) and a Chinese female nonsmoking population (OR=2.8, 95% CI=1.1-7.6) (Ng, Tan et al. 2005). A null association was reported in a US Caucasian female never-smoking population (Bennett, Alavanja et al. 1999), and a Japanese population (Sunaga, Kohno et al. 2002). Regarding joint effects, Caucasian non-smokers with combined *CYP1A1* Ile462Val variant and *GSTM1* null genotype showed a 4.67-fold increased risk of lung cancer (95% CI=2.00-10.9) as compared with those carrying *CYP1A1* wild type and *GSTM1* null genotype (Hung, Boffetta et al. 2003). The significant findings for *CYP1A1* Ile462Val reflect that the polymorphism Ile462Val maybe a potential risk factor for SHS-related lung cancer.

As described in the "Biomarkers of biologically effective does/early effect", genetic polymorphisms of *CYP1A1* MspI and A2455G, the combination of *CYP1A1* MspI/*GSTM1* null, *CYP1A1* MspI /*GSTP1* (Ile/Val), and *CYP1A1* MspI /*EPHX* slow phenotype were not significantly associated with the level of PAH-DNA adducts and aberrant chromosome after SHS exposure (Georgiadis, Demopoulos et al. 2004; Georgiadis, Topinka et al. 2005). SHS exposure and maternal genotypes of *CYP1A1 MspI* and Ile462Val and *CYP2E1 PstI* did not affect the level of neonatal oxidative damage MDA and 8-OHdG (Hong, Kim et al. 2001).

For childhood ALL, increased but not significant risk were found for children carrying the *CYP1A1**4 (C2453A) allele at high levels of maternal smoking in the last trimesters and at low level of paternal postnatal smoking (Infante-Rivard, Krajinovic et al. 2000). Decreased ALL risk was observed for the *CYP1A1**2B (A2455G) allele, which appeared to confer a protective advantage at low levels of maternal prenatal smoking and at high levels for paternal postnatal smoking (Infante-Rivard, Krajinovic et al. 2000). However, another study could not replicate these findings (Canalle, Burim et al. 2004).

CYP1B1

In an analyses of data from Surveillance, Epidemiology and End Results (SEER) database, Caucasian never-smokers carrying *CYP1B1* variant (Val) were found to have an increased risk of lung cancer (OR=2.87, 95% CI=1.63-5.07) (Wenzlaff, Cote et al. 2005). Gene-gene interactions have also been investigated. Never smokers carrying variant alleles of both *CYP1B1* Leu432Val and *NQO1* C609T had an elevated risk of lung cancer (OR=4.14, 95% CI=1.60-10.74), findings remained significant among those carrying *CYP1B1* Leu432Val and *GSTM1* null genotypes (OR=2.62, 95% CI=1.18-5.81), or *CYP1B1* Leu432Val and *GSTP1* Ile105Val (OR=3.21, 95% CI=1.34-7.74) (Wenzlaff, Cote et al. 2005). The consistent findings supported the contention that genetic polymorphisms of *CYP1B1* may play a role in lung carcinogenesis due to SHS exposure. As detailed in the "Biomarkers of biologically effective does/early effect", sequence variants of *CYP1B1*

(Arg486Gly+Ala119Ser, Leu432Val, or Asn453Ser) were significantly associated with higher level of DNA adducts among SHS exposed individuals (Schoket, Papp et al. 2001; Georgiadis, Demopoulos et al. 2004).

GSTs (Glutathione-S-Transferase)

STT1

Though several studies have investigated the relationship between *GSTT1* and lung cancer risk among nonsmokers, most findings did not reach significance. Null findings were observed in a European Caucasian non-smoking population (Malats, Camus-Radon et al. 2000), a US Caucasian non-smoking female population (Bennett, Alavanja et al. 1999), two US Caucasian-predominant populations (Nazar-Stewart, Vaughan et al. 2003; Wenzlaff, Cote et al. 2005), nonsmokers in a pooled analysis of 14 Caucasian case-control studies (Hung, Boffetta et al. 2003), a Japanese non-smoking population (Sunaga, Kohno et al. 2002), and a Greek nonsmoking population (Georgiadis, Demopoulos et al. 2004). For joint effects, in a Chinese population of female nonsmokers, the combination of *GSTT1* null and *CYP1A1* MspI variant was significantly associated with increased risk of lung cancer (OR=2.7, 95% CI=1.1-6.9) (Ng, Tan et al. 2005), but not in a Greek nonsmoking population (Georgiadis, Demopoulos et al. 2004). However, the combination of *GSTT1* null and *CYP1A1* Ile462Val variants showed null association (Georgiadis, Demopoulos et al. 2004; Ng, Tan et al. 2005). In summary, *GSTT1* null genotype may not be a risk factor of lung cancer from SHS exposure.

As mentioned in the "Biomarkers of biologically effective does/early effect", *GSTT1* null genotype was not associated with significant change of urinary 1-OHP level among PAH exposed Italian police officers (Merlo, Andreassen et al. 1998). No significant association was observed for the maternal genotype, SHS exposure and the levels of neonatal oxidative damages (8-OHdG and MDA) (Hong, Kim et al. 2001).

GSTM1

GSTM1 null is a common polymorphism in Caucasians (Georgiadis, Demopoulos et al. 2004). Elevated risk of lung cancer was significantly linked to *GSTM1* null genotype in a US Caucasian non-smoking female population (OR=2.6, 95% CI=1.1-6.1) (Bennett, Alavanja et al. 1999), in Japanese nonsmokers (lung adenocarcinoma: OR=3.32, 95% CI=1.41-7.84) (Sunaga, Kohno et al. 2002), in another Japanese lifetime nonsmoking population (OR=2.27, 95% CI=1.13-4.57, high-dose SHS+*GSTM1* null vs. low-dose SHS +*GSTM1* present) (Kiyohara, Wakai et al. 2003), in nonsmokers from the SEER database (OR=2.32, 95% CI= 1.05-5.13, ≧20 household SHS years +*GSTM1* null vs. no household SHS +*GSTM1* present) (Wenzlaff, Cote et al. 2005), and in a Chinese female population of never smokers (Ng, Tan et al. 2005). The magnitude of OR reported among nonsmokers was higher than those among smokers. For example, in a meta-analysis, *GSTM1* deficiency was associated with a 1.4-fold increased risk of lung cancer among smokers (95% CI=1.2-1.6) and accounted for 17% of all lung cancers because of its high prevalence (McWilliams, Sanderson et al. 1995). Insignificant association was observed in a Swedish nonsmoking population (Nyberg, Hou et al. 1998), a European Caucasian population (Malats, Camus-Radon et al. 2000), and two

Caucasian-predominant populations (Tang, Rundle et al. 1998; Nazar-Stewart, Vaughan et al. 2003). Gene-gene interactions were observed in some studies. Among Swedish never-smokers, individual with *NAT2* slow acetylator and *GSTM1* present genotype had a 3.1-fold risk of lung cancer (95% CI=1.1-8.6), but no clear pattern was observed among smokers (Nyberg, Hou et al. 1998). In a pooled analysis of Caucasian nonsmokers, individuals carrying *GSTM1* null and *CYP1A1* Ile 462 Val variant were significantly associated with lung cancer risk (OR=4.67, 95% CI=1.00-10.9) (Hung, Boffetta et al. 2003). In a Caucasian-predominant population, significant association was detected among nonsmokers carrying *GSTM1* null and *GSTP1* Val (OR=4.67, 95% CI=1.00-10.9) (Wenzlaff, Cote et al. 2005). *GSTM1* null genotype is a sensitive marker for nonsmokers, it could be important for assessing the association between SHS exposure and lung cancer risk.

The *GSTM1* genotype may also play a role in asthma and wheezing because xenobiotic metabolism and antioxidant pathways are involved in asthma pathogenesis (Gilliland, McConnell et al. 1999; Hayes and Stange 2000; Ivashchenko, Sideleva et al. 2001; Piirila, Wikman et al. 2001). In a Caucasian-predominant population (61% Caucasian and 24.5% Hispanics), *in utero* tobacco smoke exposure was associated with increased risk of early onset of asthma (OR=1.6, 95% CI=1.0-2.5), asthma with current symptoms (OR=1.7, 95%CI=1.1-2.8), persistent asthma (OR=1.6, 95% CI=1.1-2.4), lifetime history of wheezing (OR=1.8, 95% CI=1.3-2.5), wheezing with exercise (OR=1.2, 95% CI=1.4-3.4), and emergency room visit in the past year (OR=3.7, 95% CI=1.4-3.4) among children carrying *GSTM1* null genotype (Gilliland, Li et al. 2002). The association between *GSTM1* and asthma has been limited and more studies are necessary to confirm these findings.

As mentioned in the "Biomarkers of biologically effective does/early effect", the *GSTM1* null genotype was not associated with elevated level of 1-OHP (Merlo, Andreassen et al. 1998) or DNA adducts (Butkiewicz, Grzybowska et al. 2000), but significantly associated with the neonatal oxidative damage (8-OHdG, but not MDA) when SHS-exposed mothers carrying the null genotype (P=0.007) (Hong, Kim et al. 2001). Genetic polymorphisms of the combination of *GSTM1* null and *CYP1A1* MspI were significantly associated with increased level of DNA adduct in one study (Georgiadis, Demopoulos et al. 2004) but not in the other (Butkiewicz, Grzybowska et al. 2000).

GSTP1

GST class p, encoded by *GSTP1* gene, is the most abundant isoform in the lung. It is highly expressed in many tissues (including the lung) and is one of the main detoxifiers of the activated form of BP (Awasthi, Sharma et al. 1994; Nakajima, Elovaara et al. 1995; Fields, Morrow et al. 1998; Hecht 1999). A common nonsynonymous SNP in exon 5 of the *GSTP1* lead to amino acid exchange (Ile3Val) in codon 105 and reduced enzyme activity (Ali-Osman, Akande et al. 1997; Johansson, Stenberg et al. 1998). This SNP was in linkage disequilibrium with the other nonsynonymous SNP at codon 114 (Ala114Val) (Harris, Coggan et al. 1998). In a US Caucasian population, they found that SHS exposure among individuals carrying the *GSTP1* GG genotype was not significantly associated with lung cancer risk as compared with those without SHS exposure and carrying AA genotype (Miller, De Vivo et al. 2003). For joint effects, in the SEER database, individuals carrying the *GSTM1* null and *GSTP1* Val allele and exposed to SHS had a significantly elevated risk of lung cancer (OR=4.6, 95% CI=1.21-17.21) (Wenzlaff, Cote et al. 2005). Conflict results and limited studies make it difficult to reach any conclusion.

As detailed in the "Biomarkers of biologically effective does/early effect", DNA adducts levels were not affected by *GSTP1* variant genotype or the combination of genotypes of *GSTM1* and *GSTP1* genotypes among nonsmokers (Butkiewicz, Grzybowska et al. 2000; Georgiadis, Demopoulos et al. 2004).

NQO1 (NAD(P)H:Quinone Oxidoreductase 1)

The enzyme encoded by the gene *NAD(P)H:quinone oxidoreductase 1 (NQO1)* is a flavoprotein that catalyzes the reduction of quinones and activates compounds like antitumor quinones and some procarcinogens present in cigarette smoke (Bock, Wenzlaff et al. 2005). *NQO1* is highly expressed in normal lung tissue and overexpressed in non-small-cell lung cancer (Siegel, Franklin et al. 1998). In a Caucasian-predominant population, no significant protective effect was observed for the *NQO1* T allele among those either with or without SHS exposure (Bock, Wenzlaff et al. 2005). In a Japanese population, the same polymorphism was not associated with lung adenocarcinoma risk among non-smokers (Sunaga, Kohno et al. 2002). Among nonsmokers, individuals with the combined genotype of *NQO1* Pro/Pro and *GSTT1* null were not at significantly higher risk of lung adenocarcinoma compared with those who carried *NQO1* Ser/Ser and *GSTT1* positive (Sunaga, Kohno et al. 2002). Few studies have explored the association between sequence variants in *NQO1* and health effects related to SHS exposure; more studies are warranted.

EPHX (Microsomal Epoxide Hydrolase)

As detailed in the "Biomarkers of biologically effective does/early effect", *EPHX* "slow" phenotype (Arg139Arg) and its combination with *CYP1A1* MspI variant were significantly associated with higher DNA adduct levels among nonsmokers (Georgiadis, Demopoulos et al. 2004).

NAT2 (N-Acetyltransferase 2)

In a Chinese female population, nonsmokers carrying *NAT2* slow acetylator had a 2-fold higher risk of lung cancer than non-carriers (95% CI=1.1-3.7), but no effect was observed among smokers (Seow, Zhao et al. 1999). The association remained significant for adenocarcinoma (OR=2.1, 95% CI=1.1-4.0) (Seow, Zhao et al. 1999). In a Swedish population, there was a higher but insignificant increase of lung cancer risk when comparing *NAT2* slow to rapid acetylator genotypes among nonsmokers, but a lower risk was observed among smokers (Nyberg, Hou et al. 1998). In the same population, individuals carrying the combination of *NAT2* slow acetylator and *GSTM1* null genotype were significantly associated with lung cancer risk among nonsmokers (Nyberg, Hou et al. 1998). Results have been conflicting for studies without considering SHS exposure. Although there were few prior studies, these interesting findings indicate that variants of *NAT2* maybe a sensitive marker and is able to differentiate the metabolism profiles between smokers and nonsmokers. More studies are needed to assess this association.

DNA repair

MGMT (O-6-Methylguanine-DNA Methyltransferase)/AGT (O6-Alkylguanine DNA Alkyltransferase)

Some nosynonymous SNPs (e.g. Gly160Arg, Ile143Val, and Lys178Arg) are located in exon 5 of *MGMT*. Among them, Ile143Val and Lys178Arg are in high linkage disequilibrium with each other (Deng, Xie et al. 1999). Other polymorphisms have been found in the promoter, exon 1, and exon 3 (Egyhazi, Ma et al. 2002). In a Caucasian population, *MGMT* 143Val and 178Arg variant carriers had a significantly higher risk of lung cancer (OR=2.05, 95% CI=1.03-4.07) (Cohet, Borel et al. 2004). The risk remained significant for adenocarcinoma (OR=2.67, 95% CI=1.21-5.87) but not for small cell carcinoma and squamous cell carcinoma (Cohet, Borel et al. 2004). However, SHS exposure did not modify this association (Cohet, Borel et al. 2004). This is the only association study explored the relationship between sequence variants of *MGMT* and the risk of lung cancer by SHS exposure. However, more studies are needed to replicate this association.

XPD (Xeroderma Pigmentosum Complementation Group D)

XPD is a DNA repair gene. Some nonsynonymous SNPs have been reported for the *XPD* gene, they are located at codons 312 (Asp>Asn, exon 10, G>A) and 751 (Lys>Gln, exon 23, A>C) (Shen, Jones et al. 1998). A Swedish study reported that *XPD* variant carriers were associated with an elevated risk of lung cancer among younger (<70 years) never smokers (exon 10: OR=2.6, 95% CI =1.1-6.5; exon 23: 3.2, 95% CI=1.3-8.0) (Hou, Falt et al. 2002). Sequence variants of *XPD* may affect its ability to repair DNA damage resulting from SHS exposure. However, only one study has assessed this association.

OGG1 (8-Oxoguanine DNA Glycosylase)

OGG1 is a DNA repair gene and encodes the enzyme responsible for the excision of a mutagenic base byproduct, 8-oxoguanine, after exposure to reactive oxygen (Hill, Hazra et al. 2001). There are two splice variants resulting from the alternative splicing of the C-terminal region. In a Japanese population, nonsmokers carrying the *OGG1* Cys was not associated with an increased risk of lung adenocarcinoma as compared to those carrying two Ser alleles (Sunaga, Kohno et al. 2002). However, no other studies have explored this association.

Immune Response

TNF (Tumor Necrosis Factor)

Tumor necrosis factor (TNF) is mainly secreted by macrophage and is involved in SHS-related inflammatory response and disease susceptibility (Vernooy, Kucukaycan et al. 2002; Churg, Wang et al. 2003). *TNF* G-308A is a common variant in the promoter region and has been associated with asthma (Noguchi, Yokouchi et al. 2002; Di Somma, Charron et al. 2003; Mitsuta, Matsuse et al. 2003).

In a population of US children (54% Caucasians, 32% Latino, 14% others), *TNF* G-308 variant carriers exposed to household SHS had an elevated risk of school absence due to respiratory illness (OR=2.13, 95% CI=1.34-3.40) or lower-respiratory illness-related school absence (OR=4.15, 95% CI=2.57-6.71) as compared to those without SHS exposure and carrying zero copies of variant (Wenten, Berhane et al. 2005). However, no other studies have explored this association.

IL-1 (Interleukin 1)

IL-1, produced by monocytes and macrophages, is involved in various immune responses, inflammatory processes, and hematopoiesis. About 30% of European adults are affected by periodontitis (Hugoson, Norderyd et al. 1998), of which smoking is a major environmental risk factors (Burgan 1997; Salvi, Lawrence et al. 1997; Gelskey 1999; Kinane and Chestnutt 2000). When compared with genotype-negative nonsmokers, increased risk of periodontitis was observed for genotype-negative smokers (OR=2.37, 95% CI=1.96-2.87) and genotype-positive smokers (OR=4.50, 95% CI=2.30-8.82) but not for genotype-positive non-smokers (Meisel, Schwahn et al. 2004). Therefore, little evidence showed that genetic polymorphisms of *IL-1* were associated with periodontitis among SHS-exposed nonsmokers.

CD14

In a Latino population, asthma patients who had *CD14* +1437 GG or GC genotypes and exposed to SHS had 8.6% lower mean baseline forced expiratory volume in the first second (FEV_1) than those without SHS exposure (p=0.03), significant changes of asthma severity and IgE level were observed for individuals carrying CD14 -159 variant genotype, and only IgE level significantly changed for those who carrying CD14 -810 variant genotype (Choudhry, Avila et al. 2005). As described in the "Biomarkers of biologically effective does/early effect", the *CD14* -159 TT genotype was significantly associated with lower level of IgE among SHS exposed individuals (Choudhry, Avila et al. 2005). This is the only study explored the interaction. Studies without stratification by smoking status and SHS exposure were conflicting (Baldini, Lohman et al. 1999; Koppelman, Reijmerink et al. 2001; Heinzmann, Dietrich et al. 2003; Leung, Tang et al. 2003; Sengler, Haider et al. 2003; Kabesch, Hasemann et al. 2004; O'Donnell, Toelle et al. 2004). Therefore, more studies will be needed to confirm these findings.

Nrf2-Dependent Antioxidant and Cytoprotective Genes

Nuclear factor, erythroidderived 2, like 2 (Nrf2) is a redox-sensitive basic leucine zipper protein transcription factor involving in the regulation of several many detoxification and antioxidant genes, which may counteract the oxidative stress and inflammation resulting from SHS exposure. Mice study showed that disruption or deficiency of the *Nrf2* gene was related to SHS-induced emphysema, bronchoalveolar inflammation, and alveolar cell apoptosis (Rangasamy, Cho et al. 2004). No association studies have been reported before.

Others

α1-AT (Alpha1-Antitrypsin)

Alpha-1-antitrypsin is a plasma protease inhibitor (Gadek and Crystal 1982) and is encoded by the *PI* gene located on chromosome 14q. The pleomorphic protein inhibitor (Pi) α1-AT locus codes for several deficiency alleles with Z and S mutations, which are the most common in Northern Europeans (Gadek and Crystal 1982; Brantly, Nukiwa et al. 1988). Deficiency in *α1-AT* (homozygous PiZZ genotype) has been associated with emphysema, rapid decline in lung function among patients with COPD, and liver disease (Janus, Phillips et al. 1985; Burrows 1990). In a German population, children exposed to SHS who had low levels of α1-AT (≦116 $mg*dL^{-1}$) showed small but significant decrements in baseline lung function (e.g., mid- to end-expiratory flow rates) as compared to SHS-exposed children with normal levels of α1-AT (von Ehrenstein, von Mutius et al. 2002). However, the genetic polymorphisms in *α1-AT* have not been linked to health effects related to SHS exposure.

ARG1 and ARG2 (Arginase)

Arginase catalyzes the hydrolysis of arginine to ornithine and urea. ARG1 and ARG2 are two isoforms of mammalian arginase, which differ in tissue distribution, subcellular localization, immunologic cross-reactivity, and physiologic function. Arginase is thought to play a role in nitric oxide and polyamine metabolism, which may contribute to asthma pathogenesis (Meurs, Maarsingh et al. 2003; Vercelli 2003). *ARG1* and *ARG2* are expressed in lung tissue; and *ARG1* was highly expressed in human asthmatic lung tissue (Zimmermann, King et al. 2003). The *ARG2* gene was shown in a linkage study to be close to chromosome 14q24.4, which has been linked to asthma (Hakonarson, Bjornsdottir et al. 2002).

In a Mexican case-parent triad population, *ARG1* SNPs and haplotypes were not associated with asthma risk, but *ARG1* SNPs were significantly associated with the number of positive skin tests ($P<0.05$)(Li, Romieu et al. 2006). For *ARG2*, childhood asthma was significantly increased among those who had smoking parents and were carrying two copies of variant arg2s2 (CC vs. TT: relative risk (RR) = 2.39, 95% CI = 1.48-3.86), but the result was insignificant for those with nonsmoking parents (P for gene*environment interaction =0.025 under recessive model). A similar result was observed for arg2s1 (CC vs.GG: RR = 2.1, 95% CI = 1.2-3.9) (Li, Romieu et al. 2006). However, we are unable to estimate the association between sequence variants in *ARG1* and *ARG2* and SHS-related health effects based on the single study.

Conclusion

In summary, for different health effects, significant associations have been observed in genetic markers, including risk modification by germline polymorphisms, gene expression changes, and somatic alterations. For lung cancer, genetic polymorphisms of *CYP1B1* MspI, *GSTM1* null, *NAT2* slow acetylator, *MGMT* variants (143Val and 178Arg) and its methylation level has been significantly related to SHS-related lung cancer. Lung adenocarcinoma is the most common histological type among nonsmoking females. *GSTT1* null and the level of *MGMT* methylation have been significantly linked to this histological type among nonsmokers. In addition, *α1-AT* PiMS genotype was significantly associated with change of lung function. For asthma, *GSTM1* null, sequence variants *ARG2* (G→G, T→C) and *CD14* (+1437, -159) were related to SHS exposure. The levels of two neonatal oxidative damage markers (8-OHdG and MDA) and deletion in exon 2-3 of *HPRT* were significantly modified by *GSTM1* null genotype and SHS exposure. Childhood ALL was significantly related to *GSTP1* Ile/Val genotype and SHS exposure status. The association between DNA adducts and SHS exposure were modified by sequence variants of *CYP1A1* (MspI, MspI in combination of *GSTM1* null, *GSTP1* Ile/Val, or EPHX slow phenotype), *CYP1B1* (Arg48Gly + Ala119Ser, Leu432Val, and Asn453Ser), *EPHX* (His139Arg), and *NAT2* slower acetylator. Besides the markers identified above, it is important to find markers that can distinguish between exposure from SHS and active smoke. For example, *NAT2* slow acetylator was associated with "increased" risk of lung cancer, while there was "decreased" risk for fast acetylator carriers. In addition, levels of DNA adducts were significantly higher among those with *NAT2* slow acetylator and are high at low nicotine-cotinine levels.

Some gaps in our knowledge of SHS health effects remain. The associations between sequence variants of genes involved in phase I and II metabolism and cell cycle pathways and the risk of lung cancer have been widely explored for SHS exposure and conclusive findings are not yet available. Chronic inflammation (an innate immune response) has been associated with some cancers (e.g., cervix, breast, primary liver, bladder, and prostate cancers) (Kinlen 2004; Chen, Giovannucci et al. 2005). However, very few studies have assessed genes involved in angiogenesis and immune response and other pathways. Other than lung cancer and asthma, the association between genetic polymorphisms of genes discussed above and the risk of other health effects due to SHS exposure remains unclear.

The other point is that most association studies focused on the relationship between a few genotypes and SHS-related health effects or cytogenetic endpoints, and therefore failed to include other confounding factors (e.g., the level of personal exposure to genotoxic compounds, age, gender and nutritional habits) (Georgiadis, Demopoulos et al. 2004). In addition to SHS, ambient air pollution (e.g., traffic exhaust) is an important source of low-dose exposure to airborne carcinogens for large segments of the general population and may therefore influence cancer risk (1989; Woodward and McMichael 1991; Georgiadis, Topinka et al. 2005). In the occupational settings, exposure to components exist in SHS, e.g., PAHs, is common (Perera, Hemminki et al. 2002; Teixeira, Gaspar et al. 2002; Pavanello and Clonfero 2004). However, it is difficult to get individual exposure information. Other environmental or occupational factors may interact with SHS and lead to health effects (e.g., arsenic, asbestos, chromium, nickel, vinyl chloride, ionizing radiation, dietary aflatoxin, and infection). Abundant evidence showed that environmental factors are major contributors to human carcinogenesis and that the risk of developing cancer is strongly influenced by genetically determined differences (Nebert, McKinnon et al. 1996; Perera and Weinstein 2000). Therefore, twin studies (Redline, Tishler et al. 1989; Schmitt, Prescott et al. 2005) provide another approach to explore environmental and genetic influences on health effects related to SHS.

The findings from previous association studies have been inconsistent due to (1) cancer risk differs between histological types, (2) small sample size, (3) population stratification, (4) small genetic effect of individual SNP, and (5) different approaches for outcome ascertainment. Lung adenocarcinoma incidence has increased and become the most frequent histological type of lung cancer (Wynder and Hoffmann 1994; Charloux, Quoix et al. 1997; Gazdar and Minna 1997; Thun, Lally et al. 1997), especially among non-smokers. However, few SHS-related studies have performed statistical analyses by histological subtypes. Past studies mainly assessed Caucasian populations, but results of association studies focused on genetic polymorphisms and the risk of health effects varied greatly according to ethnicity. For example, Puerto Ricans and Mexicans are both Latinos, but asthma morbidity and mortality were 4-fold higher among Puerto Ricans than among Mexicans (Carter-Pokras and Gergen 1993; Homa, Mannino et al. 2000). Therefore, it is important to consider the effect of population stratification in genetic epidemiologic studies.

Besides association and experimental studies, some other approaches are useful to resolve the mystery of pathogenesis of SHS-related health effects. Large regions in the human genome have not been investigated for SHS exposure. Linkage study is a nice tool to identify genomic regions related to SHS exposure. For example, chromosome 1p at 97 cM, 5q at 135 cM, and 9q at 106 cM were significant ly related to SHS exposure ($P<0.01$)(Colilla, Nicolae et al. 2003). From the region identified, we could explore genes harbor in these area. Currently, SNP and haplotype analyses are two popular ways to investigate the association between SHS exposure and the risk of an outcome. But haplotype analyses (Taioli, Crofts et al. 1995), which capture more genetic variations as compared to SNP analyses, have not been widely used. Because of the importance of gene-gene interaction, pathway analyses have recently become important. However, such analyses are very complicated. In addition, microarray analyses (Izzotti, Cartiglia et al. 2004; Landi, Gemignani et al. 2005) is a promising method to find susceptibility genes associated with SHS exposure. This approach can help us to find the genetic differences resulting from different histological types or ethnic groups. Once we find these susceptibility genes, they could be used to identify the populations susceptible to SHS exposure, develop drugs to treat related diseases or conditions, and produce gene chips for disease screening purposes. As a whole, more studies using various approaches are needed to access genetic susceptibility to SHS in order to better understand the pathogenesis of related health effects.

References

Abdel-Rahman, S. Z. and R. A. El-Zein (2000). "The 399Gln polymorphism in the DNA repair gene XRCC1 modulates the genotoxic response induced in human lymphocytes by the tobacco-specific nitrosamine NNK." *Cancer Lett 159(1)*: 63-71.

Adgent, M. A. (2006). "Environmental tobacco smoke and sudden infant death syndrome: a review." *Birth Defects Res B Dev Reprod Toxicol 77(1)*: 69-85.

Ahijevych, K. L., R. F. Tyndale, et al. (2002). "Factors influencing cotinine half-life during smoking abstinence in African American and Caucasian women." *Nicotine Tob Res* 4(4): 423-31.

Al-Delaimy, W., T. Fraser, et al. (2001). "Nicotine in hair of bar and restaurant workers." *N Z Med J 114(1127)*: 80-3.

Alavanja, M. C. R., R. C. Brownson, et al. (1992). "Preexisting lung disease and lung cancer among nonsmoking women." *Am J Epidemiol 136*: 623-632.

Ali-Osman, F., O. Akande, et al. (1997). "Molecular cloning, characterization, and expression in Escherichia coli of full-length cDNAs of three human glutathione S-transferase Pi gene variants. Evidence for differential catalytic activity of the encoded proteins." *J Biol Chem 272(15)*: 10004-12.

Amos, C. I., W. Xu, et al. (1999). "Is there a genetic basis for lung cancer susceptibility?" *Recent Results Cancer Res 151*: 3-12.

Arredondo, J., V. T. Nguyen, et al. (2001). "A receptor-mediated mechanism of nicotine toxicity in oral keratinocytes." *Lab Invest 81(12)*: 1653-68.

Arshad, S. H., R. J. Kurukulaaratchy, et al. (2005). "Early life risk factors for current wheeze, asthma, and bronchial hyperresponsiveness at 10 years of age." *Chest 127(2)*: 502-8.

Attvall, S., J. Fowelin, et al. (1993). "Smoking induces insulin resistance--a potential link with the insulin resistance syndrome." *J Intern Med 233(4)*: 327-32.

Awasthi, Y. C., R. Sharma, et al. (1994). "Human glutathione S-transferases." *Int J Biochem 26(3)*: 295-308.

Bai, T. R., D. Zhou, et al. (1995). "Substance P (NK1)- and neurokinin A (NK2)-receptor gene expression in inflammatory airway diseases." *Am J Physiol 269(3 Pt 1)*: L309-17.

Baker, J. A., O. O. Odunuga, et al. (2006). "Active and passive smoking and risk of ovarian cancer." *Int J Gynecol Cancer 16 Suppl 1*: 211-8.

Baldini, M., I. C. Lohman, et al. (1999). "A Polymorphism* in the 5' flanking region of the CD14 gene is associated with circulating soluble CD14 levels and with total serum immunoglobulin E." *Am J Respir Cell Mol Biol 20(5)*: 976-83.

Baldwin, R. T. and S. Preston-Martin (2004). "Epidemiology of brain tumors in childhood--a review." *Toxicol Appl Pharmacol 199(2)*: 118-31.

Barnes, K. C. (1999). "Gene-environment and gene-gene interaction studies in the molecular genetic analysis of asthma and atopy." *Clin Exp Allergy 29 Suppl 4*: 47-51.

Bartsch, H., N. Caporaso, et al. (1990). "Carcinogen hemoglobin adducts, urinary mutagenicity, and metabolic phenotype in active and passive cigarette smokers.[comment]." *Journal of the National Cancer Institute. 82(23)*: 1826-31.

Bennett, W. P., M. C. Alavanja, et al. (1999). "Environmental tobacco smoke, genetic susceptibility, and risk of lung cancer in never-smoking women." *J Natl Cancer Inst 91(23)*: 2009-14.

Besaratinia, A., L. M. Maas, et al. (2002). "A molecular dosimetry approach to assess human exposure to environmental tobacco smoke in pubs." *Carcinogenesis 23(7)*: 1171-6.

Bianchini, F., F. Donato, et al. (1998). "Urinary excretion of 5-(hydroxymethyl) uracil in healthy volunteers: effect of active and passive tobacco smoke." *Int J Cancer 77(1)*: 40-6.

Blum, M., A. Demierre, et al. (1991). "Molecular mechanism of slow acetylation of drugs and carcinogens in humans." *Proc Natl Acad Sci U S A 88(12)*: 5237-41.

Bock, C. H., A. S. Wenzlaff, et al. (2005). "NQO1 T allele associated with decreased risk of later age at diagnosis lung cancer among never smokers: results from a population-based study." *Carcinogenesis 26(2)*: 381-6.

Boffetta, P. (1993). *Occupational factors of lun cancer. Prevention of respiratory disease.* A. Hirsh, M. Goldberg, J. P. Martin and R. Massw. New York, Marcek Dekker: 37-63.

Boffetta, P., A. Agudo, et al. (1998). "Multicenter case-control study of exposure to environmental tobacco smoke and lung cancer in Europe." *J Natl Cancer Inst 90(19)*: 1440-50.

Bohr, V. A., C. A. Smith, et al. (1985). "DNA repair in an active gene: removal of pyrimidine dimers from the DHFR gene of CHO cells is much more efficient than in the genome overall." *Cell 40(2)*: 359-69.

Bonassi, S., L. Hagmar, et al. (2000). "Chromosomal aberrations in lymphocytes predict human cancer independently of exposure to carcinogens. European Study Group on Cytogenetic Biomarkers and Health." *Cancer Res 60(6)*: 1619-25.

Borchers, M. T., M. P. Carty, et al. (1999). "Regulation of human airway mucins by acrolein and inflammatory mediators." *Am J Physiol 276(4 Pt 1)*: L549-55.

Borchers, M. T., S. E. Wert, et al. (1998). "Acrolein-induced MUC5ac expression in rat airways." *Am J Physiol 274(4 Pt 1)*: L573-81.

Borchers, M. T., S. Wesselkamper, et al. (1999). "Monocyte inflammation augments acrolein-induced Muc5ac expression in mouse lung." *Am J Physiol 277(3 Pt 1)*: L489-97.

Brantly, M., T. Nukiwa, et al. (1988). "Molecular basis of alpha-1-antitrypsin deficiency." *Am J Med 84(6A)*: 13-31.

Burgan, S. W. (1997). "The role of tobacco use in periodontal diseases: a literature review." *Gen Dent 45(5)*: 449-60; quiz 469-70.

Burns, D. M. (1994). *Tobacco smoking. Epidemiology of Lung Cancer.* J. M. Samet. New York, NT, Marcel Dekker Inc.: 15-50.

Burrows, B. (1990). "Airways obstructive diseases: pathogenetic mechanisms and natural histories of the disorders." *Med Clin North Am 74(3)*: 547-59.

Butkiewicz, D., E. Grzybowska, et al. (2000). "Polymorphisms of the GSTP1 and GSTM1 genes and PAH-DNA adducts in human mononuclear white blood cells." *Environ Mol Mutagen 35(2)*: 99-105.

Butler, M. A., N. P. Lang, et al. (1992). "Determination of CYP1A2 and NAT2 phenotypes in human populations by analysis of caffeine urinary metabolites." *Pharmacogenetics 2(3)*: 116-27.

Byrd, R. S. and C. R. Howard (1995). "Children's passive and prenatal exposure to cigarette smoke." *Pediatr Ann 24(12)*: 640-2, 644-5.

Byun, D.-S., M.-G. Lee, et al. (2001). "Frequent Epigenetic Inactivation of RASSF1A by Aberrant Promoter Hypermethylation in Human Gastric Adenocarcinoma." *Cancer Res 61(19)*: 7034-7038.

Canalle, R., R. V. Burim, et al. (2004). "Genetic polymorphisms and susceptibility to childhood acute lymphoblastic leukemia." *Environ Mol Mutagen 43(2)*: 100-9.

Cardenas, V. M., M. J. Thun, et al. (1997). "Environmental tobacco smoke and lung cancer mortality in the American Cancer Society's Cancer Prevention Study. II." *Cancer Causes Control 8(1)*: 57-64.

Carrano, A. V. (1986). "Chromosomal alterations as markers of exposure and effect." *J Occup Med 28(10)*: 1112-6.

Carter-Pokras, O. D. and P. J. Gergen (1993). "Reported asthma among Puerto Rican, Mexican-American, and Cuban children, 1982 through 1984." *Am J Public Health 83(4)*: 580-2.

Catusse, J., A. Liotard, et al. (2003). "Characterization of the molecular interactions of interleukin-8 (CXCL8), growth related oncogen alpha (CXCL1) and a non-peptide antagonist (SB 225002) with the human CXCR2." *Biochem Pharmacol 65(5)*: 813-21.

Charloux, A., E. Quoix, et al. (1997). "The increasing incidence of lung adenocarcinoma: reality or artifact? A review of the epidemiology of lung adenocarcinoma." International *Journal of Epidemiology 26*: 14-23.

Chen, Y., D. C. Rennie, et al. (1998). "Evidence for major genetic control of wheeze in relation to history of respiratory allergy: Humboldt family study." *Am J Med Genet 75(5)*: 485-91.

Chen, Y. C., J. H. Chen, et al. (2004). "Lung adenocarcinoma and human papillomavirus infection." *Cancer 101(6)*: 1428-36.

Chen, Y. C., E. Giovannucci, et al. (2005). "Sequence Variants of Toll-Like Receptor 4 (TLR4) and Susceptibility to Prostate Cancer." *Cancer Research 65(24)*: 11771-11778.

Chen, Y. C., H. J. Su, et al. (2005). "Interaction between environmental tobacco smoke and arsenic methylation ability on the risk of bladder cancer." *Cancer Causes Control 16(2)*: 75-81.

Cherpillod, P. and P. A. Amstad (1995). "Benzo[a]pyrene-induced mutagenesis of p53 hot-spot codons 248 and 249 in human hepatocytes." *Mol Carcinog 13(1)*: 15-20.

Choudhry, S., P. C. Avila, et al. (2005). "CD14 tobacco gene-environment interaction modifies asthma severity and immunoglobulin E levels in Latinos with asthma." *Am J Respir Crit Care Med 172(2)*: 173-82.

Churg, A., R. D. Wang, et al. (2003). "Macrophage metalloelastase mediates acute cigarette smoke-induced inflammation via tumor necrosis factor-alpha release." *Am J Respir Crit Care Med 167(8)*: 1083-9.

Clearing the air: asthma and indoor exposure. Washington, DC, Committee on the assessment of Asthma and Indoor Air, National Academy of Sciences (2000).

Cohet, C., S. Borel, et al. (2004). "Exon 5 polymorphisms in the O6-alkylguanine DNA alkyltransferase gene and lung cancer risk in non-smokers exposed to second-hand smoke." *Cancer Epidemiol Biomarkers Prev 13(2)*: 320-3.

Colilla, S., D. Nicolae, et al. (2003). "Evidence for gene-environment interactions in a linkage study of asthma and smoking exposure." *J Allergy Clin Immunol 111(4)*: 840-6.

Collier, A. C. and C. A. Pritsos (2003). "Environmental tobacco smoke in the workplace: markers of exposure, polymorphic enzymes and implications for disease state." *Chem Biol Interact 146(3)*: 211-24.

Cook, D. G. and D. P. Strachan (1997). "Health effects of passive smoking. 3. Parental smoking and prevalence of respiratory symptoms and asthma in school age children." *Thorax 52(12)*: 1081-94.

Crawford, F. G., J. Mayer, et al. (1994). "Biomarkers of environmental tobacco smoke in preschool children and their mothers." *J Natl Cancer Inst 86(18)*: 1398-402.

Cribb, A. E., R. Isbrucker, et al. (1994). "Acetylator phenotyping: the urinary caffeine metabolite ratio in slow acetylators correlates with a marker of systemic NAT1 activity." *Pharmacogenetics 4(3)*: 166-70.

Dammann, R., U. Schagdarsurengin, et al. (2003). "Epigenetic inactivation of the Ras-association domain family 1 (RASSF1A) gene and its function in human carcinogenesis." *Histol Histopathol 18(2)*: 665-77.

Daniel, V. (1993). "Glutathione S-transferases: gene structure and regulation of expression." *Crit Rev Biochem Mol Biol 28(3)*: 173-207.

Daube, H., G. Scherer, et al. (1997). "DNA adducts in human placenta in relation to tobacco smoke exposure and plasma antioxidant status." *J Cancer Res Clin Oncol 123(3)*: 141-51.

Dautzenberg, B. (2004). "[Tobacco-related diseases]." *Rev Prat 54(17)*: 1877-82.

de Boer, J. and J. H. Hoeijmakers (2000). "Nucleotide excision repair and human syndromes." *Carcinogenesis 21(3)*: 453-60.

De Flora, S., R. M. Balansky, et al. (2003). "Molecular alterations and lung tumors in p53 mutant mice exposed to cigarette smoke." *Cancer Res 63(4)*: 793-800.

De Flora, S., A. Izzotti, et al. (2005). "Induction and modulation of lung tumors: genomic and transcriptional alterations in cigarette smoke-exposed mice." *Exp Lung Res 31(1)*: 19-35.

Dejin-Karlsson, E., B. S. Hanson, et al. (1998). "Does passive smoking in early pregnancy increase the risk of small-for-gestational-age infants?" *Am J Public Health 88(10)*: 1523-7.

Deng, C., D. Xie, et al. (1999). "Genetic polymorphism of human O6-alkylguanine-DNA alkyltransferase: identification of a missense variation in the active site region." *Pharmacogenetics 9(1)*: 81-7.

Denissenko, M. F., A. Pao, et al. (1996). "Preferential formation of benzo[a]pyrene adducts at lung cancer mutational hotspots in P53." *Science 274(5286)*: 430-2.

Di Somma, C., D. Charron, et al. (2003). "Atopic asthma and TNF-308 alleles: linkage disequilibrium and association analyses." *Hum Immunol 64(3)*: 359-65.

Divine, K. K., L. C. Pulling, et al. (2005). "Multiplicity of abnormal promoter methylation in lung adenocarcinomas from smokers and never smokers." *Int J Cancer 114(3)*: 400-5.

Dockery, D. W. and D. Trichopoulos (1997). "Risk of lung cancer from environmental exposures to tobacco smoke." *Cancer Causes Control 8(3)*: 333-45.

Dogliotti, E., P. Hainaut, et al. (1998). "Mutation spectra resulting from carcinogenic exposure: from model systems to cancer-related genes." *Recent Results Cancer Res 154*: 97-124.

Egyhazi, S., S. Ma, et al. (2002). "Novel O6-methylguanine-DNA methyltransferase SNPs: a frequency comparison of patients with familial melanoma and healthy individuals in Sweden." *Hum Mutat 20(5)*: 408-9.

Ehrlich, R., E. Jordaan, et al. (2001). "Household smoking and bronchial hyperresponsiveness in children with asthma." *J Asthma 38(3)*: 239-51.

Environmental Tobacco Smoke. *Measuring Exposures and Assessing Health Effects*. National Research Council. Board on Environmental Studies and Toxicology. Committee on Passive Smoking. Washington, DC, National Academy Press (1986).

Esteller, M., S. R. Hamilton, et al. (1999). "Inactivation of the DNA repair gene O6-methylguanine-DNA methyltransferase by promoter hypermethylation is a common event in primary human neoplasia." *Cancer Res 59(4)*: 793-7.

Esteller, M., M. Toyota, et al. (2000). "Inactivation of the DNA repair gene O6-methylguanine-DNA methyltransferase by promoter hypermethylation is associated with G to A mutations in K-ras in colorectal tumorigenesis." *Cancer Res 60(9)*: 2368-71.

Exposure to Environmental Tobacco Smoke and Cotinine Levels ? Fact Sheet. National Center for Chronic Disease Prevention and Health Promotion, Centers for Disease Control and Prevention, US Department of Health and Human Services (2006).

Faraglia, B., S. Y. Chen, et al. (2003). "Evaluation of 4-aminobiphenyl-DNA adducts in human breast cancer: the influence of tobacco smoke." *Carcinogenesis 24(4)*: 719-25.

Fields, W. R., C. S. Morrow, et al. (1998). "Overexpression of stably transfected human glutathione S-transferase P1-1 protects against DNA damage by benzo[a]pyrene diol-epoxide in human T47D cells." *Mol Pharmacol 54(2)*: 298-304.

Finette, B. A., J. P. O'Neill, et al. (1998). "Gene mutations with characteristic deletions in cord blood T lymphocytes associated with passive maternal exposure to tobacco smoke." *Nat Med 4(10)*: 1144-51.

Fontham, E. T. (1990). "Protective dietary factors and lung cancer." *Int J Epidemiol 19 Suppl 1*: S32-42.

Fontham, E. T., P. Correa, et al. (1994). "Environmental tobacco smoke and lung cancer in nonsmoking women. A multicenter study." *Jama 271(22)*: 1752-9.

Frederickson, S. M., E. M. Messing, et al. (1994). "Relationship between in vivo acetylator phenotypes and cytosolic N-acetyltransferase and O-acetyltransferase activities in human uroepithelial cells." *Cancer Epidemiol Biomarkers Prev 3(1)*: 25-32.

Gadek, J. E. and R. G. Crystal (1982). *Alpha1Antitrypsin deficiency. The metabolic basis of inherited disease.* J. B. Stanbury, J. B. Wyngaarden, D. S. Fredrickson, J. L. Goldstein and M. S. Brown. New York, McGraw Hill Book Company: 1450-1467.

Gao, Y. T. (1996). "Risk factors for lung cancer among nonsmokers with emphasis on lifestyle factors." *Lung Cancer 14 Suppl 1*: S39-45.

Gazdar, A. F. and J. D. Minna (1997). "Cigarettes, sex, and lung adenocarcinoma." *J Natl Cancer Inst 89(21)*: 1563-5.

Gealy, R., L. Zhang, et al. (1999). "Comparison of mutations in the p53 and K-ras genes in lung carcinomas from smoking and nonsmoking women." *Cancer Epidemiol Biomarkers Prev 8(4 Pt 1)*: 297-302.

Gebremichael, A., K. Tullis, et al. (1996). "Ah-receptor-dependent modulation of gene expression by aged and diluted sidestream cigarette smoke." *Toxicol Appl Pharmacol 141(1)*: 76-83.

Gelskey, S. C. (1999). "Cigarette smoking and periodontitis: methodology to assess the strength of evidence in support of a causal association." *Community Dent Oral Epidemiol 27(1)*: 16-24.

General, U. S. S. (1986). The health consequences of involuntary smoking. A report of the surgeon general Rockville, Maryland, Office of Smoking and Health.

Georgiadis, P., N. A. Demopoulos, et al. (2004). "Impact of phase I or phase II enzyme polymorphisms on lymphocyte DNA adducts in subjects exposed to urban air pollution and environmental tobacco smoke." *Toxicol Lett 149(1-3)*: 269-80.

Georgiadis, P., J. Topinka, et al. (2001). "Biomarkers of genotoxicity of air pollution (the AULIS project): bulky DNA adducts in subjects with moderate to low exposures to airborne polycyclic aromatic hydrocarbons and their relationship to environmental tobacco smoke and other parameters." *Carcinogenesis 22(9)*: 1447-57.

Georgiadis, P., J. Topinka, et al. (2005). "Interactions between CYP1A1 polymorphisms and exposure to environmental tobacco smoke in the modulation of lymphocyte bulky DNA adducts and chromosomal aberrations." *Carcinogenesis 26(1)*: 93-101.

Gerde, P., B. A. Muggenburg, et al. (1998). "A relevant dose of 4-(methylnitrosamino)-1-(3-pyridyl)-1-butanone is extensively metabolized and rapidly absorbed in the canine tracheal mucosa." *Cancer Res 58(7)*: 1417-22.

Gerde, P., B. A. Muggenburg, et al. (1997). "Benzo[a]pyrene at an environmentally relevant dose is slowly absorbed by, and extensively metabolized in, tracheal epithelium." *Carcinogenesis 18(9)*: 1825-32.

Gergen, P. J., J. A. Fowler, et al. (1998). "The burden of environmental tobacco smoke exposure on the respiratory health of children 2 months through 5 years of age in the United States: Third National Health and Nutrition Examination Survey, 1988 to 1994." *Pediatrics 101(2)*: E8.

Gilliland, F. D., Y. F. Li, et al. (2002). "Effects of glutathione S-transferase M1, maternal smoking during pregnancy, and environmental tobacco smoke on asthma and wheezing in children." *Am J Respir Crit Care Med 166(4)*: 457-63.

Gilliland, F. D., Y. F. Li, et al. (2001). "Effects of maternal smoking during pregnancy and environmental tobacco smoke on asthma and wheezing in children." *Am J Respir Crit Care Med 163(2)*: 429-36.

Gilliland, F. D., R. McConnell, et al. (1999). "A theoretical basis for investigating ambient air pollution and children's respiratory health." *Environ Health Perspect 107 Suppl 3*: 403-7.

Girod, C. E. and T. E. King, Jr. (2005). "COPD: a dust-induced disease?" *Chest 128(4)*: 3055-64.

Gold, D. R. (2000). "Environmental tobacco smoke, indoor allergens, and childhood asthma." *Environ Health Perspect 108 Suppl 4*: 643-51.

Hackshaw, A. K., M. R. Law, et al. (1997). "The accumulated evidence on lung cancer and environmental tobacco smoke." *Bmj 315(7114)*: 980-8.

Hainaut, P. and G. P. Pfeifer (2001). "Patterns of p53 G-->T transversions in lung cancers reflect the primary mutagenic signature of DNA-damage by tobacco smoke." *Carcinogenesis 22(3)*: 367-74.

Hakonarson, H., U. S. Bjornsdottir, et al. (2002). "A major susceptibility gene for asthma maps to chromosome 14q24." *Am J Hum Genet 71(3)*: 483-91.

Hammond, E. C. and H. Seidman (1980). "Smoking and cancer in the United States." *Prev Med 9(2)*: 169-74.

Hammond, S. K., J. Coghlin, et al. (1993). "Relationship between environmental tobacco smoke exposure and carcinogen-hemoglobin adduct levels in nonsmokers." *J Natl Cancer Inst 85(6)*: 474-8.

Hanke, W., J. Kalinka, et al. (1999). "Passive smoking and pregnancy outcome in central Poland." *Hum Exp Toxicol 18(4)*: 265-71.

Harris, M. J., M. Coggan, et al. (1998). "Polymorphism of the Pi class glutathione S-transferase in normal populations and cancer patients." *Pharmacogenetics 8(1)*: 27-31.

Harris, R. E., E. A. Zang, et al. (1993). "Race and sex differences in lung cancer risk associated with cigarette smoking." *Int J Epidemiol 22(4)*: 592-9.

Hasday, J. D., R. Bascom, et al. (1999). "Bacterial endotoxin is an active component of cigarette smoke." *Chest 115(3)*: 829-35.

Hassett, C., L. Aicher, et al. (1994). "Human microsomal epoxide hydrolase: genetic polymorphism and functional expression in vitro of amino acid variants." *Hum Mol Genet 3(3)*: 421-8.

Hayashi, S., J. Watanabe, et al. (1991). "Genetic linkage of lung cancer-associated MspI polymorphisms with amino acid replacement in the heme binding region of the human cytochrome P450IA1 gene." *J Biochem (Tokyo) 110(3)*: 407-11.

Hayes, J. D. and R. C. Stange (2000). "Glutathione S-transferase polymorphisms and their biological consequences." *Pharmacology 61*: 154-166.

Hayes, R. B., W. Bi, et al. (1993). "N-acetylation phenotype and genotype and risk of bladder cancer in benzidine-exposed workers." *Carcinogenesis 14(4)*: 675-8.

Health effects of exposure to environmental tobacco smoke. Sacramento, CA, California Environmental Protection Agency (1997).

Hecht, S. S. (1998). "Biochemistry, biology, and carcinogenicity of tobacco-specific N-nitrosamines." *Chem Res Toxicol 11(6)*: 559-603.

Hecht, S. S. (1999). "Tobacco smoke carcinogens and lung cancer." *J Natl Cancer Inst 91(14)*: 1194-210.

Hecht, S. S. (2002). "Human urinary carcinogen metabolites: biomarkers for investigating tobacco and cancer." *Carcinogenesis 23(6)*: 907-22.

Hecht, S. S., S. G. Carmella, et al. (2006). "4-(methylnitrosamino)-1-(3-pyridyl)-1-butanol and its glucuronides in the urine of infants exposed to environmental tobacco smoke." *Cancer Epidemiol Biomarkers Prev 15(5)*: 988-92.

Hecht, S. S., S. G. Carmella, et al. (1993). "A tobacco-specific lung carcinogen in the urine of men exposed to cigarette smoke." *N Engl J Med 329(21)*: 1543-6.

Heeschen, C., J. J. Jang, et al. (2001). "Nicotine stimulates angiogenesis and promotes tumor growth and atherosclerosis." *Nat Med 7(7)*: 833-9.

Hein, D. W. (1988). "Acetylator genotype and arylamine-induced carcinogenesis." *Biochim Biophys Acta 948(1)*: 37-66.

Hein, D. W., M. A. Doll, et al. (1993). "Metabolic activation and deactivation of arylamine carcinogens by recombinant human NAT1 and polymorphic NAT2 acetyltransferases." *Carcinogenesis 14(8)*: 1633-8.

Heinzmann, A., H. Dietrich, et al. (2003). "Promoter polymorphisms of the CD14 gene are not associated with bronchial asthma in Caucasian children." *Eur J Immunogenet 30(5)*: 345-8.

Hernandez-Boussard, T. M. and P. Hainaut (1998). "A specific spectrum of p53 mutations in lung cancer from smokers: review of mutations compiled in the IARC p53 database." *Environ Health Perspect 106(7)*: 385-91.

Hill, J. W., T. K. Hazra, et al. (2001). "Stimulation of human 8-oxoguanine-DNA glycosylase by AP-endonuclease: potential coordination of the initial steps in base excision repair." *Nucl. Acids Res. 29(2)*: 430-438.

Hoffjan, S., D. Nicolae, et al. (2003). "Association studies for asthma and atopic diseases: a comprehensive review of the literature." *Respir Res 4*: 14.

Hoffjan, S. and C. Ober (2002). "Present status on the genetic studies of asthma." *Curr Opin Immunol 14(6)*: 709-17.

Hoffmann, D. and I. Hoffmann (2001). The changing cigarette: chemical studies and bioassays. Risks associated with smoking cigarettes with low machine-measured yields of tar and nicotine. D. R. Shopland, D. M. Burns and N. L. Benowitz, National Cancer Institute.

Holt, P. G., P. D. Sly, et al. (1997). "Atopic versus infectious diseases in childhood: a question of balance?" *Pediatr Allergy Immunol 8(2)*: 53-8.

Holz, O., R. Meissner, et al. (1993). "Detection of DNA single-strand breaks in lymphocytes of smokers." *Int Arch Occup Environ Health 65(2)*: 83-8.

Homa, D. M., D. M. Mannino, et al. (2000). "Asthma mortality in U.S. Hispanics of Mexican, Puerto Rican, and Cuban heritage, 1990-1995." *Am J Respir Crit Care Med 161(2 Pt 1)*: 504-9.

Hong, Y. C., H. Kim, et al. (2001). "Maternal genetic effects on neonatal susceptibility to oxidative damage from environmental tobacco smoke." *J Natl Cancer Inst 93(8)*: 645-7.

Hong, Y. C., K. H. Lee, et al. (2003). "Effects of the GSTM1 and GSTT1 polymorphisms on the relationship between maternal exposure to environmental tobacco smoke and neonatal birth weight." *J Occup Environ Med 45(5)*: 492-8.

Hou, S. M., S. Falt, et al. (2002). "The XPD variant alleles are associated with increased aromatic DNA adduct level and lung cancer risk." *Carcinogenesis 23(4)*: 599-603.

Houston, T. K., T. K. Houston, et al. (2006). "Active and passive smoking and development of glucose intolerance among young adults in a prospective cohort: CARDIA study." *BMJ*: *bmj*.38779.584028.55.

Hu, W., Z. Feng, et al. (2004). "Chromium(VI) enhances (+/-)-anti-7beta,8alpha-dihydroxy-9alpha,10alpha-epoxy-7,8,9,10-tetrahydro benzo[a]pyrene-induced cytotoxicity and mutagenicity in mammalian cells through its inhibitory effect on nucleotide excision repair." *Biochemistry 43(44)*: 14282-9.

Hugoson, A., O. Norderyd, et al. (1998). "Distribution of periodontal disease in a Swedish adult population 1973, 1983 and 1993." *J Clin Periodontol 25(7)*: 542-8.

Humble, C., J. Croft, et al. (1990). "Passive smoking and 20-year cardiovascular disease mortality among nonsmoking wives, Evans County, Georgia." *Am J Public Health 80(5)*: 599-601.

Hung, R. J., P. Boffetta, et al. (2003). "CYP1A1 and GSTM1 genetic polymorphisms and lung cancer risk in Caucasian non-smokers: a pooled analysis." *Carcinogenesis. 24(5)*: 875-82.

Husgafvel-Pursiainen, K., P. Boffetta, et al. (2000). "p53 mutations and exposure to environmental tobacco smoke in a multicenter study on lung cancer." *Cancer Res 60(11)*: 2906-11.

IARC *Monographs on The Evaluation of Carcinogenic Risk to Human.* Lyon, IARC. 46 (1989).

IARC, Ed. (2004). Tobacco smoke and involuntary smoking. *IARC Monographs on the Evaluation of Carocinogenic Risks to Humans.* Lyon, France, IARC.

Infante-Rivard, C., M. Krajinovic, et al. (2000). "Parental smoking, CYP1A1 genetic polymorphisms and childhood leukemia (Quebec, Canada)." *Cancer Causes Control 11(6)*: 547-53.

Ivashchenko, T. E., O. G. Sideleva, et al. (2001). "[Genetic factors in predisposition to bronchial asthma]." *Genetika 37(1)*: 107-11.

Izzotti, A., C. Cartiglia, et al. (2004). "Gene expression in the lung of p53 mutant mice exposed to cigarette smoke." *Cancer Res 64(23)*: 8566-72.

Jaakkola, J. J., P. Nafstad, et al. (2001). "Environmental tobacco smoke, parental atopy, and childhood asthma." *Environ Health Perspect 109(6)*: 579-82.

Janerich, D. T., W. D. Thompson, et al. (1990). "Lung cancer and exposure to tobacco smoke in the household." *N Engl J Med 323(10)*: 632-6.

Janus, E. D., N. T. Phillips, et al. (1985). "Smoking, lung function, and alpha 1-antitrypsin deficiency." *Lancet 1(8421)*: 152-4.

Janzon, L., K. Berntorp, et al. (1983). "Glucose tolerance and smoking: a population study of oral and intravenous glucose tolerance tests in middle-aged men." *Diabetologia 25(2)*: 86-8.

Jarmalaite, S., A. Kannio, et al. (2003). "Aberrant p16 promoter methylation in smokers and former smokers with nonsmall cell lung cancer." *Int J Cancer 106(6)*: 913-8.

Jemal, A., R. Siegel, et al. (2006). "Cancer statistics, 2006." *CA Cancer J Clin 56(2)*: 106-30.

Ji, B. T., X. O. Shu, et al. (1997). "Paternal cigarette smoking and the risk of childhood cancer among offspring of nonsmoking mothers." *J Natl Cancer Inst 89(3)*: 238-44.

Jindal, S. K., A. N. Aggarwal, et al. (2006). "A multicentric study on epidemiology of chronic obstructive pulmonary disease and its relationship with tobacco smoking and environmental tobacco smoke exposure." *Indian J Chest Dis Allied Sci 48(1)*: 23-9.

Johansson, A. S., G. Stenberg, et al. (1998). "Structure-activity relationships and thermal stability of human glutathione transferase P1-1 governed by the H-site residue 105." *J Mol Biol 278(3)*: 687-98.

Jordaan, E. R., R. I. Ehrlich, et al. (1999). "Environmental tobacco smoke exposure in children: household and community determinants." *Arch Environ Health 54(5)*: 319-27.

Kabat, G. C. (1996). "Aspects of the epidemiology of lung cancer in smokers and nonsmokers in the United States." *Lung Cancer 15(1)*: 1-20.

Kabesch, M., K. Hasemann, et al. (2004). "A promoter polymorphism in the CD14 gene is associated with elevated levels of soluble CD14 but not with IgE or atopic diseases." *Allergy 59(5)*: 520-5.

Kawakami, N., N. Takatsuka, et al. (1997). "Effects of smoking on the incidence of non-insulin-dependent diabetes mellitus. Replication and extension in a Japanese cohort of male employees." *Am J Epidemiol 145(2)*: 103-9.

Kharrazi, M., G. N. DeLorenze, et al. (2004). "Environmental tobacco smoke and pregnancy outcome." *Epidemiology 15(6)*: 660-70.

Kinane, D. F. and I. G. Chestnutt (2000). "Smoking and periodontal disease." *Crit Rev Oral Biol Med 11(3)*: 356-65.

Kinlen, L. (2004). "Infections and immune factors in cancer: the role of epidemiology." *Oncogene 23(38)*: 6341-8.

Kiyohara, C. (2000). "Genetic polymorphism of enzymes involved in xenobiotic metabolism and the risk of colorectal cancer." *J Epidemiol 10(5)*: 349-60.

Kiyohara, C., K. Wakai, et al. (2003). "Risk modification by CYP1A1 and GSTM1 polymorphisms in the association of environmental tobacco smoke and lung cancer: a case-control study in Japanese nonsmoking women." *Int J Cancer 107(1)*: 139-44.

Klebanoff, M. A., J. D. Clemens, et al. (1996). "Maternal smoking during pregnancy and childhood cancer." *Am J Epidemiol 144(11)*: 1028-33.

Ko, Y. C., C. H. Lee, et al. (1997). "Risk factors for primary lung cancer among non-smoking women in Taiwan." *International Journal of Epidemiology 26(1)*: 24-31.

Koo, L. C. and J. H. C. Ho (1990). "Worldwide epidemiological patterns of lung cancer in nonsmokers." *Int J Epidemiol 19(Suppl 1)*: S14-23.

Koppelman, G. H., N. E. Reijmerink, et al. (2001). "Association of a promoter polymorphism of the CD14 gene and atopy." *Am J Respir Crit Care Med 163(4)*: 965-9.

Krajinovic, M., H. Sinnett, et al. (2002). "Role of NQO1, MPO and CYP2E1 genetic polymorphisms in the susceptibility to childhood acute lymphoblastic leukemia." *Int J Cancer 97(2)*: 230-6.

Kramer, U., C. H. Lemmen, et al. (2004). "The effect of environmental tobacco smoke on eczema and allergic sensitization in children." *Br J Dermatol 150(1)*: 111-8.

Kukla, L., D. Hruba, et al. (2001). "Smoking and damages of reproduction: evidence of ELSPAC." *Cent Eur J Public Health 9(2)*: 59-63.

Kurie, J. M. and R. N. Dubois (2001). "Prostaglandin E Synthase: Another Enzyme in the Cyclooxygenase Pathway Driving Epithelial Cancer?" *Clin Cancer Res 7(9)*: 2608-2610.

Kurz, T. and C. Ober (2004). "The role of environmental tobacco smoke in genetic susceptibility to asthma." *Curr Opin Allergy Clin Immunol 4(5)*: 335-9.

Landi, S., F. Gemignani, et al. (2005). "A database of single-nucleotide polymorphisms and a genotyping microarray for genetic epidemiology of lung cancer." *Exp Lung Res 31(2)*: 223-58.

Larsson, L., B. Szponar, et al. (2004). "Tobacco smoking increases dramatically air concentrations of endotoxin." *Indoor Air 14(6)*: 421-4.

Larsson, M. L., M. Frisk, et al. (2001). "Environmental tobacco smoke exposure during childhood is associated with increased prevalence of asthma in adults." *Chest 120(3)*: 711-7.

Lee, C. Z., F. H. Royce, et al. (2000). "Effect of in utero and postnatal exposure to environmental tobacco smoke on the developmental expression of pulmonary cytochrome P450 monooxygenases." *J Biochem Mol Toxicol 14(3)*: 121-30.

Lee, J. H., S. B. Rho, et al. (2005). "Programmed Cell Death 6 (PDCD6) Protein Interacts with Death-Associated Protein Kinase 1 (DAPk1): Additive Effect on Apoptosis via Caspase-3 Dependent Pathway." *Biotechnology Letters 27(14)*: 1011-1015.

Leung, T. F., N. L. Tang, et al. (2003). "The C-159T polymorphism in the CD14 promoter is associated with serum total IgE concentration in atopic Chinese children." *Pediatr Allergy Immunol 14(4)*: 255-60.

Li, H., I. Romieu, et al. (2006). "Genetic polymorphisms in arginase I and II and childhood asthma and atopy." *J Allergy Clin Immunol 117(1)*: 119-26.

Li, Q. J., S. Lu, et al. (2000). "Isolation and characterization of a new chemokine receptor gene, the putative chicken CXCR1." *Gene 257(2)*: 307-17.

Liggett, W. H., Jr. and D. Sidransky (1998). "Role of the p16 tumor suppressor gene in cancer." *J Clin Oncol 16(3)*: 1197-1206.

Little, J., A. Cardy, et al. (2004). "Smoking and orofacial clefts: a United Kingdom-based case-control study." *Cleft Palate Craniofac J 41(4)*: 381-6.

Liu, L., J. H. Yoon, et al. (2002). "Frequent hypermethylation of the RASSF1A gene in prostate cancer." *Oncogene 21(44)*: 6835-40.

Liu, Z. (1992). "Smoking and lung cancer in China: combined analysis of eight case-control studies." *Int J Epidemiol 21(2)*: 197-201.

London, S. J., J. Smart, et al. (2000). "Lung cancer risk in relation to genetic polymorphisms of microsomal epoxide hydrolase among African-Americans and Caucasians in Los Angeles County." *Lung Cancer 28(2)*: 147-55.

Lu, K. P., N. F. Alejandro, et al. (2002). "Differential expression of ribosomal L31, Zis, gas-5 and mitochondrial mRNAs following oxidant induction of proliferative vascular smooth muscle cell phenotypes." *Atherosclerosis 160(2)*: 273-80.

MacLennan, R., J. Da Costa, et al. (1977). "Risk factors for lung cancer in Singapore Chinese, a population with high female incidence rates." *Int J Cancer 20(6)*: 854-60.

Maclure, M., R. B. Katz, et al. (1989). "Elevated blood levels of carcinogens in passive smokers." *Am J Public Health 79(10)*: 1381-4.

Mainous, A. G., 3rd and W. J. Hueston (1994). "Passive smoke and low birth weight. Evidence of a threshold effect." *Arch Fam Med 3(10)*: 875-8.

Malats, N., A. M. Camus-Radon, et al. (2000). "Lung cancer risk in nonsmokers and GSTM1 and GSTT1 genetic polymorphism." *Cancer Epidemiol Biomarkers Prev 9(8)*: 827-33.

Manna, S. K., T. Rangasamy, et al. (2006). "Long term environmental tobacco smoke activates nuclear transcription factor-kappa B, activator protein-1, and stress responsive kinases in mouse brain." *Biochem Pharmacol 71(11)*: 1602-9.

Martin, T. R. and M. B. Bracken (1986). "Association of low birth weight with passive smoke exposure in pregnancy." *Am J Epidemiol 124(4)*: 633-42.

Martinez, F. D., M. Cline, et al. (1992). "Increased incidence of asthma in children of smoking mothers." *Pediatrics 89(1)*: 21-6.

Matikainen, T., G. I. Perez, et al. (2001). "Aromatic hydrocarbon receptor-driven Bax gene expression is required for premature ovarian failure caused by biohazardous environmental chemicals." *Nat Genet 28(4)*: 355-60.

Matsuda, T., M. Kawanishi, et al. (1998). "Specific tandem GG to TT base substitutions induced by acetaldehyde are due to intra-strand crosslinks between adjacent guanine bases." *Nucleic Acids Res 26(7)*: 1769-74.

Mayer, A. S. and L. S. Newman (2001). "Genetic and environmental modulation of chronic obstructive pulmonary disease." *Respir Physiol 128(1)*: 3-11.

McWilliams, J. E., B. J. Sanderson, et al. (1995). "Glutathione S-transferase M1 (GSTM1) deficiency and lung cancer risk." *Cancer Epidemiol Biomarkers Prev 4(6)*: 589-94.

Meisel, P., C. Schwahn, et al. (2004). "Dose-effect relation of smoking and the interleukin-1 gene polymorphism in periodontal disease." *J Periodontol 75(2)*: 236-42.

Merlo, F., A. Andreassen, et al. (1998). "Urinary excretion of 1-hydroxypyrene as a marker for exposure to urban air levels of polycyclic aromatic hydrocarbons." *Cancer Epidemiol Biomarkers Prev 7(2)*: 147-55.

Meurs, H., H. Maarsingh, et al. (2003). "Arginase and asthma: novel insights into nitric oxide homeostasis and airway hyperresponsiveness." *Trends Pharmacol Sci 24(9)*: 450-5.

Meyers, D. A., D. S. Postma, et al. (2005). "Genome screen for asthma and bronchial hyperresponsiveness: interactions with passive smoke exposure." *J Allergy Clin Immunol 115(6)*: 1169-75.

Miller, D. P., I. De Vivo, et al. (2003). "Association between self-reported environmental tobacco smoke exposure and lung cancer: modification by GSTP1 polymorphism." *International Journal of Cancer. 104(6)*: 758-63.

Mitchell, K. R. and D. Warshawsky (1999). "Frequent Ha-ras mutations in murine skin and liver tumors induced by 7H-dibenzo[c,g]carbazole." *Mol Carcinog 25(2)*: 107-12.

Mitsuta, K., H. Matsuse, et al. (2003). "Production of TNF-alpha by peripheral blood mononuclear cells through activation of nuclear factor kappa B by specific allergen stimulation in patients with atopic asthma." *Allergy Asthma Proc 24(1)*: 19-26.

Mooney, L. A., R. M. Santella, et al. (1995). "Decline of DNA damage and other biomarkers in peripheral blood following smoking cessation." *Cancer Epidemiol Biomarkers Prev 4(6)*: 627-34.

Morimoto, K., K. Miura, et al. (1984). "Human health situation and chromosome alterations: sister chromatid exchange frequency in lymphocytes from passive smokers and patients with hereditary diseases." *Basic Life Sci 29 Pt B*: 801-11.

Murphy, V. E., T. Zakar, et al. (2002). "Reduced 11beta-hydroxysteroid dehydrogenase type 2 activity is associated with decreased birth weight centile in pregnancies complicated by asthma." *J Clin Endocrinol Metab 87(4)*: 1660-8.

Nakajima, T., E. Elovaara, et al. (1995). "Expression and polymorphism of glutathione S-transferase in human lungs: risk factors in smoking-related lung cancer." *Carcinogenesis 16(4)*: 707-11.

National Health Survey 1002 Highlights of Main Survey Findings (Report), Research and Evaluation Department, Ministry of Health, Singapore (1993).

National Research Council (U.S.). Committee on Passive Smoking. (1986). *Environmental tobacco smoke: measuring exposures and assessing health effects*. Washington, D.C., National Academy Press.

National Research Council, C. o. P. S. (1986). *Environmental tobacco smoke: measuring exposures and assessing health effects*. Washington, D.C., National Academy Press.

National Research Council, N. A. o. S. (1993). *Pesticides in the diets of infants and children*. Washington, DC, National Academy Press.

Nazar-Stewart, V., T. L. Vaughan, et al. (2003). "A population-based study of glutathione S-transferase M1, T1 and P1 genotypes and risk for lung cancer." *Lung Cancer 40(3)*: 247-58.

Nebert, D. W., R. A. McKinnon, et al. (1996). "Human drug-metabolizing enzyme polymorphisms: effects on risk of toxicity and cancer." *DNA Cell Biol 15(4)*: 273-80.

Nelson, H. H., D. C. Christiani, et al. (1999). "k-ras mutation and occupational asbestos exposure in lung adenocarcinoma: asbestos-related cancer without asbestosis." *Cancer Research. 59(18)*: 4570-3.

Ng, D. P., K. W. Tan, et al. (2005). "CYP1A1 polymorphisms and risk of lung cancer in non-smoking Chinese women: influence of environmental tobacco smoke exposure and GSTM1/T1 genetic variation." *Cancer Causes Control 16(4)*: 399-405.

Noguchi, E., Y. Yokouchi, et al. (2002). "Association between TNFA polymorphism and the development of asthma in the Japanese population." *Am J Respir Crit Care Med 166(1)*: 43-6.

Norppa, H. (2004). "Cytogenetic biomarkers and genetic polymorphisms." *Toxicol Lett 149(1-3)*: 309-34.

Nyberg, F., S. M. Hou, et al. (1998). "Glutathione S-transferase mu1 and N-acetyltransferase 2 genetic polymorphisms and exposure to tobacco smoke in nonsmoking and smoking lung cancer patients and population controls." *Cancer Epidemiol Biomarkers Prev 7(10)*: 875-83.

O'Donnell, A. R., B. G. Toelle, et al. (2004). "Age-specific relationship between CD14 and atopy in a cohort assessed from age 8 to 25 years." *Am J Respir Crit Care Med 169(5)*: 615-22.

Olds, D. L., C. R. Henderson, Jr., et al. (1994). "Intellectual impairment in children of women who smoke cigarettes during pregnancy." *Pediatrics 93(2)*: 221-7.

Parain, K., C. Hapdey, et al. (2003). "Cigarette smoke and nicotine protect dopaminergic neurons against the 1-methyl-4-phenyl-1,2,3,6-tetrahydropyridine Parkinsonian toxin." *Brain Res 984(1-2)*: 224-32.

Parkin, D. M., C. S. Muir, et al. (1992). Cancer incidence in five continetns Vol VI. IARC Scientific Publication No. 120. Lyon, France, International Agency of Research on Cancer.

Parkin, D. M., P. Pisani, et al. (1999). "Global cancer statistics." *CA Cancer J Clin 49(1)*: 33-64, 1.

Parsons, W. D., S. G. Carmella, et al. (1998). "A metabolite of the tobacco-specific lung carcinogen 4-(methylnitrosamino)-1-(3-pyridyl)-1-butanone in the urine of hospital workers exposed to environmental tobacco smoke." *Cancer Epidemiol Biomarkers Prev 7(3)*: 257-60.

Pavanello, S. and E. Clonfero (2004). "[Individual susceptibility to occupational carcinogens: the evidence from biomonitoring and molecular epidemiology studies]." *G Ital Med Lav Ergon 26(4)*: 311-21.

Perera, F., K. Hemminki, et al. (2002). "In utero DNA damage from environmental pollution is associated with somatic gene mutation in newborns." *Cancer Epidemiol Biomarkers Prev 11(10 Pt 1)*: 1134-7.

Perera, F. P. (1997). "Environment and cancer: who are susceptible?" *Science 278(5340)*: 1068-73.

Perera, F. P. and I. B. Weinstein (2000). "Molecular epidemiology: recent advances and future directions." *Carcinogenesis 21(3)*: 517-24.

Pershagen, G., A. Ericson, et al. (1992). "Maternal smoking in pregnancy: does it increase the risk of childhood cancer?" *Int J Epidemiol 21(1)*: 1-5.

Petruzzelli, S., A. Celi, et al. (1998). "Serum antibodies to benzo(a)pyrene diol epoxide-DNA adducts in the general population: effects of air pollution, tobacco smoking, and family history of lung diseases." *Cancer Res 58(18)*: 4122-6.

Phillips, D. H. (2002). "Smoking-related DNA and protein adducts in human tissues." *Carcinogenesis 23(12)*: 1979-2004.

Piirila, P., H. Wikman, et al. (2001). "Glutathione S-transferase genotypes and allergic responses to diisocyanate exposure." *Pharmacogenetics 11(5)*: 437-45.

Pirkle, J. L., K. M. Flegal, et al. (1996). "Exposure of the US population to environmental tobacco smoke: the Third National Health and Nutrition Examination Survey, 1988 to 1991." *Jama 275(16)*: 1233-40.

Pluth, J. M., M. J. Ramsey, et al. (2000). "Role of maternal exposures and newborn genotypes on newborn chromosome aberration frequencies." *Mutat Res 465(1-2)*: 101-11.

Pulling, L. C., K. K. Divine, et al. (2003). "Promoter hypermethylation of the O6-methylguanine-DNA methyltransferase gene: more common in lung adenocarcinomas from never-smokers than smokers and associated with tumor progression." *Cancer Res 63(16)*: 4842-8.

Raherison, C., A. Taytard, et al. (2003). "[Smoking, asthma and associated phenotypes. An epidemiological approach]." *Rev Mal Respir 20(2 Pt 1)*: 233-47.

Rangasamy, T., C. Y. Cho, et al. (2004). "Genetic ablation of Nrf2 enhances susceptibility to cigarette smoke-induced emphysema in mice." *J Clin Invest 114(9)*: 1248-59.

Redline, S., P. V. Tishler, et al. (1989). "Genotypic and phenotypic similarities in pulmonary function among family members of adult monozygotic and dizygotic twins." *Am J Epidemiol 129(4)*: 827-36.

Repace, J. L., J. Jinot, et al. (1998). "Air nicotine and saliva cotinine as indicators of workplace passive smoking exposure and risk." *Risk Anal 18(1)*: 71-83.

Report of the scientific committee on tobacco and health. UK: Her Majesty's Stationery Office, Scientific Committee on Tobacco and Health (SCPTH) (1998).

Report on carcinogens. 11th Edition. P. H. S. U.S. Department of Health and Human Services, National Toxicology Program (2005).

Respiratory health effects of passive smoking: lung cancer and other disorders. US Environmental Protection Agency. Washington, DC (1992).

Reynolds, P., S. Hurley, et al. (2004). "Active smoking, household passive smoking, and breast cancer: evidence from the California Teachers Study." *J Natl Cancer Inst 96(1)*: 29-37.

Rimm, E. B., J. Chan, et al. (1995). "Prospective study of cigarette smoking, alcohol use, and the risk of diabetes in men." *Bmj 310(6979)*: 555-9.

Rimm, E. B., J. E. Manson, et al. (1993). "Cigarette smoking and the risk of diabetes in women." *Am J Public Health 83(2)*: 211-4.

Ronmark, E., E. Jonsson, et al. (1999). "Different pattern of risk factors for atopic and nonatopic asthma among children--report from the Obstructive Lung Disease in Northern Sweden Study." *Allergy 54(9)*: 926-35.

Rushton, L., C. Courage, et al. (2003). "Estimation of the impact on children's health of environmental tobacco smoke in England and Wales." *J R Soc Health 123(3)*: 175-80.

Salvi, G. E., H. P. Lawrence, et al. (1997). "Influence of risk factors on the pathogenesis of periodontitis." *Periodontol 2000 14*: 173-201.

Samet, J. M., D. Brenner, et al. (1998). *Health effects of exposure to radon: BEIR VI.* Washington DC, National Academy Press.

Sardas, S., B. Karahalil, et al. (1995). "The effect of smoking on sister chromatid exchange rate of newborn infants born to smoking mothers." *Mutat Res 341(4)*: 249-53.

Schmitt, J. E., C. A. Prescott, et al. (2005). "The differential heritability of regular tobacco use based on method of administration." *Twin Res Hum Genet 8(1)*: 60-2.

Schoket, B., G. Papp, et al. (2001). "Impact of metabolic genotypes on levels of biomarkers of genotoxic exposure." *Mutat Res 482(1-2)*: 57-69.

Schonberger, H. J. and C. P. Van Schayck (1998). "Prevention of asthma in genetically predisposed children in primary care--from clinical efficacy to a feasible intervention programme." *Clin Exp Allergy 28(11)*: 1325-31.

Sellers, T. A., J. D. Potter, et al. (1992). "Lung cancer detection and prevention: evidence for an interaction between smoking and genetic predisposition." *Cancer Res 52(9 Suppl)*: 2694s-2697s.

Sengler, C., A. Haider, et al. (2003). "Evaluation of the CD14 C-159 T polymorphism in the German Multicenter Allergy Study cohort." *Clin Exp Allergy 33(2)*: 166-9.

Seow, A., B. Zhao, et al. (1999). "NAT2 slow acetylator genotype is associated with increased risk of lung cancer among non-smoking Chinese women in Singapore." *Carcinogenesis 20(9)*: 1877-81.

Sepkovic, D. W., N. J. Haley, et al. (1986). "Elimination from the body of tobacco products by smokers and passive smokers." *Jama 256(7)*: 863.

Shen, M. R., I. M. Jones, et al. (1998). "Nonconservative amino acid substitution variants exist at polymorphic frequency in DNA repair genes in healthy humans." *Cancer Res 58(4)*: 604-8.

Shu, X. O., J. A. Ross, et al. (1996). "Parental alcohol consumption, cigarette smoking, and risk of infant leukemia: a Childrens Cancer Group study." *J Natl Cancer Inst 88(1)*: 24-31.

Siegel, D., W. A. Franklin, et al. (1998). "Immunohistochemical detection of NAD(P)H:quinone oxidoreductase in human lung and lung tumors." *Clin Cancer Res 4(9)*: 2065-70.

Silverman, E. K. and F. E. Speizer (1996). "Risk factors for the development of chronic obstructive pulmonary disease." *Med Clin North Am 80(3)*: 501-22.

Slezak, R. and M. Sasiadek (2000). "[Poland's syndrome]." Pol Merkuriusz Lek 9(50): 568-71.

Smoking and tobacco control monograph 10: Health effects of exposure to environmental tobacco smoke. Bethesda, MD: National Cancer Institute (1999).

Song, N., W. Tan, et al. (2001). "CYP 1A1 polymorphism and risk of lung cancer in relation to tobacco smoking: a case-control study in China." *Carcinogenesis 22(1)*: 11-6.

Song, S., S. M. Lippman, et al. (2005). "Induction of cyclooxygenase-2 by benzo[a]pyrene diol epoxide through inhibition of retinoic acid receptor-beta 2 expression." *Oncogene 24(56)*: 8268-76.

Sorahan, T., P. Prior, et al. (1997). "Childhood cancer and parental use of tobacco: deaths from 1971 to 1976." *Br J Cancer 76(11)*: 1525-31.

Sorsa, M., K. Husgafvel-Pursiainen, et al. (1989). "Cytogenetic effects of tobacco smoke exposure among involuntary smokers." *Mutat Res 222(2)*: 111-6.

"State-specific prevalence of cigarette smoking among adults, and children's and adolescents' exposure to environmental tobacco smoke -- United States, 1996." *MMWR Morb Mortal Wkly Rep 46(44)*: 1038-43 (1997).

Stewart, P. M., F. M. Rogerson, et al. (1995). "Type 2 11 beta-hydroxysteroid dehydrogenase messenger ribonucleic acid and activity in human placenta and fetal membranes: its relationship to birth weight and putative role in fetal adrenal steroidogenesis." *J Clin Endocrinol Metab 80(3)*: 885-90.

Stierum, R. H., G. J. Hageman, et al. (1997). "Age-related negative associations between parameters of cytogenetic damage and ex vivo (+/-)-anti-benzo(a)pyrene diolepoxide-induced unscheduled DNA synthesis in smoking humans." *Cancer Epidemiol Biomarkers Prev 6(11)*: 943-8.

Stoney, C. M., L. M. Lentino, et al. (1998). "Environmental tobacco smoke: association with cardiovascular function at rest and during stress." *Int J Behav Med 5(3)*: 230-44.

Strachan, D. P. and D. G. Cook (1998). "Health effects of passive smoking. 6. Parental smoking and childhood asthma: longitudinal and case-control studies." *Thorax 53(3)*: 204-12.

Streissguth, A. P., P. D. Sampson, et al. (1994). *The effects of prenatal exposure to alcohol and tobacco: contributions from the Seattle Longitudinal Prospective Study and implications for public policy.* H. L. Needleman and D. Bellinger. Beltimore, The Johns Hopkins University Press: 148-183.

Sunaga, N., T. Kohno, et al. (2002). "Contribution of the NQO1 and GSTT1 polymorphisms to lung adenocarcinoma susceptibility." *Cancer Epidemiol Biomarkers Prev 11(8)*: 730-8.

Taioli, E., F. Crofts, et al. (1995). "Radical differences in CYP1A1 genotype and function." *Toxicol Lett 77(1-3)*: 357-62.

Talamini, G., C. Bassi, et al. (1999). "Alcohol and smoking as risk factors in chronic pancreatitis and pancreatic cancer." *Dig Dis Sci 44(7)*: 1303-11.

Tang, D., D. Warburton, et al. (1999). "Molecular and genetic damage from environmental tobacco smoke in young children." *Cancer Epidemiol Biomarkers Prev 8(5)*: 427-31.

Tang, D. L., A. Rundle, et al. (1998). "Associations between both genetic and environmental biomarkers and lung cancer: evidence of a greater risk of lung cancer in women smokers." *Carcinogenesis 19(11)*: 1949-53.

Tang, X., F. R. Khuri, et al. (2000). "Hypermethylation of the death-associated protein (DAP) kinase promoter and aggressiveness in stage I non-small-cell lung cancer." *J Natl Cancer Inst 92(18)*: 1511-6.

Teixeira, J. P., J. Gaspar, et al. (2002). "Aromatic DNA adduct levels in coke oven workers: correlation with polymorphisms in genes GSTP1, GSTM1, GSTT1 and CYP1A1." *Mutat Res 517(1-2)*: 147-55.

The Health Consequences of Involuntary Exposure to Tobacco Smoke: A Report of the Surgeon General. US Department of Health and Human Services (2006).

The health consequences of involuntary smoking. A report of the Surgeon General. Public Health Service. U.S. Department of Health and Human Services, Centers for Disease Control, Center for Health Promotion and Education, Office on Smoking and Health. Rockville, MD (1986).

Thorn, J., J. Brisman, et al. (2001). "Adult-onset asthma is associated with self-reported mold or environmental tobacco smoke exposures in the home." *Allergy 56(4)*: 287-92.

Thun, M. J., C. A. Lally, et al. (1997). "Cigarette smoking and changes in the histopathology of lung cancer." *J Natl Cancer Inst. 89(21)*: 1580-1586.

Tobacco free initiative: consultative report. International Consultation on Environmental Tobacco Smoke and Child Health proceedings. Geneva, Switzerland, WHO (1999).

Tucker, J. D., D. A. Eastmond, et al. (1997). *Application of Biomarkers in Cancer Epidemiology. Cytogenetic end-points as biological dosimeters and predictors of risk in epidemiological studies.* P. Toniolo, P. Boffetta, D. E. G. Shukeret al. Lyon, France, IARC: 185–200.

Ueta, E., Y. Tadokoro, et al. (2003). "The effect of cigarette smoke exposure and ascorbic acid intake on gene expression of antioxidant enzymes and other related enzymes in the livers and lungs of Shionogi rats with osteogenic disorders." *Toxicol Sci 73(2)*: 339-47.

Vahakangas, K. H., W. P. Bennett, et al. (2001). "p53 and K-ras mutations in lung cancers from former and never-smoking women." *Cancer Res 61(11)*: 4350-6.

Vatsis, K. P., W. W. Weber, et al. (1995). "Nomenclature for N-acetyltransferases." *Pharmacogenetics 5(1)*: 1-17.

Vercelli, D. (2003). "Arginase: marker, effector, or candidate gene for asthma?" *J Clin Invest 111(12)*: 1815-7.

Vercelli, D. (2004). "Genetics, epigenetics, and the environment: switching, buffering, releasing." *J Allergy Clin Immunol 113(3)*: 381-6; quiz 387.

Vernooy, J. H., M. Kucukaycan, et al. (2002). "Local and systemic inflammation in patients with chronic obstructive pulmonary disease: soluble tumor necrosis factor receptors are increased in sputum." *Am J Respir Crit Care Med 166(9)*: 1218-24.

Vineis, P., H. Bartsch, et al. (1994). "Genetically based N-acetyltransferase metabolic polymorphism and low-level environmental exposure to carcinogens." *Nature 369(6476)*: 154-6.

Vineis, P., F. Veglia, et al. (2003). "CYP1A1 T3801 C polymorphism and lung cancer: a pooled analysis of 2451 cases and 3358 controls." *Int J Cancer 104(5)*: 650-7.

Vinke, J. G., A. KleinJan, et al. (1999). "Passive smoking causes an 'allergic' cell infiltrate in the nasal mucosa of non-atopic children." *Int J Pediatr Otorhinolaryngol 51(2)*: 73-81.

von Ehrenstein, O. S., E. von Mutius, et al. (2002). "Lung function of school children with low levels of alpha1-antitrypsin and tobacco smoke exposure." *Eur Respir J 19(6)*: 1099-106.

von Mutius, E. (2002). "Environmental factors influencing the development and progression of pediatric asthma." *J Allergy Clin Immunol 109(6 Suppl)*: S525-32.

Walter, R., D. J. Gottlieb, et al. (2000). "Environmental and genetic risk factors and gene-environment interactions in the pathogenesis of chronic obstructive lung disease." *Environ Health Perspect 108 Suppl 4*: 733-42.

Wang, T. J., B. S. Zhou, et al. (1996). "Lung cancer in nonsmoking Chinese women: a case-control study." *Lung Cancer 14 Suppl 1*: S93-8.

Wang, Y., Z. Zhang, et al. (2005). "Tobacco smoke-induced lung tumorigenesis in mutant A/J mice with alterations in K-ras, p53, or Ink4a/Arf." *Oncogene 24(18)*: 3042-9.

Wannamethee, S. G., A. G. Shaper, et al. (2001). "Smoking as a modifiable risk factor for type 2 diabetes in middle-aged men." *Diabetes Care 24(9)*: 1590-5.

Weiss, W. (1997). "Cigarette smoking and lung cancer trends. A light at the end of the tunnel?" *Chest 111(5)*: 1414-6.

Wenten, M., K. Berhane, et al. (2005). "TNF-308 modifies the effect of second-hand smoke on respiratory illness-related school absences." *Am J Respir Crit Care Med 172(12)*: 1563-8.

Wenzlaff, A. S., M. L. Cote, et al. (2005). "CYP1A1 and CYP1B1 polymorphisms and risk of lung cancer among never smokers: a population-based study." *Carcinogenesis 26(12)*: 2207-12.

Wenzlaff, A. S., M. L. Cote, et al. (2005). "GSTM1, GSTT1 and GSTP1 polymorphisms, environmental tobacco smoke exposure and risk of lung cancer among never smokers: a population-based study." *Carcinogenesis 26(2)*: 395-401.

Whyatt, R. M., S. J. Garte, et al. (1995). "CYP1A1 messenger RNA levels in placental tissue as a biomarker of environmental exposure." *Cancer Epidemiol Biomarkers Prev 4(2)*: 147-53.

Whyatt, R. M., R. M. Santella, et al. (1998). "Relationship between ambient air pollution and DNA damage in Polish mothers and newborns." *Environ Health Perspect 106 Suppl 3*: 821-6.

Wilce, M. C. and M. W. Parker (1994). "Structure and function of glutathione S-transferases." *Biochim Biophys Acta 1205(1)*: 1-18.

Will, J. C., D. A. Galuska, et al. (2001). "Cigarette smoking and diabetes mellitus: evidence of a positive association from a large prospective cohort study." *Int J Epidemiol 30(3)*: 540-6.

Williams, M. D. and A. B. Sandler (2001). "The epidemiology of lung cancer." *Cancer Treatment & Research 105*: 31-52.

Witschi, H., V. I. Oreffo, et al. (1995). "Six-month exposure of strain A/J mice to cigarette sidestream smoke: cell kinetics and lung tumor data." *Fundam Appl Toxicol 26(1)*: 32-40.

Wolf, A., A. Kutz, et al. (2005). "The effect of benzo(a)pyrene on porcine urinary bladder epithelial cells analyzed for the expression of selected genes and cellular toxicological endpoints." *Toxicology 207(2)*: 255-69.

Wong, S. S., N. N. Sun, et al. (2002). "Tissue-specific patterns of neurokinin-1 receptor (NK-1R) gene expression in mice exposed to sidestream cigarette smoke." *Toxicol Ind Health 18(9-10)*: 435-44.

Woodward, A. and A. J. McMichael (1991). "Passive smoking and cancer risk: the nature and uses of epidemiological evidence." *Eur J Cancer 27(11)*: 1472-9.

World cancer report. B. W. Stewart and P. Kleihues. Lyon, IARC Press: 182 (2003).

Wu, D., X. Q. Zhang, et al. (2001). "[Analysis of association between gene polymorphisms of microsomal epoxide hydrolase (EPHX1) and infant birthweight]." *Yi Chuan Xue Bao 28(7)*: 595-600.

Wu, M. F., W. J. Wu, et al. (2004). "Increased expression of cytochrome P4501B1 in peripheral leukocytes from lung cancer patients." *Toxicol Lett 150(2)*: 211-9.

Wynder, E. L. and D. Hoffmann (1994). "Smoking and lung cancer: scientific challenges and opportunities." *Cancer Res 54(20)*: 5284-95.

Yang, K., L. Julan, et al. (2006). "Cadmium reduces 11 beta-hydroxysteroid dehydrogenase type 2 activity and expression in human placental trophoblast cells." Am J Physiol *Endocrinol Metab 290(1)*: E135-E142.

Yang, M. and M. Y. Pyo (2005). "Molecular epidemiology of lung cancer in female passive smokers." *J Environ Sci Health C Environ Carcinog Ecotoxicol Rev 23(1)*: 75-97.

Yao, R., Y. Wang, et al. (2005). "K-ras mutations in lung tumors from p53 mutant mice exposed to cigarette smoke." *Exp Lung Res 31(2)*: 271-81.

Zenzes, M. T., L. A. Puy, et al. (1998). "Immunodetection of benzo[a]pyrene adducts in ovarian cells of women exposed to cigarette smoke." *Mol Hum Reprod 4(2)*: 159-65.

Zhu, B. Q., C. Heeschen, et al. (2003). "Second hand smoke stimulates tumor angiogenesis and growth." *Cancer Cell 4(3)*: 191-6.

Zimmermann, N., N. E. King, et al. (2003). "Dissection of experimental asthma with DNA microarray analysis identifies arginase in asthma pathogenesis." *J Clin Invest 111(12)*: 1863-74.

In: Smoking and Health Research Frontiers
Editor: Calvin B. Fong, pp. 63-79
ISBN 1-60021-480-0

Chapter III

THE EFFECT OF PASSIVE SMOKE-EXPOSURE ON FERTILITY

Michael S. Neal [*] ***and Warren G. Foster***
Centre for Reproductive Care, Hamilton Health Sciences and Reproductive Biology Division, Department of Obstetrics and Gynecology, McMaster University, Hamilton, Ontario, Canada.

ABSTRACT

Although tobacco smoking is a widely recognized health hazard and a major cause of preventable mortality, smoking remains prevalent in our society. Approximately 30% of women and 35% of men of reproductive age smoke. But more importantly, the incidence of smoking is increasing among adolescents and specifically teenage girls. Environmental tobacco smoke (ETS), or passive smoke, is a significant source of exposure to a large number of substances known to be hazardous to human health. Recently, substantial harmful effects of cigarette smoke on the ability to become pregnant have become apparent. The deleterious effect of passive smoke exposure is similar to active smoking with respect to fertility. Women who smoke take longer to achieve a natural pregnancy, require more hormonal stimulation during IVF treatment with reduced success, and reach menopause earlier than their non-smoking counterparts. Toxicants found in passive smoke have been isolated at higher levels in the serum and follicular fluid of women exposed to ETS compared to non-smokers implying that cigarette smoke may act as an ovarian toxicant as one mechanism to disrupt fertility. However, the male contribution to infertility cannot be excluded. The paternal effect on infertility is largely dependant on sperm function. The effect of cotinine, for example, has

[*] Correspondence concerning this article should be addressed to Michael S. Neal, Laboratory Director, Centre for Reproductive Care, Hamilton Health Sciences, 690 Main St.West, West End Clinic, Hamilton, Ontario, Canada L8S 1A4. Phone: 905-521-2100 ext 76515; E-mail: nealm@hhsc.ca

been shown to alter sperm function, and may be an underlying mechanism of impaired fertility. Paternal smoking is associated with sperm with a higher incidence of DNA abnormalities that may account for higher implantation failures and miscarriage rates. Both the female and male gamete are sensitive to toxic exposure(s) and slight alterations to either the sperm or oocyte may be lethal at the peri-implantation stage of embryo development leading to sub-fertility. Passive smoke exposure may induce toxic effects and compromise fertility through several direct or indirect mechanisms.

INTRODUCTION

Reproductive function in humans can be compromised by exposure to toxic chemicals. With the recent trend for couples to delay the start of a family, there has been an enhanced awareness of chemicals in the environment that impact the reproductive function of men and women. Considerations that affect fertility include a reduced quality of the gametes from the male (sperm) and female (oocyte). As couples wait longer to attempt conception, age and the increase in the number of years of exposure to environmental influences becomes more apparent. The habit of cigarette smoking is a major source of exposure to toxicants and has been shown to have an effect on fertility and pregnancy outcomes.

Despite the fact that tobacco smoking is a widely recognized as a health hazard and a major cause of preventable mortality, smoking remains prevalent in society. While there has been a decrease in the incidence of smoking in the general population, the percentage of adolescent smokers has increased. What is even more troubling is the incidence of smoking among young women. A recent survey of high school students in southwestern Ontario revealed that 36.2% of teenage girls smoke [1] and a study from the United Kingdom reports that, at the age of 15, 33% of girls are regular smokers [2].

The reproductive health effects of cigarette smoke exposure for women are far-reaching [3]. Several comprehensive reviews of the literature have been published summarizing the cumulative data supporting an association between cigarette smoking and diminished male and female fertility [2, 4-6]. Smoking has been associated with longer time to pregnancy, decreased pregnancy success using assisted reproductive techniques [7, 8] and menstrual changes including early menopause [9]. The risk of being unable to conceive within one year of trying is increased 2- to 3-fold among smokers [10]. Consistent with earlier studies, Van Voorhis et al. [11] reported a dose-related decrease in ovarian function and a 50% reduction in pregnancy rate among current smokers tying to achieve a pregnancy. Furthermore, the impact of cigarette smoking on early spontaneous abortion has been an important addition to the cause of reduced fecundity. Increased pregnancy loss coupled with a higher risk of ectopic pregnancies attributed to smoking adds to the overall adverse reproductive impact of the smoking habit [12-14]. This evidence led Joffe [15] to describe smoking as the foremost reproductive poison of the 20th Century.

Epidemiology

Smokers inhale toxic, carcinogenic and mutagenic substances known to be prevalent in cigarette smoke, and many non-smokers are regularly exposed by inhalation of side-stream smoke from the smoldering end of the burning cigarette and/or from the passive smoke exhaled by smokers into the environment. Cumulative data reported in the literature on cigarette smoking and fertility all support the conclusion that cigarette smoke has a negative impact [2, 4, 6, 7, 16]. Due to the fact that these studies include diverse populations, there is considerable concern about confounding variables from multiple sources [2, 7]. However, the first large scale population based study to demonstrate that smoking negatively affects fecundity, independent of other factors, was recently published [17]. The investigators studied nearly 15,000 pregnancies to determine time to conception. In addition to smoking, factors such as parental age, ethnicity, education, employment, housing, pre-pregnancy body mass index (BMI), and alcohol consumption were considered for their possible influence(s). Active smoking was associated with failure to conceive in both 6- and 12-month duration of the study. Delay in time to pregnancy (TTP) was correlated with increasing cigarette consumption. Conception delay for over 12 months was 54% higher among smokers compared to nonsmokers. Furthermore, active smoking by either partner elicited an effect, and the impact of passive cigarette exposure was only slightly smaller than that seen for active smoking by either partner [6].

ETS and Assisted Reproductive Technology

The field of assisted reproductive technology (ART) has provided a unique opportunity to measure and observe the adverse effects of constituents of cigarette smoke on the seminal and follicular microenvironments. Cotinine, the metabolite of nicotine; cadmium, a heavy metal in cigarette smoke; and benzo-[a]-pyrene, a carcinogenic polycyclic aromatic hydrocarbon, have all been detected in the follicular fluid of women undergoing IVF treatment [8, 18]. This demonstrates that these toxicants found in cigarette smoke are present at the target tissue, the developing follicle. Furthermore, the estradiol concentration in follicular fluid [19] or serum [20] have been shown to be significantly lower in female smokers compared to their non-smoking counterparts. This implies that the cigarette smoke toxicants found in the follicular fluid of IVF patients may be acting to impair steroidogenesis. In addition to this, the estradiol:testosterone ratio in follicles is predictive of maturity and quality of the oocytes retrieved [21]. Thus, introduction of these toxicants may impair estradiol production, which may in turn adversely affect oocyte maturity and quality that would ultimately decrease the chance of a successful IVF pregnancy outcome. Impaired follicular steroidogenesis may be only one mechanism leading to sub-fertility. Paszowski et al., [19] have reported that active smoking alters the pro-oxidant/anti-oxidant balance in follicular fluid such that there is oxidative stress in the growing follicle. Oxidative stress may in turn lead to cell damage and cytotoxicity in the oocyte and companion granulosa cells.

Cigarette smoke has also been shown to adversely affect oocyte quality [8]. Plachot [22] observed that approximately 25% of oocytes that fail to successfully fertilize after *in vitro* fertilization possess chromosome abnormalities. Moreover, women who smoke have a higher incidence of oocytes with a diploid chromosome complement to oocytes from non-smokers [8].

Ovarian Function

Folliculogenesis

Follicular development begins during fetal life with the transformation of primordial germ cells into oocytes and their enclosure in structures called follicles. In mammals, primordial follicles form either before, or in the first few days after birth. Primordial follicles give rise to primary follicles which transform into preantral (secondary follicles) and then antral follicles (tertiary follicles) and finally pre-ovulatory, Graafian follicles, in a co-ordinated series of transitions regulated by hormones and local intra-ovarian factors. The growth and differentiation of follicles from the primordial population is termed folliculogenesis. With the LH surge, Graafian follicles rupture and oocytes are released, leaving the follicular cells to luteinize and form a corpus luteum. Sex steroids play important roles in the growth and differentiation of reproductive tissues and in the maintenance of fertility.

Steroidogenesis

Steroid production in the ovary is a tightly regulated and complex process that involves several different signaling pathways in multiple types of cells. The mammalian ovary consists of four cell types. Each follicle contains an oocyte surrounded by cumulus granulosa cells. These cells are then bound by outer mural granulosa cells, which in turn are surrounded by theca cells [23, 24]. Steroidogenesis in most mammals (including humans) occurs via the two cell/two gonadotropin model whereby androgens are synthesized from cholesterol in LH-stimulated theca cells, followed by conversion to estrogens in follicle stimulating hormone (FSH)-exposed granulosa cells. LH receptors and the enzyme CYP17, which converts pregnenolone and progesterone to dehydroepiandrosterone (DHEA) and adrostenedione, respectively, are expressed primarily in the theca cells. FSH receptors, and aromatase (CYP19), which converts androgens to estrogens, are expressed mainly in the granulosa cells. Both theca and granulosa cells express steroidogenic acute regulatory protein (StAR), CYP11A1 (side chain cleavage enzyme), and 3β-HSD and are capable of making prenenolone and/or progesterone from cholesterol. However, in the follicular phase, the relatively avascularized granulosa cells see limited oxygen or cholesterol, and thus small amounts of steroids are produced. In contrast, after exposure to gonadotropins, the granulosa cells become luteinized, and then are able to synthesize large amounts of prenenolone and progesterone from cholesterol [23, 24].

Effect of ETS Constituents on Steroidogensis

Cigarette smoke is composed of more than 4000 chemical compounds including hundreds of reproductive toxicants and carcinogens [25, 26]. The majority (~50%) of tobacco consists of carbohydrates and proteins. Other significant constituents are alkaloids (0.5 – 5.5%) with nicotine being the predominant compound (~95% of the total alkaloids), polyphenols (0.5 – 4.5%), phytoteoles (0.1 – 2.5%), carboxilic acids (0.1 – 0.7%), alkanes (0.1 – 0.4%), aromatic hydrocarbons, aldehydes, ketones, amines, nitriles, pesticides, alkali nitrates (0.01 – 5.0%) and at least 30 metallic compounds [8, 27]. three components, cadmium, nicotine, and benzo-[a]-pyrene, are discussed below in relation to their effect on fertility.

Cadmium

Cadmium (Cd^{2+}) is a heavy metal and a major constituent of cigarette smoke [28] that accumulates in various organs, including the ovaries [29] and has been measured at higher concentrations in follicular fluid from women exposed to cigarette smoke. The concentration of cadmium in seminal plasma of smokers is almost twice the amount found in nonsmokers [30, 31]. Several studies propose that Cd^{2+} exerts a dual, concentration dependant effect on steroidogenesis. At low concentrations (0.6 – 3 μM), Cd^{2+} stimulates transcription of the P450scc gene and the steroidogenic pathway in the ovary [32]. At higher concentrations (over 2-5 μM), Cd^{2+} inhibits activity of the P450scc gene [32], progesterone synthesis [33], and facilitates changes in cell morphology and cell death [32, 34]. Therefore, the changes induced by Cd^{2+} on the P450scc gene expression in granulosa cells could affect the synthesis of all steroid hormones in the ovary.

Nicotine

Nicotine is quickly absorbed from cigarette smoke into the organism through the respiratory tract. Cotinine, a major metabolite of nicotine, is regularly used as a marker of smoke exposure because of its longer half-life of ~ 20 h compared to the 2 h half-life of nicotine [35]. Cotinine has been detected in the follicular fluid of women undergoing assisted conception at a concentration of 2 μM [8, 36]. The effect of smoking on the function of human granulosa-lutein cells have been contradictory. Barberi et al., [37] reported that *in vitro* exposure to nicotine inhibited granulosa cell aromatase. Another study showed that neither cotinine or nicotine altered progesterone or estradiol secretion by human granulosa cells in the presence of serum [36] while in serum-free medium a dose-dependant increase in the secretion of estradiol and decrease in the secretion of progesterone was observed [38]. Therefore the mechanism(s) of nicotine or cotinine effect on steroidogenesis seems to be, at least in part, indirect. Miceli et al., [39] showed that nicotine negatively affected basal luteal steroidogenesis at all tested concentrations (0.01 nM to 1 μM) while it was not able to affect hCG-induced progesterone release. Furthermore, nicotine was able to significantly increase mRNA expression of vascular endothelial growth factor (VEGF), which is strictly involved with luteal pathophysiology and may induce a sort of luteal insufficiency by inhibiting progesterone release [39]. Another indirect mechanism has been suggested by Gocze and Freeman [40] who concluded from their study that inhibition of progesterone synthesis by cigarette smoke alkaloids is largely exerted by preventing the growth and/or killing the steroid synthesizing cell.

Benzo-[a]-pyrene

Benzo-[a]-pyrene (B[a]P) belongs to a group of environmental pollutants called polycyclic aromatic hydrocarbons (PAHs). PAHs are chemicals produced from incomplete combustion of fossil fuels and are found in air pollution, tobacco smoke, and the diet (barbecued foods or cereal grains) and have the ability to bind covalently to DNA, giving rise to DNA adducts [8]. B[a]P is primariliy produced from the smoldering end of the cigarette in amounts of 6 – 40 ng per cigarette; someone consuming 20 cigarettes in an 8 hr day (pack a day smoker) would be expected to inhale 0.07 to 0.57 μg of B[a]P [41].

Gametogenesis

The ability to reproduce depends largely on the meiotic maturation of germinal cells, or gametogenesis. Gametogenesis, involves two cell divisions: meiosis I and meiosis II. Meiosis I is reductional and results in oocytes and spermatocytes with a haploid complement of chromosomes (23 instead of 46 chromosomes). During meiosis II the two sister chromatids of each chromosome separate, leading to four haploid cells. Gametogenesis is a vulnerable period of development and is a time that the risk of damage to cigarette smoking is high [42]. Sensitivity to external insults and the ablitity to repair damage in male and female germinal cells is very different and is explained in more detail below.

Oogenesis

Female meiotic maturation of germ cells (oogenesis) results in one haploid oocyte arrested at metaphase II, which completes meiosis at the time of fertilization. Three dysfunctional polar bodies (the first polar body divides shortly after extrusion) are the bi-products of oogenesis. This process involves not only nuclear but cytoplasmic maturation. During oogenesis there is a long period of meiotic arrest of the primary (meiosis I) oocytes which begins during fetal life and lasts until puberty and sexual maturation. Oocytes are very vulnerable when they divide during meiosis I and II and become metabolically active: firstly, during fetal life at the diplotene stage in prophase I; and secondly, during the pre-ovulatory stage of the menstrual cycle when oocytes resume and complete meiotic maturation into metaphase II [43].

During post-natal life, ovarian follicles grow, mature and either ovulate or regress. Follicles are recruited continuously with each menstrual cycle in humans until the original store is exhausted and menopause ensues. Of the estimated 500,000 follicles present at birth in females, only 400 or so actually reach the preovulatory stage and ovulate. During the late pre-antral to early antral period, oocytes synthesize molecules necessary for the resumption of meiosis, and the production of developmentally competent oocytes. Fluid accumulates within the small spaces between the granulosa cells layers and these colexnar bodies eventually coalesce to form the large fluid filled antral cavity. Follicular fluid is formed by filtered blood supply that penetrates the thecal layers of the follicle. Follicles acquire the ablility to sythesize steroid hormones during this pre-antral stage of oogenesis. The oocyte, surrounded by granulosa cells, becomes bathed in follicular fluid, and is vulnerable to toxicants that reach the follicular fluid.

Ovarian Depletion

Onset of menopause occurs one to four years earlier in women who smoke compared to their non-smoking counterparts [17]. The dose-dependant nature of this effect supports the contention that smoking may accelerate ovarian follicular depletion. Chemicals in cigarette smoke appear to hasten follicular depletion and the loss of reproductive function. Mean basal FSH levels are significantly higher in young smokers compared to non-smokers [7, 44]. Basal FSH levels were 66% higher in active smokers than in non-smokers and 39% higher in passive smokers than non-smokers [7]. Furthermore, urinary estrogen excretion during the luteal phase in smokers is only about one third that tobacco smoke inhibit granulosa cell aromatase [8].

The fact that women who smoke cigarettes are two and a half times more likely than non-smokers to have a dimished ovarian reserve [45] implies that accelerated loss of oocytes is at the heart of the problem. Tobacco smoke also has long term effects on the developing fetus, with reports of impaired fertility in women whose mothers smoked during pregnancy [46]. Identification of the chemical(s) in tobacco smoke responsible for altering fertility and accelerating menopause is complicated by several factors. The first is the complex chemical composition of cigarette smoke, which contains more than 50 carcinogens, such as polycyclic aromatic hydrocarbons (PAH), aromatic amines and N-nitrosomines [27]. The second is the lack of suitable approaches for the detection and monitoring of cytotoxic responses of human ovaries *in vivo*, which has limited extrapolation of results from animal models in female reproductive toxicology studies.

There is evidence to support the argument that PAHs are the key culprits that accelerate oocyte death promoting pre-mature depletion of ovarian reserves leading to an earlier onset of menopause in women who smoke. Computer simulations using data from animal studies have determined that it would take destruction of 25% of the follicle pool to account for a 2-year advance in the age of menopause [47]. Almost 30 years ago Mattison et al., [48] reported that oocytes are rapidly depleted from the ovaries of young female mice that were exposed to PAHs *in vitro*. Further studies [47] supported this finding and also showed that *in utero* exposure of female mouse fetuses to PAH or cigarette smoke is cytotoxic to the developing germ line. More recent studies have focussed on the mechanism(s) leading to PAH induced follicle loss. The first important observation came from studies that show that a cytoplasmic receptor for PAH, called the aromatic hydrocarbon receptor (Ahr) is abundantly expressed in oocytes [49]. The Ahr belongs to the PER-ARNT-SIM (PAS) family of transcription factors that evolved in multi-cellular organisms over 450 million years ago [50]. The natural ligand(s) for the Ahr remain elusive, but the receptor is known to bind, and be activated by a number of chemicals including members of the PAH family. Once activated the Ahr translocates to the nucleus and interacts with genes that contain a common nucleotide sequence (known as the Ahr reponse element, AHRE) resulting in altered gene expression [50]. Ahr-mutant mice have a two-fold greater number of oocytes at birth due to attenuated fetal germ-cell apoptosis [51]. Furthermore, oocytes in fetal mouse ovaries increase Bax production and undergo apoptosis in an Ahr-dependant fashion following PAH exposure [49].

Expansion of the Cumulus Oocyte Complex (COC)

During the latter part of folliculogenesis, a population of follicular granulosa cells (called cumulus cells) form the cumulus oocyte complex (COC). The pre-ovulatory surge of gonadotropins induces a cascade of processes culminating in ovulation. One of the most marked of these events is cumulus expansion. The pre-ovulatory deposition of hyaluronic acid in the COC matrix causes a dramatic increase in volume of the COC, dissociation of the COC form the follicle wall and the resumption of meiosis occurs. The expanded cumulus cells continue to provide nutrients and hormones to the developing oocyte as it travels through the oviduct and for several hours after fertilization. Optimal expansion of the cumulus cells has been linked to normal ovulation, fertilization and subsequent development [52, 53] and the aromatase activity of these cells has been correlated with pregnancy success when using *in vitro* fertilization techniques [54].

Effects of ETS Constituents on the COC

The effect of cigarette smoke components on COC expansion has been studied by observing follicles isolated from the porcine ovary [55]. More than 60% of the control COCs culutre in the presence of FSH alone, had fair expansion. In contrast, in the presence of cadmium and nicotine (each in concentrations of 1, 10, or 100 μM), only 30% of the COCs had comparable expansion [55]. High concentrations of cadmium and nicotine (100 μM) also exerted significant suppression of hyaluronic acid synthesis by the cumulus cells. Furthermore, the effects of ETS constituents on the COC related processes were accompanied by a significant inhibition of progesterone synthesis [55].

Benzo-[a]-pyrene (B[a]P) has been shown to attenuate follicle growth and COC expansion in an isolated follicle culture [18]. It is well known that oocytes and cumulus cells exchange numerous factors and communicate through gap junction channels [56, 57]. Environmental toxicants may exert their deleterious effect by disrupting the flow of communication and nutrients from the granulosa cells to the oocyte. A break in this pathway results in subtle changes in cytoplasmic maturation. Thus, perturbation of gap junction communication and cummulus expansion allows for the oocyte to ovulate, fertilize and appear to have normal pre-implantation embyro development but does not provide the framework to sustain proper implantation leading to a viable pregnancy. Taken together these studies have shown that COC expansion is another reproduction event that is potentially disrupted by the effects of cigarette smoke constituents.

Oocyte Maturation and Competence

Successful initiation of a pregnancy relies not only requires a nuclear mature oocyte but it is critical to have an oocyte that possesses cytoplasmic maturation and competence. Mammalian oocytes are arrested in the prophase of the first meiotic divison and oocytes resume meiosis in response to the preovulatory gonadotropin surge. Oocyte maturation involves resumption of meiosis, progression to metaphase II (MII), and the accompanying cytoplasmic changes that prepare the oocyte for proper fertilization and subsequent embryonic development. Despite extensive investigation, the regulatory mechanisms for oocyte maturation remains poorly understood.

ETS and Oocyte Quality

Cigarette smoking has been shown to alter the meiotic spindle of oocytes, leading to chromosome errors which affect reproductive outcomes [8]. In patients undergoing assisted conception, a significant decrease in the number of retrieved oocytes in association with smoking has been observed [11, 58]. Oocyte elimination occurs preferentially during meiosis I, a period sensitive to genetic damage by external insults [59]. It has been reported that, of the oocytes that fail to fertilize after *in vitro* fertlization, approximately 25% have chromosome abnormalities [22]. Zenzes et al., [8] have reported that women who are exposed to cigarette smoke have and increased frequency of oocytes with a diploid chromosome complement compared to non-smokers. They suggested that this difference occurred due to the prevention of the first polar body extrusion, suggesting that there is an effect of maternal cigarette smoking on oocyte maturation [8]. Similarly, Neal et al., [54] have shown that the percentage of oocytes that were meiotically mature as determined by the presence of the first polar body at the time of ICSI was lower in female patients who were smoking at the time of assisted reproduction treatment. The effect on oocyte maturity was more pronounced in smoking women aged > 30 years [8]. Furthermore, ETS has been linked to an increased risk of DNA damage.

Benzo-[a]-pyrene, has been shown to induce DNA adduct formation in granulosa-lutein cells which results in higher DNA damage [8, 60]. DNA-adduct formation has been demonstrated in the ovarian cells of smokers [8]. Furthermore, passive smoke exposure at home is associated with DNA adduct formation in leucocytes [61]. In granulosa-lutein cells, the mean number of DNA adducts were correlated in a dose-dependant fashion with cotinine levels measured in follicular fluid [8]. DNA adduct concentrations were 3-times higher among active smokers and 2-times higher among passive smokers relative to the levels in nonsmokers [8]. The presence of DNA adducts represents an increased risk for chromosomal and cellular damage. B[a]P has been shown to elicit cytogenetic damage in hamster cell lines including structural and numerical chromosome aberrations and spindle disturbances [62]. The higher the level of DNA adducts in the resulting embryo may contribute to normal appearing pre-implantation embryo development, but results in failed implantation.

Spermatogenesis

In contrast to oogenesis, spermatogenesis involves a continuous production of male germ cells from puberty until old age. Once germinal cells enter meiosis (I and II) they become vulnerable to environmental insults [63].

ETS and Sperm Quality

Increased environmental pollution and ETS are potential explanations for an apparent decline in sperm counts over the last 50 years [64]. The deleterious effect of ETS on male fertility manifests as reduced sperm concentration, increased abnormal cells, and chromosome abnormalities [5]. Cigarette smoking has been associated with an increased risk of aneuploidy in sperm, and this affect appears to be chromosome specific [65]. ETS also increases the risk for DNA and apoptosis in sperm damage [60, 66, 67]. Apoptosis may, therefore, be involved in the occurrence of oligospermia after exposure to various environmental toxicants. Moreover, apoptosis of damaged pre-meiotic germ cells may serve a critical role in protecting subsequent generations from the diverse genotoxic effects of environmental toxicants.

Since ejaculated sperm lacks any repairing capability DNA adducts in sperm, formed from toxicants in cigarette smoke, present a potential vehicle to transport damaged genetic material to the zygote. Parental transmission of DNA adducts has been shown to occur at a higher rate (3.7 fold increase in mean number of DNA adducts) in embryos derived from a smoking couple (either mainstream or sidestream smoke exposure) than in embryos from nonsmoking parents [68]. Fertilization and pregnancy rates using assisted conception were decreased not only in women who smoked but in women exposed who were exposed to cigarette smoke because their partner actively smoked at home [54].

UTERINE ENVIRONMENT

Implantation

There is growing evidence that smoking disrupts fertility by altering uterine-fallopian tube functions that mediates gamete and embryo transport. Smoking has been shown to increase the resting tone of the uterus and the amplitude of uterine contractions in women [69]. Moreover, nicotine administered to rhesus monkeys significantly altered oviductal tone and uterine contraction amplitude [70]. Talbot et al., further demonstrated that an *in vivo* effect of both mainstream and sidestream smoke exposure on oviductal cilia cells and corpora lutea in hamsters [71]. Additional *in vitro* studies demonstrate an inhibitory effect of smoke solutions, and more specifically potassium cyanide, on ciliary beat frequency and oocyte pick-up rate [72]. The evidence that smoking may impair fertility through alterations in utero-tubal motility, or the rate of oocyte, sperm, or embryo transport may be one underlying reason for the increased risk of ectopic pregnancies in women who smoke [13].

Little is understood about the effects of smoking on the response of the human uterine endometrium to steroid hormones, or about the ability of an embryo to undergo proper implantation. Smokers have an approximately 50 per cent lower risk of endometrial cancer, and decreased incidence of endometriosis and uterine fibroids compared with their non-smoking counterparts [73, 74]. Although factors such as weight, diet, parity, alcohol consumption and early menopause in smokers may exert an anti-estrogenic effect, post-menopausal women who smoke still exhibit a substantially lower risk of endometrial cancer [75]. It is intriguing to question how cigarette smoke is protective against benign and malignant tumors, while being associated with impaired implantation and pregnancy success. Some studies have shown that infertility among women who smoke has been linked to fallopian tube dysfunction and pelvic inflammation [76]. In addition to this there is some evidence of direct effects of constituents of cigarette smoke on uterine tissue. Nicotine administered to rats caused an adverse effect on the decidualization process, and was manifested as delayed implantation and altered spacing of implantation sites [77, 78]. Furthermore, exposure of human RL95-2 endometrial adenocarcinoma cells to benzo-[a]-pyrene markedly decreased proliferation, cell attachment and invasion of basement membrane [65]. Shiverick et al., [65] have further shown that B[a]P mediated alterations in endometrial cell attachment appear to be correlated with a loss of cell surface expression of receptors for epidermal growth factor (EGF) and decreased levels of E-cadherin, a cell adhesion molecule essential for cell to cell communication. Therefore, B[a]P mediated loss of cell adhesion molecules may serve as a biomarker for alterations in uterine receptivity that impacts trophoblast implantation.

Increased miscarriage rates among mothers who smoke have been documented to be as high as 33 per cent [79]. During early pregnancy, stem cells fuse to form the syncytium or aggregate to form cell columns that first adhere to and then invade the uterus. Experimental data indicate that smoking causes a generalized dysfunction of both villous and invasive trophoblasts in early pregnancy. Biochemical markers of placental function such as maternal levels of estradiol, human chorionic gonadotropin (hCG), and human placental lactogen (hPL) are lower in smokers compared to non-smokers [80]. Furthermore, placental aromatase activity is decreased *in vivo* in smokers as well as *in vitro* by exposure to nicotine and continine [81, 82]. Also, levels of the heavy metal cadmium, a known placental toxin in both animals and humans, are increased in smokers [65]. Using the perfused human placenta model, Wier et al., [83], showed that cadmium produced ultrastructural changes and resulted in decrease secretion of hCG. Cadmium was further found to inhibit cell interactions with calmodulin, an intracellular calcium binding protein [84].

A consistent finding has been the presence of smoking related alterations in placental receptor for EGF, a potent mitogen and differentiation factor for trophoblasts. Exposure of human placental cells in primary culture to PAHs directly resulted in concentration-dependant loss of EGF-receptor binding and kinase activity, which was greatest in cells from first trimester placenta [85]. In first trimester placental villus explants grown on Matrigel, B[a]P significantly decreased EGF receptor levels as well as hGG secretion [65]. Further studies with human trophoblastic choriocarcinoma cell lines have shown that the B[a]P mediated loss of EGF receptors is linked not only with decreased trophoblast proliferation and hCG secretion [86], but also with decreased expression of the proto-oncogene c-myc, whereas TGF-β1expression is increased [87]. Taken together, this evidence supports the notion that constituents of tobacco smoke have the potential to alter trophoblast gene expression in the direction of down regulation of positive regulators (EGF-receptors, c-myc) and up regulation of negative factors (TGF-β1) of normal trophoblast function.

Conclusion

Studying infertility is complicated by the fact that reproduction is a multi-step process that relies on proper gametogenesis, fertilization, pre-implantation embryo development, implantation and early placentation. Any one of these steps may be influenced by environmental tobacco smoke exposure. Furthermore, the entire reproductive process is orchestrated by hormones, so an alteration in their production or metabolism caused by constituents in cigarette smoke could impair fertility. Animal and human studies have suggested an effect of tobacco smoke on tubal function, which supports the association between smoking and tubal infertility. Further animal studies suggest that exposure to tobacco smoke or its constituent's nicotine and polycyclic aromatic hydrocarbons, results in oocyte and/or follicle destruction, which in turn could lead to, reduced fertility.

In summary, the mechanism(s) by which smoking may affect fertility has not been definitively identified, but such an effect is plausible. Indeed the epidemiological evidence is supportive of a negative effect of both active and passive smoking on fertility.

REFERENCES

[1] Cohen B, Evers S, Manske S, Bercovitz K, Edward HG. Smoking, physical activity and breakfast consumption among secondary school students in a southwestern Ontario community. *Can J Public Health* 2003; 94: 41-44.

[2] Augood C, Duckitt K, Templeton AA. Smoking and female infertility: a systematic review and meta-analysis. *Hum Reprod* 1998; 13: 1532-1539.

[3] Seltzer V. Smoking as a risk factor in the health of women. *Int J Gynaecol Obstet* 2003; 82: 393-397.

[4] Stillman RJ, Rosenberg MJ, Sachs BP. Smoking and reproduction. *Fertil Steril* 1986; 46: 545-566.

[5] Vine MF. Smoking and male reproduction: a review. *Int J Androl* 1996; 19: 323-337.

[6] Weisberg E. Smoking and reproductive health. *Clin Reprod Fertil* 1985; 3: 175-186.

[7] Cooper GS, Baird DD, Hulka BS, Weinberg CR, Savitz DA, Hughes CL, Jr. Follicle-stimulating hormone concentrations in relation to active and passive smoking. *Obstet Gynecol* 1995; 85: 407-411.

[8] Zenzes MT. Smoking and reproduction: gene damage to human gametes and embryos. *Hum Reprod Update* 2000; 6: 122-131.

[9] Jick H, Porter J. Relation between smoking and age of natural menopause. Report from the Boston Collaborative Drug Surveillance Program, Boston University Medical Center. *Lancet* 1977; 1: 1354-1355.

[10] Werler MM. Teratogen update: smoking and reproductive outcomes. *Teratology* 1997; 55: 382-388.

[11] Van Voorhis BJ, Syrop CH, Hammitt DG, Dunn MS, Snyder GD. Effects of smoking on ovulation for assisted reproductive techniques. *Fertil Steril* 1992; 58: 981-985.

[12] Stergachis A, Scholes D, Daling JR, Weiss NS, Chu J. Maternal cigarette smoking and the risk of tubal pregnancy. *Am J Epidemiol* 1991; 133: 332-337.

[13] Saraiya M, Berg CJ, Kendrick JS, Strauss LT, Atrash HK, Ahn YW. Cigarette smoking as a risk factor for ectopic pregnancy. *Am J Obstet Gynecol* 1998; 178: 493-498.

[14] Coste J, Job-Spira N, Fernandez H. Increased risk of ectopic pregnancy with maternal cigarette smoking. *Am J Public Health* 1991; 81: 199-201.

[15] Joffe M, Key J, Best N, Keiding N, Scheike T, Jensen TK. Studying time to pregnancy by use of a retrospective design. *Am J Epidemiol* 2005; 162: 115-124.

[16] Fredricsson B, Gilljam H. Smoking and reproduction. Short and long term effects and benefits of smoking cessation. *Acta Obstet Gynecol Scand* 1992; 71: 580-592.

[17] Hull MG, North K, Taylor H, Farrow A, Ford WC. Delayed conception and active and passive smoking. The Avon Longitudinal Study of Pregnancy and Childhood Study Team. *Fertil Steril* 2000; 74: 725-733.

[18] Neal MS, Zhu JP, Foster WG. Quantification of benzo-[a]-pyrene (B[a]P) in serum and follicular fluid and its effect on follicle growth in an isolated follicle culture assay. . Canadian Fertility and Adrology Society Annual Meeting, Montreal. 2005.

[19] Paszkowski T. [The influence of smoking on the estradiol level in the preovulatory follicular fluid]. *Ginekol Pol* 2001; 72: 989-992.

[20] Sterzik K, Strehler E, De Santo M, Trumpp N, Abt M, Rosenbusch B, Schneider A. Influence of smoking on fertility in women attending an in vitro fertilization program. *Fertil Steril* 1996; 65: 810-814.

[21] Xia P, Younglai EV. Relationship between steroid concentrations in ovarian follicular fluid and oocyte morphology in patients undergoing intracytoplasmic sperm injection (ICSI) treatment. *J Reprod Fertil* 2000; 118: 229-233.

[22] Plachot M. Chromosomal abnormalities in oocytes. *Mol Cell Endocrinol* 2001; 183 Suppl 1: S59-63.

[23] Havelock JC, Rainey WE, Carr BR. Ovarian granulosa cell lines. *Mol Cell Endocrinol* 2004; 228: 67-78.

[24] Wood JR, Strauss JF, 3rd. Multiple signal transduction pathways regulate ovarian steroidogenesis. *Rev Endocr Metab Disord* 2002; 3: 33-46.

[25] Swauger JE, Steichen TJ, Murphy PA, Kinsler S. An analysis of the mainstream smoke chemistry of samples of the U.S. cigarette market acquired between 1995 and 2000. *Regul Toxicol Pharmacol* 2002; 35: 142-156.

[26] Rustemeier K, Stabbert R, Haussmann HJ, Roemer E, Carmines EL. Evaluation of the potential effects of ingredients added to cigarettes. Part 2: chemical composition of mainstream smoke. *Food Chem Toxicol* 2002; 40: 93-104.

[27] Lodovici M, Akpan V, Evangelisti C, Dolara P. Sidestream tobacco smoke as the main predictor of exposure to polycyclic aromatic hydrocarbons. *J Appl Toxicol* 2004; 24: 277-281.

[28] Staessen J, Yeoman WB, Fletcher AE, Markowe HL, Marmot MG, Rose G, Semmence A, Shipley MJ, Bulpitt CJ. Blood cadmium in London civil servants. *Int J Epidemiol* 1990; 19: 362-366.

[29] Varga B, Zsolnai B, Paksy K, Naray M, Ungvary G. Age dependent accumulation of cadmium in the human ovary. *Reprod Toxicol* 1993; 7: 225-228.

[30] Telisman S, Jurasovic J, Pizent A, Cvitkovic P. Cadmium in the blood and seminal fluid of nonoccupationally exposed adult male subjects with regard to smoking habits. *Int Arch Occup Environ Health* 1997; 70: 243-248.

[31] Saaranen M, Kantola M, Saarikoski S, Vanha-Perttula T. Human seminal plasma cadmium: comparison with fertility and smoking habits. *Andrologia* 1989; 21: 140-145.

[32] Smida AD, Valderrama XP, Agostini MC, Furlan MA, Chedrese J. Cadmium stimulates transcription of the cytochrome p450 side chain cleavage gene in genetically modified stable porcine granulosa cells. *Biol Reprod* 2004; 70: 25-31.

[33] Massanyi P, Bardos L, Oppel K, Hluchy S, Kovacik J, Csicsai G, Toman R. Distribution of cadmium in selected organs of mice: effects of cadmium on organ contents of retinoids and beta-carotene. *Acta Physiol Hung* 1999; 86: 99-104.

[34] Kondoh M, Araragi S, Sato K, Higashimoto M, Takiguchi M, Sato M. Cadmium induces apoptosis partly via caspase-9 activation in HL-60 cells. *Toxicology* 2002; 170: 111-117.

[35] Benowitz NL, Kuyt F, Jacob P, 3rd, Jones RT, Osman AL. Cotinine disposition and effects. *Clin Pharmacol Ther* 1983; 34: 604-611.

[36] Weiss T, Eckert A. Cotinine levels in follicular fluid and serum of IVF patients: effect on granulosa-luteal cell function in vitro. *Hum Reprod* 1989; 4: 482-485.

[37] Barbieri RL, McShane PM, Ryan KJ. Constituents of cigarette smoke inhibit human granulosa cell aromatase. *Fertil Steril* 1986; 46: 232-236.

[38] Bodis J, Torok A, Tinneberg HR, Hanf V, Hamori M, Cledon P. Influence of serotonin on progesterone and estradiol secretion of cultured human granulosa cells. *Fertil Steril* 1992; 57: 1008-1011.

[39] Miceli F, Minici F, Tropea A, Catino S, Orlando M, Lamanna G, Sagnella F, Tiberi F, Bompiani A, Mancuso S, Lanzone A, Apa R. Effects of nicotine on human luteal cells in vitro: a possible role on reproductive outcome for smoking women. *Biol Reprod* 2005; 72: 628-632.

[40] Gocze PM, Freeman DA. Cytotoxic effects of cigarette smoke alkaloids inhibit the progesterone production and cell growth of cultured MA-10 Leydig tumor cells. *Eur J Obstet Gynecol Reprod Biol* 2000; 93: 77-83.

[41] Kaiserman MJ, Rickert WS. Carcinogens in tobacco smoke: benzo[a]pyrene from Canadian cigarettes and cigarette tobacco. *Am J Public Health* 1992; 82: 1023-1026.

[42] Mattison DR, Nightingale MS, Shiromizu K. Effects of toxic substances on female reproduction. *Environ Health Perspect* 1983; 48: 43-52.

[43] Mattison DR. Sites of female reproductive vulnerability: implications for testing and risk assessment. *Reprod Toxicol* 1993; 7 Suppl 1: 53-62.

[44] El-Nemr A, Al-Shawaf T, Sabatini L, Wilson C, Lower AM, Grudzinskas JG. Effect of smoking on ovarian reserve and ovarian stimulation in in-vitro fertilization and embryo transfer. *Hum Reprod* 1998; 13: 2192-2198.

[45] Sharara FI, Beatse SN, Leonardi MR, Navot D, Scott RT, Jr. Cigarette smoking accelerates the development of diminished ovarian reserve as evidenced by the clomiphene citrate challenge test. *Fertil Steril* 1994; 62: 257-262.

[46] Weinberg CR, Wilcox AJ, Baird DD. Reduced fecundability in women with prenatal exposure to cigarette smoking. *Am J Epidemiol* 1989; 129: 1072-1078.

[47] Mattison DR, Thomford PJ. The mechanisms of action of reproductive toxicants. *Toxicol Pathol* 1989; 17: 364-376.

[48] Mattison DR, Thorgeirsson SS. Genetic differences in mouse ovarian metabolism of benzo [a]pyrene and oocyte toxicity. *Biochem Pharmacol* 1977; 26: 909-912.

[49] Robles R, Morita Y, Mann KK, Perez GI, Yang S, Matikainen T, Sherr DH, Tilly JL. The aryl hydrocarbon receptor, a basic helix-loop-helix transcription factor of the PAS gene family, is required for normal ovarian germ cell dynamics in the mouse. *Endocrinology* 2000; 141: 450-453.

[50] Tilly JL. Commuting the death sentence: how oocytes strive to survive. *Nat Rev Mol Cell Biol* 2001; 2: 838-848.

[51] Schmidt JV, Bradfield CA. Ah receptor signaling pathways. *Annu Rev Cell Dev Biol* 1996; 12: 55-89.

[52] Vanderhyden BC, Armstrong DT. Role of cumulus cells and serum on the in vitro maturation, fertilization, and subsequent development of rat oocytes. *Biol Reprod* 1989; 40: 720-728.

[53] Ball GD, Leibfried ML, Lenz RW, Ax RL, Bavister BD, First NL. Factors affecting successful in vitro fertilization of bovine follicular oocytes. *Biol Reprod* 1983; 28: 717-725.

[54] Neal MS, YoungLai EV, Holloway AC, Foster WG. Aromatase activity in granulosa cells as a predictor of pregnancy potential. *Int Congress Series* 2004; 1271: 139-142.

[55] Vrsanska S, Nagyova E, Mlynarcikova A, Fickova M, Kolena J. Components of cigarette smoke inhibit expansion of oocyte-cumulus complexes from porcine follicles. *Physiol Res* 2003; 52: 383-387.

[56] Mori K, Noguchi M, Matsuo M, Nomata K, Suematsu T, Kanetake H. Decreased cellular membrane expression of gap junctional protein, connexin 43, in rat detrusor muscle with chronic partial bladder outlet obstruction. *Urology* 2005; 65: 1254-1258.

[57] Atef A, Francois P, Christian V, Marc-Andre S. The potential role of gap junction communication between cumulus cells and bovine oocytes during in vitro maturation. *Mol Reprod Dev* 2005; 71: 358-367.

[58] Pattinson HA, Taylor PJ, Pattinson MH. The effect of cigarette smoking on ovarian function and early pregnancy outcome of in vitro fertilization treatment. *Fertil Steril* 1991; 55: 780-783.

[59] Racowsky C, Kaufman ML. Nuclear degeneration and meiotic aberrations observed in human oocytes matured in vitro: analysis by light microscopy. *Fertil Steril* 1992; 58: 750-755.

[60] Zenzes MT, Bielecki R, Reed TE. Detection of benzo(a)pyrene diol epoxide-DNA adducts in sperm of men exposed to cigarette smoke. *Fertil Steril* 1999; 72: 330-335.

[61] Mooney LA, Santella RM, Covey L, Jeffrey AM, Bigbee W, Randall MC, Cooper TB, Ottman R, Tsai WY, Wazneh L, et al. Decline of DNA damage and other biomarkers in peripheral blood following smoking cessation. *Cancer Epidemiol Biomarkers Prev* 1995; 4: 627-634.

[62] Sbrana I, Puliti A, Seidel A, Glatt H, Turchi G. Induction of chromosomal aberrations and spindle disturbances in Chinese hamster epithelial liver cells in culture by pyrene and benzo[a]pyrene quinones. *Mutagenesis* 1995; 10: 505-512.

[63] Wyrobek AJ. Application of human sperm parameters for monitoring. *Prog Clin Biol Res* 1986; 207: 101-120.

[64] Skakkebaek NE, Keiding N. Changes in semen and the testis. *Bmj* 1994; 309: 1316-1317.

[65] Shiverick KT, Salafia C. Cigarette smoking and pregnancy I: ovarian, uterine and placental effects. *Placenta* 1999; 20: 265-272.

[66] Fraga CG, Motchnik PA, Wyrobek AJ, Rempel DM, Ames BN. Smoking and low antioxidant levels increase oxidative damage to sperm DNA. *Mutat Res* 1996; 351: 199-203.

[67] Shen HM, Chia SE, Ni ZY, New AL, Lee BL, Ong CN. Detection of oxidative DNA damage in human sperm and the association with cigarette smoking. *Reprod Toxicol* 1997; 11: 675-680.

[68] Zenzes MT, Puy LA, Bielecki R, Reed TE. Detection of benzo[a]pyrene diol epoxide-DNA adducts in embryos from smoking couples: evidence for transmission by spermatozoa. *Mol Hum Reprod* 1999; 5: 125-131.

[69] Neri A, Eckerling B. Influence of smoking and adrenaline (epinephrine) on the uterotubal insufflation test (Rubin test). *Fertil Steril* 1969; 20: 818-828.

[70] Neri A, Marcus SL. Effect of nicotine on the motility of the oviducts in the rhesus monkey: a preliminary report. *J Reprod Fertil* 1972; 31: 91-97.

[71] Magers T, Talbot P, DiCarlantonio G, Knoll M, Demers D, Tsai I, Hoodbhoy T. Cigarette smoke inhalation affects the reproductive system of female hamsters. *Reprod Toxicol* 1995; 9: 513-525.

[72] Knoll M, Talbot P. Cigarette smoke inhibits oocyte cumulus complex pick-up by the oviduct in vitro independent of ciliary beat frequency. *Reprod Toxicol* 1998; 12: 57-68.

[73] Baron JA. Beneficial effects of nicotine and cigarette smoking: the real, the possible and the spurious. *Br Med Bull* 1996; 52: 58-73.

[74] Baron JA, La Vecchia C, Levi F. The antiestrogenic effect of cigarette smoking in women. *Am J Obstet Gynecol* 1990; 162: 502-514.

[75] Franks AL, Kendrick JS, Tyler CW, Jr. Postmenopausal smoking, estrogen replacement therapy, and the risk of endometrial cancer. *Am J Obstet Gynecol* 1987; 156: 20-23.

[76] Phipps WR, Cramer DW, Schiff I, Belisle S, Stillman R, Albrecht B, Gibson M, Berger MJ, Wilson E. The association between smoking and female infertility as influenced by cause of the infertility. *Fertil Steril* 1987; 48: 377-382.

[77] Card JP, Mitchell JA. The effects of nicotine administration on deciduoma induction in the rat. *Biol Reprod* 1978; 19: 326-331.

[78] Yoshinaga K, Rice C, Krenn J, Pilot RL. Effects of nicotine on early pregnancy in the rat. *Biol Reprod* 1979; 20: 294-303.

[79] Wang X, Tager IB, Van Vunakis H, Speizer FE, Hanrahan JP. Maternal smoking during pregnancy, urine cotinine concentrations, and birth outcomes. A prospective cohort study. *Int J Epidemiol* 1997; 26: 978-988.

[80] Bernstein L, Pike MC, Lobo RA, Depue RH, Ross RK, Henderson BE. Cigarette smoking in pregnancy results in marked decrease in maternal hCG and oestradiol levels. *Br J Obstet Gynaecol* 1989; 96: 92-96.

[81] Barbieri RL, Gochberg J, Ryan KJ. Nicotine, cotinine, and anabasine inhibit aromatase in human trophoblast in vitro. *J Clin Invest* 1986; 77: 1727-1733.

[82] Kitawaki J, Inoue S, Tamura T, Yamamoto T, Honjo H, Higashiyama T, Osawa Y, Okada H. Cigarette smoking during pregnancy lowers aromatase cytochrome P-450 in the human placenta. *J Steroid Biochem Mol Biol* 1993; 45: 485-491.

[83] Wier PJ, Miller RK, Maulik D, DiSant'Agnese PA. Toxicity of cadmium in the perfused human placenta. *Toxicol Appl Pharmacol* 1990; 105: 156-171.

[84] Powlin SS, Keng PC, Miller RK. Toxicity of cadmium in human trophoblast cells (JAr choriocarcinoma): role of calmodulin and the calmodulin inhibitor, zaldaride maleate. *Toxicol Appl Pharmacol* 1997; 144: 225-234.

[85] Guyda HJ, Mathieu L, Lai W, Manchester D, Wang SL, Ogilvie S, Shiverick KT. Benzo(a)pyrene inhibits epidermal growth factor binding and receptor autophosphorylation in human placental cell cultures. *Mol Pharmacol* 1990; 37: 137-143.

[86] Zhang L, Connor EE, Chegini N, Shiverick KT. Modulation by benzo[a]pyrene of epidermal growth factor receptors, cell proliferation, and secretion of human chorionic gonadotropin in human placental cell lines. *Biochem Pharmacol* 1995; 50: 1171-1180.

[87] Zhang L, Shiverick KT. Benzo(a)pyrene, but not 2,3,7,8-tetrachlorodibenzo-p-dioxin, alters cell proliferation and c-myc and growth factor expression in human placental choriocarcinoma JEG-3 cells. *Biochem Biophys Res Commun* 1997; 231: 117-120.

In: Smoking and Health Research Frontiers
Editor: Calvin B. Fong, pp. 81-96

ISBN 1-60021-480-0

Chapter IV

Cardiovascular Effects of Passive Smoking in Adults and Children

Judith A. Groner*, Mandar Joshi, Hong Huang and John A. Bauer

The Ohio State University Department of Pediatrics Investigator, Center for Cardiovascular Medicine, The Columbus Children's Research Institute, Columbus Children's Hospital, 700 Children's Drive Columbus, Ohio 43205.

Abstract

Multiple sources of evidence have linked secondhand smoke to cardiovascular disease (CVD) in adults. While the prevalence of this exposure has decreased in the past 20 years, a substantial proportion of the population (43%) still remains exposed. The relative risk of CVD in passive smokers is approximately 1.25 when controlled for confounding variables. Potential mechanisms appear to be oxidant gas exposure, which leads to endothelial dysfunction, resulting in multiple abnormalities of the vascular system (arterial thickening, and the pro-inflammatory, pro-thrombotic, and pro-atherogenic state). Additional mechanisms accounting for the causal relationship between secondhand smoke exposure and CVD include mitochondrial damage leading to energy perturbations and alterations in autonomic function, leading to decreased heart rate variability, a risk factor for higher mortality rates in patients with chronic heart failure. Children are at high risk due to home exposure, but there is has been limited research in this area, with most research on the effects of tobacco smoke exposure in childhood focusing on the respiratory system. Non-invasive diagnostic research tools will be useful in determining the effects of tobacco smoke exposure during childhood on the developing cardiovascular system.

* Correspondence concerning this article should be addressed to Judith A. Groner, MD, Clinical Professor of Pediatrics, The Ohio State University Department of Pediatrics Investigator, Center for Cardiovascular Medicine, The Columbus Children's Research Institute, Columbus Children's Hospital, 700 Children's Drive Columbus, Ohio 43205. Phone: 614-722-4957; Fax: 614-722-4966; e-mail: *jgroner@chi.osu.edu*.

INTRODUCTION

The response of the cardiovascular system in adults to environmental tobacco smoke exposure has been well documented. Between 30,000 to 60,000 deaths in the U.S. from CVD per year in non-smokers have been attributed to secondhand smoke [1]. The 2006 Surgeon General's Report stated that evidence is sufficient to infer a "causal relationship between exposure to secondhand smoke and increased risks of coronary heart disease morbidity and mortality among both men and women" [2]. The Report additionally noted that there is no risk-free level of exposure to secondhand smoke. The purpose of this review is to summarize the significance of passive smoke in relation to CVD, describe potential mechanisms of increased cardiovascular risk with passive smoke exposure, and discuss unique aspects of these phenomena as they relate to children.

PREVALENCE OF PASSIVE SMOKE EXPOSURE IN ADULTS AND CHILDREN

Although there has been a recent decrease in the prevalence of passive smoking, a substantial proportion of both adults and children in the United States continue to be exposed to tobacco smoke. Since 1988, researchers have used serum cotinine measurements to assess exposures to secondhand smoke within the NHANES (National Health and Nutrition Examination Survey), which is designed to examine a nationally representatives sample of the U.S. civilian population. The percent of people over four years old who were exposed to tobacco smoke (defined by detectable serum cotinine levels greater than 0.050 ng/ml) dropped from 88% in the 1991-1994 survey to 43% in the 2001-2002 survey [3]. Overall, between 1988 – 2002, a substantial decrease in mean serum cotinine in the population has been noted (approximately 70%), most likely due to smoking bans required in public places and voluntary bans in the home. However, in absolute numbers, many American non-smokers are still exposed to tobacco smoke. Based on the NHANES data, in 2002 over 86 million non-smoking adults aged 20, over 18 million nonsmoking youth aged 12-19 years, and over 22 million children from 3 -11 years were exposed to secondhand smoke [2].

Approximately 25% of U.S. children are exposed to tobacco smoke, with higher prevalence rates (30%–70%) among children from low-income families. According to the most recent NHANES survey, mean serum cotinine is higher in children between 4-11 years than in adolescents or adults [3]. Cotinine levels representing the 95% in adults have dropped about 40% over the past 14 years, but there has been no change in the 95% level among children or adolescents [3]. This means that there continues to be a group of highly exposed children regardless of the decreased exposure of the rest of the population. The home is the site of the most significant tobacco smoke exposure for children [4,5]. While home exposure has decreased between 1992 and 2000 from 36% to 25%, this change has been more marked in families with higher parental education and income [6]. Secondhand smoke exposure, along with smoking prevalence, varies inversely with family income, maternal and paternal education [6]. Biochemically verified (urinary cotinine) rates as high as 79% have been reported in high risk urban low income neighborhoods [7].

Worldwide, tobacco smoke exposure is increasing in the developing world as more adults, particularly men, are becoming smokers. In China, a recent survey revealed that over 60% of men and 7% of women were smokers, and that over 100 million women who were non-smokers were exposed in the home to tobacco smoke [8,9]. The massive exposure to tobacco smoke is likely to cause widespread cardiovascular morbidity and mortality in the coming years.

Components of Passive Smoke

Tobacco smoke is composed of sidestream smoke from burning cigarettes (85%) and exhaled mainstream smoke (15%) [9]. Sidestream smoke is emitted off the end of a burning cigarette between puffs; mainstream smoke is first inhaled by an active smoker and then exhaled [9]. The chemical composition of mainstream smoke has been more extensively characterized than that of sidestream smoke. Over 4,000 individual constituents have been identified in mainstream smoke, and approximately 400 compounds have been measured quantitatively in both. Constituents of both components include eye and respiratory irritants, systemic toxicants, mutagens, and carcinogens [10] but sidestream smoke contains a relatively higher concentration of the toxic gaseous component than mainstream smoke [11].

Evidence Linking Secondhand Smoke to Cardiovascular Disease

Evidence supporting the causal relationship between passive smoking in non-smokers and the development of CVD comes from a variety of sources - epidemiological studies, animal models, and non-invasive assessments of cardiovascular function in humans. The epidemiological evidence includes both cohort and case/control studies; non-invasive assessment includes imaging of arterial thickness and vascular reactivity along with determinations of plasma markers of the pro-inflammatory and pro-thrombotic states such as C-reactive protein, fibrinogen, and homocysteine. All of these diverse sources of evidence demonstrate a consistent relationship between passive smoking and cardiovascular risk.

Epidemiological Data on Passive Smoking and Cardiovascular Risk in Adults

Both longitudinal cohort and case/control studies, performed over the last 25 years in multiple settings and countries support the fact that passive exposure to tobacco smoke is a known risk factor for the development of adult CVD. Estimates of excessive risk of CVD for tobacco smoke exposed non-smokers range from 25%-30% [2] Based on a meta-analysis of

18 epidemiological studies of CVD risk and secondhand smoke exposure in adults, including only studies which controlled for potential confounding factors, He and colleagues reported that the relative risk of atherosclerotic heart disease in exposed non-smokers was 1.25 [12]. An updated meta-analysis of 16 epidemiological studies (nine cohort and seven case-control) published subsequent to this analysis was included in the 2006 Surgeon General's Report [2]; this analysis showed a similar relative risk of 1.27.

Other researchers have found greater risk for acute cardiac events. In the CARDIO 2000 Study, the relative risk of developing acute cardiac syndrome was found to be increased by 50% among tobacco smoke exposed non-smokers [13]. The authors estimated that 34 coronary events per 134 subjects would occur as a result of passive smoke exposure during their lifetime. In a "natural observational experiment" in Billings Montana, while a smoking ban was enforced in all public places, hospital admissions for myocardial infarctions decreased by nearly 50% and returned to baseline when the ban was repealed [14]. A recent case control study [15] examining the relationship of all types of tobacco exposure (active smoking, past smoking, secondhand smoke exposure, and chewing tobacco) and acute non-fatal myocardial infarction (MI) showed that secondhand smoke exposure was associated with a graded increase in risk related to exposure. The odds ratio of acute MI was 1.24 in those exposed the least (1-7 hours per week) and increased to 1.62 in those who were most exposed (>21 hours per week).

Methodological Issues in Epidemiological Studies

Bias may be introduced into epidemiological research in this area due to two main methodological "threats" - the presence of uncontrolled confounding factors associated with both passive smoke exposure and CVD, and the misclassification of tobacco smoke exposure. People who are exposed to tobacco smoke may also eat unhealthy diets, exercise less, and in general lead a less heart-healthy life than those unexposed to tobacco smoke, leading to a misattribution of their cardiac risk to the tobacco exposure rather than other lifestyle issues. Indeed, there have been several studies which have shown that women exposed to smoke from their spouses more likely than other women to be less educated, report more alcohol consumption eat more fried foods, be more overweight, and eat fewer fruits and salads [16,17]. However, other studies [18], using a large 1988-1992 NHANES III data set, did not find baseline differences between secondhand smoke exposed and unexposed groups in thirteen potential cardiovascular risk factors after adjustment for age, gender, race and education. Other investigators have described a modest attenuation in relative risk of CVD in studies which controlled for potential confounding cardiovascular risk factors. For example, in the Nurses Health Study, the relative risk of CVD attributed to secondhand smoke exposure was 1.97. After controlling for a wide range of multiple confounders, including BMI, alcohol consumption, physical activity, and hypertension, this risk diminished only slightly to 1.71 [19]. Steenland and colleagues [18] described the same minor attenuation of relative risk from 1.31 to 1.19 in men and 1.25 to 1.23 in women. It is therefore accepted that while controlling for potential confounders may slightly decrease the relative risk of CVD, this procedure by no means diminishes the relative risk entirely.

The second methodological issue is potential bias which is due to misclassification of secondhand smoke exposure. In case control studies, non-smokers who develop heart disease may selectively recall their exposure to secondhand smoke while control non-smokers may not. In their meta-analysis [12], He and colleagues reported a higher pooled odds ratio in eight case control studies (1.51) compared to the pooled relative risk of 1.21 in ten pooled cohort studies. However, even if this difference is due to recall bias, it would not account for the elevated relative risk in the pooled cohort studies.

Conversely, epidemiological research may actually underestimate the cardiovascular risk of tobacco smoke exposure for non-smokers [20]. This has occurred because the research definition for a "secondhand smoke exposed non-smoker" was marriage to a smoker. This definition did not capture other possible tobacco smoke exposures, including the workplace and public places such as restaurants or bars. As a result, in epidemiologic research, relatively more exposed people were compared to relatively less exposed people, but not to those without any exposure at all. This would bias the epidemiological data toward the null hypothesis. This concept was confirmed by Whincup and colleagues who reported on a 20 year prospective study of tobacco smoke and CVD using serum cotinine as an objective marker of exposure. Non-smokers with the highest quartile of cotinine concentration were found to have 50%-60% increased risk of CVD [21].

Potential Mechanisms for Observed Association Between Secondhand Smoke and CVD

While secondhand-exposed non-smokers have a considerable risk of CVD, their exposure to tobacco smoke is less than 1% of the exposure of an active smoker of 20 cigarettes per day [22]. Some researchers have noted that unlike lung cancer, the risk of acute myocardial infarction and CVD with tobacco smoke exposure is non-linear, increasing rapidly even with the relatively small exposures in the environment. This finding is similar to the relatively high cardiovascular risk of individuals who smoke only one or two cigarettes per day [23]. On the other hand, other investigators [15] have described a dose-response relationship with increasing cardiovascular risk noted with increased secondhand smoke exposure. However, the fact remains that cardiovascular risk for secondhand smoke exposed non-smokers is surprisingly high considering their low levels of exposure compared to active smokers and warrants explanation.

Effects of Secondhand Smoke on the Cellular Level

There have been multiple effects noted at the cellular level which affect the cardiovascular system due to secondhand smoke exposure (Table 1). Potential agents include carbon monoxide, nicotine, polycyclic aromatic hydrocarbons, reactive oxygen products, and particulate matter. Blood levels of nicotine and carbon monoxide are low in tobacco smoke exposed non-smokers, so it is unlikely that these substances are significant factors in causing

CVD [22]. The most likely cause of the increased cardiac risk among non-smokers exposed to tobacco smoke appears to be exposure to reactive oxygen species [22], which can be significant with secondhand smoke [22,24]. Cigarette smoking is an abundant source of free radicals [24]. Oxidant stress, causing endothelial dysfunction, is likely to be the pathway linking secondhand smoke exposure with cardiovascular morbidity and mortality (Figure 1). The linkage between oxidative stress, endothelial dysfunction, and the various abnormalities observed in secondhand smoke exposure (arterial thickening, pro-inflammatory, thombotic and atherogenic states) is both biologically plausible and explains why low levels of exposure can cause significant cardiovascular damage, corresponding to the epidemiologic evidence of higher than expected risk due to the exposure.

Table 1. Direct effects of secondhand smoke components on the cardiovascular system.

Tobacco components	**Signaling/Mechanisms**	**Cellular Events**	**Clinical Outcomes**
Carbon monoxide	$\downarrow$ O_2 supply by $\uparrow$carboxyhemoglobin	Platelet adhesion and aggregation	Coronary ischemia Coronary thrombosis Acute myocardial infarction
Nicotine	Release of catecholamines	Platelet aggregation Vasoconstriction	
Polycyclic aromatic hydrocarbons (PAHs)	DNA damage Oncogene activation	Endothelial injury SMC proliferation	Atherosclerosis
Reactive oxygen products	Inflammatory responses Inactivation of nitric oxide Oxidation of lipoproteins	Endothelial injury/activation EC-leukocyte interaction Endothelial dysfunction Foam cell formation	Atherosclerosis
Particulate matter	Systemic inflammation Modulation of the autonomic function	EC injury, activation, and dysfunction	Ischemic heart disease Heart failure Cardiac arrest

Other Effects on the Cellular Level - Mitochondrial Damage and Energy Perturbations

Another cellular global effect of secondhand smoke is inhibition of energy production by the mitochondria. Animal studies have shown that secondhand smoke impairs the ability of the heart muscle to convert oxygen into ATP [25,26]. Researchers have described a time-dependent decrease in the enzymatic activity of cytochrome oxidase after exposure to secondhand smoke [27]. There is also evidence for reduced antioxidant activity in mitochondria exposed to secondhand smoke [28]. In addition, exposure resulted in higher levels of aortic mitochondrial DNA (mtDNA) damage compared with unexposed mice. Increased duration of exposure resulted in even higher levels of mtDNA damage, and high cholesterol accentuated the effects of secondhand smoke [28].

These alterations in the mitochondrial function may affect the energy utilization by the cardiac muscle. The insufficient energy production may also lead to a metabolic switch to anaerobic respiration by cardiac myocytes, leading to increased intracellular lactate levels. This can cause a perturbation in the energy utilization by the myocytes. This imbalance in the cardiac energy management after exposure to secondhand smoke may lead to increased cardiac work and ultimately lead to heart failure.

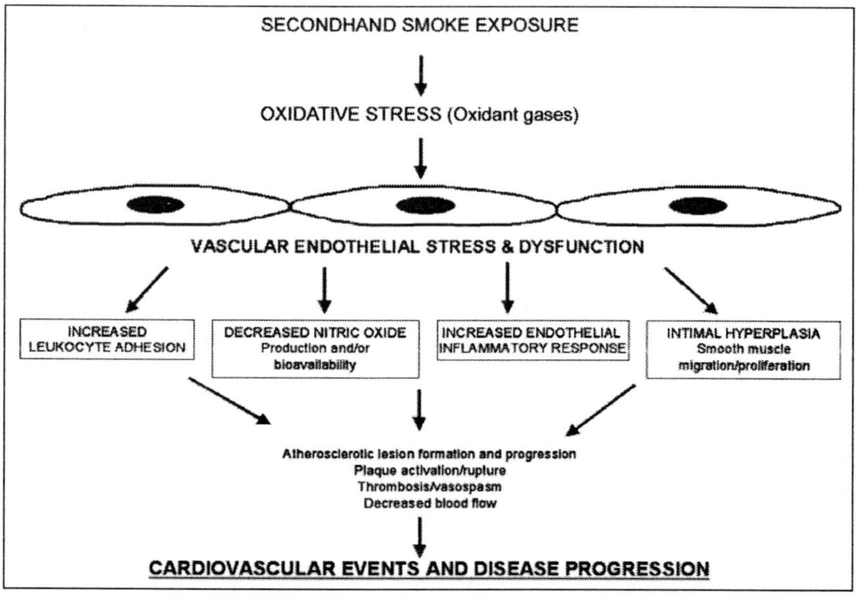

Figure 1. Hypothesized mechanism for causal relationship between secondhand smoke and cardiovascular disease.

ENDOTHELIAL DYSFUNCTION

Endothelial dysfunction appears to be the key feature which links tobacco smoke exposure to cardiovascular disease. Studies in humans suggest that the endothelium plays a key role in vascular health and that endothelial dysfunction is directly involved in secondhand smoke induced cardiovascular damage. Far from being inert, endothelial cells regulate thrombosis, leukocyte interactions and adhesion, and modulate vasodilation or vasoconstriction via release of nitric oxide (NO), prostacyclin and endothelin [29,30]. An essential component of normal endothelial cell function is the production of NO via metabolism of arginine which provides local modulation of vascular tone and inhibits blood cell adhesion. An impaired capacity of the endothelium dependent and NO-mediated relaxant response has been observed in a wide variety of patients with vascular risk factors, including diabetes, smoking history, male gender, elevated cholesterol, and family history of cardiovascular disease. Thus it appears that the phenomenon of early endothelial cell dysfunction is a common and unifying feature of vascular disease development. In the particular case of secondhand smoke induced CVD, oxidative stress plays a key role; superoxide inactivates NO, and thereby produces endothelial dysfunction [31].

Animal models support the link between exposure to tobacco smoke, endothelial dysfunction, and abnormal vasoconstrictor activity. Using a rat model of acute myocardial ischemia and reperfusion, Zhu and colleagues [32] demonstrated that rats exposed to tobacco smoke in exposure chambers during the neonatal to adolescent period had significantly larger infarct sizes than unexposed rats. Levels of endothelin-1 (a potent vasoconstrictor) were significantly increased among exposed rats. The microenvironment for the exposed rats was composed of fresh and aged sidestream smoke and was equivalent to four passengers in a car smoking four cigarettes per hour. Hutchison and colleagues reported abnormally increased vasoconstrictor sensitivity in response to phenylephrine among rats exposed to smoke in the early neonatal period as compared with unexposed rats [33]. Similar findings were reported by Torok and colleagues [34] using the adult rabbit model. Rabbits that were exposed to three weeks of secondhand smoke showed impaired endothelium-dependent relaxation induced by acetylcholine in the carotid artery and the thoracic aorta as compared with unexposed rabbits. In 1997 Hutchison and colleagues [35] demonstrated endothelial dysfunction in healthy rats exposed to smoke for 10 weeks; by administering l-arginine, a substrate for nitric oxide synthase (NOS), this effect was blocked.

Physiologic Changes: Flow- Mediated Dilation

Noninvasive ultrasound measurements of flow-mediated dilation (FMD) have been extensively used as a method to assess endothelial functional integrity. The physiological principle underlying this test is a phenomenon known as shear-stress induced vasorelaxation. This response is known to be endothelium mediated and governed by the endothelium mono-layer's ability to produce NO (via shear stress activation of the endothelial isoform of NOS). In 1996, Celermajer and colleagues reported that FMD was impaired among healthy subjects ages 15-30 years who were exposed to tobacco smoke for at least one hour per day, as compared to controls who were non-exposed non-smokers [36]. Passive smokers were no different from active smokers in the degree of impairment in the FMD response detected. The FMD response was inversely related to the intensity of tobacco smoke exposure as measured by structured questionnaire. Nitroglycerin-induced FMD was no different in the three groups. This is significant because nitroglycerin-induced vasodilation is not mediated by NO. In 1999 Raitakari and colleagues [37] showed that endothelial dysfunction among tobacco smoke exposed non-smokers may be potentially reversible. Former passive smokers had FMD function that was higher than current passive smokers, but not as high as never exposed non-smokers. This link between passive smoking and endothelial dysfunction is suggestive of a causative role for passive smoke in the early stages of atherogenesis.

ANATOMIC CHANGES: INTIMA-MEDIAL THICKENING

Dysfunction of the endothelium over time leads to measurable thickening of the intima and media of the vessel wall of large and medium sized muscular arteries and large elastic arteries such as the aorta, carotid and iliac arteries [38]. This thickening is the earliest anatomical change of atherosclerosis. These changes are known as intima-medial thickening (IMT) and can be imaged by B-mode, high resolution ultrasound. IMT, which precedes clinical cardiovascular events by decades, is considered a marker of generalized atherosclerosis in adults [39]. Carotid IMT in adults is associated with arteriographically documented lesions and subsequent myocardial infarction and stroke, and also with the presence of known cardiovascular risk factors such as diabetes and obesity [40].

In a landmark study, Howard & Wagenknecht and colleagues demonstrated the adverse effects of passive tobacco smoke exposure on the progression of atherosclerosis as indicated by intimal thickening [41]. Over 10,000 adults between 45 and 64 years had common carotid arterial IMT measured at baseline and then three years later. After adjustment for demographic variables, other cardiovascular risk factors and lifestyle variables, a consistent relationship between passive tobacco smoke exposure and progression of atherosclerosis was noted. Secondhand smoke exposure was estimated to be associated with an increase of approximately 20% or 5.9 micrometers over three years [41]. The difference in progression between those least exposed to smoke (never smokers who were never exposed to tobacco smoke) and those most exposed (current smokers) was 17.1 micrometers per 3 years. Therefore, the impact of tobacco smoke exposure was 34% (5.9/17.1), as great as the impact of active smoking on the progression of IMT [41].

PRO-INFLAMMATORY CHANGES

Endothelial dysfunction was initially identified as impaired vasodilation to specific stimuli, but recent investigations have broadened the term to include not only reduced vasodilation, but also a pro-inflammatory and pro-thrombotic state. In the past several years, the role of inflammation in the development of CVD has been appreciated, and resultant processes leading to increased cellular oxidation have been implicated [42]. The presence of cytokines and inflammatory factors such as C-reactive protein (CRP) induce important phenotypic changes in the endothelium, including a decrease in the production and/or biological activity of endothelium-derived NO (eNO). Decreased NO activity promotes leukocyte adhesion, thrombosis, vasoconstriction, and cellular proliferation and thus plays a role in endothelial dysfunction [43, 44].

Tobacco smoke exposure has been linked with increased inflammatory markers. Panagiotakis and colleagues demonstrated [45] that tobacco smoke exposed adult non-smokers had higher levels of inflammatory markers than non-exposed non-smokers. Non-smokers exposed to tobacco smoke more than three days per week had higher WBC counts, homocysteine and fibrinogen, even after adjusting for age, gender, physical activity status, BMI, and food consumption. The level of inflammatory markers was positively and consistently associated with years of tobacco exposure. This effect was as high as that of current smokers, and showed a significant dose-response relationship when evaluating years of exposure. The mechanism for observed tobacco smoke-related cardiovascular effects may therefore be mediated at least partially through chronic inflammation.

Pro-Atherogenic Changes

Oxidation of LDL has been recognized to confer many pro-atherogenic properties to lipoproteins in vitro [24] by enhancing its penetration into arterial intima, binding to intimal cells, and increasing uptake by macrophages. Tobacco smoke exposure has been associated with increased LDL oxidation in vivo [45], after controlling for multiple potential confounders. The effects of secondhand smoke exposure were similar to the effects of current active smoking in terms of LDL oxidation. Additionally, an animal model also suggests the existence of a relationship between tobacco smoke exposure and LDL accumulation in the arterial wall. Using a rat model, Roberts and colleagues [46] reported that after a single exposure to tobacco smoke, LDL accumulation in the carotid artery wall increased significantly

HDL is thought to play a critical role in preventing atherosclerosis and reduce the risk of CVD [47,48]. It mediates cholesterol efflux from macrophage cells, inhibits foam cell formation, restores and protects from endothelial dysfunction, and prevents the oxidation of LDL. Many clinical reports demonstrate that exposure to secondhand smoke has been consistently linked with lower levels of HDL in adults. After an acute 6 hour exposure to tobacco smoke, male non-smokers showed an acute reduction in HDL, which was sustained 24-hours post exposure [49]. In a larger epidemiological study from Japan, investigators reported on data from over 3000 non-smokers from 27 offices with few smoking restrictions. After adjusting for multiple confounders, they found an inverse linear relationship between workplace tobacco exposure and HDL levels, more strikingly in women [50].

Pro-Thrombotic Changes

The initial evidence explaining the association between tobacco smoke exposure and cardiovascular disease came from studies on platelet activity. Secondhand smoke activates blood platelets, increasing the risk of thrombus formation. Over 20 years ago, Burghuber & colleagues [51] reported that 20 minutes of exposure to tobacco smoke in non-smokers activated platelets to the extent that their platelet activity was not discernible from that of the active smokers. In an in vitro experiment, researchers [52] exposed human platelets to both sidestream and mainstream smoke extract from one cigarette. Platelet activation was evaluated under static and flow conditions, since blood flow increases platelet activation. Under both conditions, sidestream smoke was about 1 ½ times more potent than mainstream smoke in activating platelets.

Other substances involved in platelet activity are also increased are increased after exposure to tobacco smoke. Thromboxane, a marker of platelet activation, is increased in passive smokers, almost to the level of active smokers after repeated exposure [53].

Fibrinogen, a mediator of platelet activation is chronically elevated in non-smokers exposed to tobacco smoke. This has been demonstrated in both adults and adolescents [54,55].

Additional Mechanisms - Arrhythmias and Heart Rate Variability

Decreased heart rate variability has been demonstrated to be an independent predictor of death in patients with congestive heart failure [56]. Secondhand smoke is known to stimulate sympathetic nervous activity (measured as muscle sympathetic nerve activity) and to inhibit vagal efferents to the heart [57]. Nicotine may partly be responsible for these effects. These alterations in the autonomic nervous function result in a decreased heart rate variability (the beat-to-beat variations in heart rate reflected in the R-R interval variation in the ECG) in passive smokers. Decreased heart rate variability is a predictor of ventricular arrhythmias and cardiac death and has been linked to an increased risk of ventricular fibrillation or ventricular tachycardia in patients after a myocardial infarction or in those with chronic heart failure.

Multiple Mechanisms Link Secondhand Smoke Exposure and CVD in Adults

Thus, secondhand smoke exposure leads to atherosclerosis through multiple mechanisms, including abnormal lipid profile (low HDL and high LDL), endothelial dysfunction, the pro-inflammatory and pro-thrombotic states – leading to stenosis of coronary arteries, and plaque instability [57]. Myocardial infarction is usually precipitated as a result of vascular stenosis and or the development of an atherosclerotic plaque. As a consequence of MI, the left ventricle undergoes remodeling resulting in ventricular dysfunction. Some of the known physiological changes in vascular thickness and reactivity in individuals exposed to secondhand smoke enhance their susceptibility to increased risk for a secondary MI. Moreover, after the infarction has occurred, secondhand smoke renders the myocardium more susceptible to a larger area of infarction and greater risk of ventricular hypertrophy. These physiological effects of secondhand smoke increase the risk of secondary events or lead to heart failure.

Special Issues in the Pediatric Population

Children bear a heavy burden of tobacco smoke exposure. In fact, mean serum cotinine is higher in children ages 4-11 than in adolescents or adults [3] according to NHANES data. Unlike adults, young children cannot exert control over their own home environments. Our research has shown that children younger than three years old and living with mothers who smoke, are in fact 'smoking cigarettes' via inhalation of secondhand smoke in their immediate environment. Their hair cotinine levels, which measure long-term exposure to tobacco, are essentially the same as their mothers' levels [58]. We hypothesized that our findings were due to higher respiratory rates of young children leading to greater respiratory exposure, deposition, and absorption of tobacco smoke. Current research on childhood morbidity related to tobacco smoke exposure has focused primarily on the respiratory system because this is where the symptoms from their exposure are seen clinically. Since children do not show obvious signs and symptoms of acquired cardiovascular disease during childhood, there has been limited research in this area. The atherosclerotic process develops silently for decades during childhood and adolescence, before cardiovascular complications such as myocardial infarction and stroke occur in adulthood. Therefore, when investigating childhood antecedents of adult cardiovascular disease, it is important to determine the effects of tobacco smoke exposure on the cardiovascular system of children.

The research reported to date in cardiovascular risk to children and adolescents exposed to tobacco smoke has focused on the association between exposure and lower HDL levels. In 1990, Moskowitz and colleagues reported that preadolescent children who were exposed to tobacco smoke had lower HDL levels then unexposed children, after adjustment for age, weight, height and gender [59]. Later Moskowitz reported that this relationship persisted when examining the same cohort of children during their adolescence [60]. Another research group reported that adolescents exposed to tobacco smoke, confirmed by serum cotinine levels, had decreased HDL levels (between 7%-9%) than unexposed teens, even when controlled for potential confounders (BMI and triglyceride level) [61]. Other investigators reported on the association between low HDL levels and tobacco smoke exposure among a group of children ages 2-18 years old who were referred to a tertiary hyperlipidemia clinic. After adjustment for BMI, age, sex, exercise, and dietary fat intake, passive smoking remained a significant risk factor for decreased HDL [62].

A significant proportion of children in the United States are still exposed to tobacco smoke in the home. Non-invasive imaging, in particular IMT and FMD, which has been used in adults to assess cardiovascular risk, has great potential for application to address this issue during childhood and adolescents. FMD and IMT have been used extensively in pediatric research to examine relationships between obesity, exercise, inflammation, diabetes, and cardiovascular risk [63]. Similarly, plasma markers of the pro-thombotic and pro-atherogenic state such as CRP are easy to obtain in children and have been studied in other conditions which are associated with adult CVD [63]. These tools can be applied to investigate the relationships between childhood exposure to tobacco smoke and cardiovascular risk.

Conclusion

There is sufficient evidence from decades of epidemiological, animal model, laboratory, and clinical human research to state that secondhand smoke exposure in non-smokers causes CVD in adult men and women. The relative risk of CVD, based on epidemiological data, is approximately 1.25, after adjustment for potential confounders. Endothelial dysfunction, most likely caused by oxidant gas exposure from the burning cigarette, appears to be the key feature which links tobacco smoke exposure to CVD. Dysfunctional endothelium results in multiple abnormalities of the vascular system including arterial thickening, and the pro-inflammatory, pro-atherogenic, and pro- thrombotic states. Since levels of oxidizing gases are high even in secondhand smoke exposure, the linkage between oxidative damage to the endothelium from exposure is both biologically plausible and explains why low levels of exposure can cause significant cardiovascular damage, corresponding to the epidemiologic evidence. Additional mechanisms accounting for the causal relationship between secondhand smoke exposure and CVD include mitochondrial damage leading to energy perturbations and alterations in autonomic function leading to decreased heart rate variability, a risk factor for cardiovascular complications and death.

While these changes are well described in adults, children remain a special population. Some children remain highly exposed to tobacco smoke and are not able to control their home environments to decrease their own exposure. Because cardiovascular changes do not clinically manifest until many decades later, there has been little research in children on the effects of secondhand smoke exposure to their developing cardiovascular system. Non-invasive cardiovascular measures which have been used to study other clinical issues during childhood can be applied to determine the effects of secondhand smoke exposure for children.

REFERENCES

[1] Puranik R and Celermajer D. Smoking and endothelial function. *Progress in Cardiovascular Diseases.* 2003;45(6):443-58

[2] U.S. Department of Health and Human Services. *The health consequences of involuntary exposure to tobacco smoke: A report of the Surgeon General.* Atlanta, GA: U.S. Department of Health and Human Services, Centers of Disease Control and Prevention, Coordinating Center for Health Promotion, National Center for Chronic Disease Prevention and Health Promotion, Office on Smoking and Health, 2006

[3] Pirkle J, et al. Trends in the exposure of non-smokers in the U.S. population to secondhand smoke: 1988-2002. *Environmental Health Perspectives.* 2006;114(6):853-8

[4] Okah FA, et al. Effect of children on home smoking restriction by inner-city smokers. *Pediatrics.* 2002;244-9

[5] Pirkle, JL, et al. Exposure of the US population to environmental tobacco smoke: the Third National Health and Nutrition Examination Survey, 1988 to 1991. *Journal of the American Medical Association.* 1996;1233-40

[6] Soliman S, Pollack HA, and Warner KE. Decrease in the prevalence of environmental tobacco smoke exposure in the home during the 1990s in families with children. *American Journal of Public Health.* 2004;314-20

[7] Cornelius MD, Goldschmidt L, and Dempsey DA. Environmental tobacco smoke exposure in low-income 6-year-olds: Parent report and urine cotinine measures. *Nicotine & Tobacco Research.* 2003;5(3):333-9

[8] Gu D, et al. Cigarette smoking and exposure to environmental tobacco smoke in China: the international collaborative study of cardiovascular disease in Asia. *American Journal of Public Health.* 2004;1972-6

[9] Witschi H, Joad JP, and Pinkerton KE. The toxicology of environmental tobacco smoke. *Annual Review of Pharmacology and Toxicology* 1997; 37:29-52

[10] National Cancer Institute. *Health effects of exposure to environmental tobacco smoke: The Report of the California Environmental Protection Agency*. Bethesda, MD:1999

[11] Glantz SA and Parmley WW. Passive smoking and heart disease. *Epidemiology, Physiology and Biochemistry.* 1991;83:1-12

[12] He J, et al. Passive smoking and the risk of coronary heart disease -- A meta-analysis of epidemiologic studies. *New England Journal of Medicine.* 1999;340(12):920-6

[13] Pitsavos C, et al. Association between passive cigarette smoking and the risk of developing acute coronary syndromes: the CARDIO 2000 study. *Heart and Vessels.* 2002;16(4):127-30

[14] Sargent RP, Shepard RM, and Glantz SA. Reduced incidence of admissions for myocardial infarction associated with public smoking ban: before and after study. *British Medical Journal.* 2004;328(7446):977-80

[15] Teo KK, et al. Tobacco use and risk of myocardial infarction in 52 countries in the INTERHEART study: a case-control study. *Lancet.* 2006;647-58

[16] Matanoski G, et al. Characteristics of nonsmoking women in NHANES I and NHANES I epidemiologic follow-up study with exposure to spouses who smoke. *American Journal of Epidemiology.* 1995;142 (2):149-57

[17] Thornton A, Lee P, and Fry J. Differences between smokers, ex-smokers, passive smokers and non-smokers. *Journal of Clinical Epidemiology.* 1994;47(10):1143-62

[18] Steenland K, et al. Environmental tobacco smoke and coronary heart disease in the American Cancer Society CPS-II Cohort. *Circulation.* 1996; 94(4):622-8

[19] Kawachi I, et al. A prospective study of passive smoking and coronary heart disease. *Circulation.* 1997;95(10):2374-9

[20] Barnoya J and Glantz SA. Cardiovascular effects of secondhand smoke: nearly as large as smoking. *Circulation.* 2005;111(20):2684-98

[21] Whincup PH, et al. Passive smoking and risk of coronary heart disease and stroke: prospective study with cotinine measurement. *British Medical Journal* 2004;329(7459):200-5

[22] Benowitz N. Cigarette smoking and cardiovascular disease: pathophysiology and implications for treatment. *Progress in Cardiovascular Diseases.* 2003; 46(1):91-111

[23] Law M. and Wald N. Environmental tobacco smoke and ischemic heart disease. *Progress in Cardiovascular Diseases.* 2003;46(1):31-8

[24] Burke A. and Fitzgerald GA. Oxidative stress and smoking-induced vascular injury. *Progress in Cardiovascular Diseases.* 2003;46(1):79-90

[25] Ambrose JA and Barua R S. The pathophysiology of cigarette smoking and cardiovascular disease: An update. *Journal of the American College of Cardiology.* 2004;43(10):1731-7

[26] Glantz, S. and Parmley W. Passive smoking and heart disease. Mechanisms and risk. *Journal of the American Medical Association.* 1995;273(13):1047-53

[27] Gvozdjak, J, et al. The effect of smoking on myocardial metabolism. *Czech Med,* 1987;10(1):47-53

[28] Knight-Lozano CA, et al. Cigarette smoke exposure and hypercholesterolemia increase mitochondrial damage in cardiovascular tissues. *Circulation.* 2002;849-54

[29] Landmesser U, Hornig B, and Drexler H. Endothelial function: a critical determinant in atherosclerosis? *Circulation.* 2004;109(21 Suppl 1):II 27-33

[30] Ross R. The pathogenesis of atherosclerosis: a perspective for the 1990s. *Nature.* 1993;362(6423):801-9

[31] Heistad, D. Oxidative stress and vascular disease: 2005 Duff lecture. *Arteriosclerosis, Thrombosis, and Vascular Biology.* 2006;26(4):689-95

[32] Zhu B, et al. Effects of second-hand smoke and gender on infarct size of young rats exposed in utero and in the neonatal to adolescent period. *Journal of the American College of Cardiology.* 1997;30(7):1878-85

[33] Hutchison S, et al. In-utero and neonatal exposure to secondhand smoke causes vascular dysfunction in newborn rats. *Journal of the American College of Cardiology.* 1998;32(5):1463-7

[34] Torok J, et al. Passive smoking impairs endothelium-dependent relaxation of isolated rabbit arteries. *Physiological Research.* 2000;49(1):135-41

[35] Hutchison S, et al. Chronic dietary L-arginine prevents endothelial dysfunction secondary to environmental tobacco smoke in normocholesterolemic rabbits. *Hypertension.* 1997;29(5):1186-91

[36] Celermajer D, et al.Passive smoking and impaired endothelium-dependent arterial dilatation in healthy young adults. *New England Journal of Medicine.* 1996;334(3): 150-54

[37] Raitakari O.T, et al. Arterial endothelial dysfunction related to passive smoking is potentially reversible in healthy young adults. *Annals of Internal Medicine.* 1999;578-81

[38] Slyper A. Clinical review 168: What vascular ultrasound testing has revealed about pediatric atherogenesis, and a potential clinical role for ultrasound in pediatric risk assessment. *The Journal of Clinical Endocrinology and Metabolism.* 2004;89(7):3089-95

[39] O'Leary D, et al. Carotid-artery intima and media thickness as a risk factor for myocardial infarction and stroke in older adults. Cardiovascular Health Study Collaborative Research Group. *New England Journal of Medicine.* 1999;340(1):14-22

[40] Hansson G.K. Inflammation, atherosclerosis, and coronary artery disease. *New England Journal of Medicine.* 2005;352(16):1685-95

[41] Howard G, et al. Cigarette smoking and progression of atherosclerosis: The Atherosclerosis Risk in Communities (ARIC) Study. *Journal of the American Medical Association.* 1998;279(2):119-24

[42] Libby P, Ridker P, and Maseri A. Inflammation and atherosclerosis. *Circulation.* 2002;105(9):1135-43

[43] Verma S, et al. A self-fulfilling prophecy: C-reactive protein attenuates nitric oxide production and inhibits angiogenesis. *Circulation*. 2002;106(8):913-9

[44] Cai H and Harrison D. Endothelial dysfunction in cardiovascular diseases: the role of oxidant stress. *Circulation Research.* 2000; 87(10):840-4

[45] Panagiotakos D, et al. Effect of exposure to secondhand smoke on markers of inflammation: the ATTICA study. *American Journal of Medicine*. 2004;116(3):145-50

[46] Roberts KA, et al. Effect of environmental tobacco smoke on LDL accumulation in the artery wall. *Circulation*. 1996;94(9):2248-53

[47] Gotto AM Jr. and Brinton EA. Assessing low levels of high-density lipoprotein cholesterol as a risk factor in coronary heart disease: a working group report and update. *Journal of the American College of Cardiology*. 2004;717-24

[48] Wang X, et al. Effects of nicotine on the number and activity of circulating endothelial progenitor cells. *Journal of Clinical Pharmacology*. 2004;44(8):881-9

[49] Moffatt RJ, et al. Acute exposure to environmental tobacco smoke reduces HDL-C and HDL2-C. *Preventive Medicine*. 2004;38(5):637-41

[50] Mizoue T, et al. Workplace exposure to environmental tobacco smoke and high density lipoprotein cholesterol among non-smokers. *American Journal of Epidemiology*. 1999;150(10):1068-72

[51] Burghuber O, et al. Platelet sensitivity to prostacyclin in smokers and non-smokers. *Chest*. 1986;90(1):34-38

[52] Rubenstein D, Jesty J, and Bluestein D. Differences between mainstream and sidestream cigarette smoke extracts and nicotine in the activation of platelets under static and flow conditions. *Circulation*. 2004;109(1):78-83

[53] Schmid P, et al. Passive smoking and platelet thromboxane. *Thrombosis Research*. 1996;81(4):451-60

[54] Iso H, et al. Passive Smoking and Plasma Fibrinogen Concentrations. *American Journal of Epidemiology*. 1996;144(12):1151-54

[55] Stavroulakis G, et al. Passive smoking adversely affects the haemostasis/fibrinolytic parameters in healthy non-smoker offspring of healthy smokers. *Thrombosis and Haemostasis*. 2000;84(5):923-4

[56] Nolan J, et al. Prospective study of heart rate variability and mortality in chronic heart failure: results of the United Kingdom Heart Failure Evaluation and Assessment of Risk Trial (UK-HEART). *Circulation*. 1998;1510-16

[57] Raupach T, et al. Secondhand smoke as an acute threat for the cardiovascular system: a change in paradigm. *European Heart Journal*. 2006;386-92

[58] Groner J, et al. Active and passive tobacco smoke exposure: a comparison of maternal and child hair cotinine levels. *Nicotine & Tobacco Research*. 2004;789-95

[59] Moskowitz W, et al. Lipoprotein and oxygen transport alterations in passive smoking preadolescent children. The MCV Twin Study. *Circulation*. 1990; 81(2): 586-92

[60] Moskowitz W, Schwartz P, and Schieken R. Childhood passive smoking, race, and coronary artery disease risk: the MCV Twin Study. Medical College of Virginia. *Archives of Pediatrics & Adolescent Medicine*.1999; 153(5):446-53

[61] Feldman J, et al. Passive smoking alters lipid profiles in adolescents. *Pediatrics*. 1991; 88(2):259-64

[62] Neufeld E, et al. Passive cigarette smoking and reduced HDL cholesterol levels in children with high-risk lipid profiles. *Circulation*. 1997; 96(5):1403-7

[63] Groner JA, Joshi M, Bauer J. Pediatrics precursors of adult cardiovascular disease - non-invasive assessment of early vascular changes in children and adolescents. *Pediatrics*. 2006; 118:1681-91

In: Smoking and Health Research Frontiers
Editor: Calvin B. Fong, pp. 97-118
ISBN 1-60021-480-0

Chapter V

Maternal Smoking Influences Health and Development of a Child

Drahoslava Hrubá[1] and Lubomír Kukla[2]
[1]Institute of Preventive Medicine, Medical Faculty, Brno, Czech Republic;
[2]Department of Preventive and Social Pediatrics, Medical Faculty, Brno, Czech Republic.

Abstract

The influence of passive smoking on human health has been studied for several decades. Currently a wide range of damaging effects due to chronical involuntary exposure of nosmokers to secondhand smoke is commonly accepted. Infants and children are the most vulnerable target population. A specific interest is focused on the antenatal exposure of fetuses. As smoking is associated with many other social, behavioral and habitual factors, the national studies involving different populations are needed for better understanding of the passive smoking and health problem.

The European Longitudinal Study of Pregnancy and Childhood (ELSPAC) includes 6 countries with the total cohort of 40.000 children and their parents. In the Czech Republic, all women in the urban city of Brno and the rural district Znojmo who were pregnant in the period between 1990/91 (cca 6.000 persons) were asked to participate in this study.

The data about parents life style, family history, education, social and living conditions, stress events and health are repeatedly collected from the second trimester (first time at 18th month of women pregnancy) through the rest of pregnancy and delivery. The follow-up measurements of newborns, infants and children include the data about many conditions influencing the child´s physical, psychical and behavioral development, skills and health. The sources of data are parents, physicians, later on teachers and children themselves as well. Within the Czech cohort, about 40% of women reported the smoking history in their life, 25% of them smoked during 9 months before pregnancy. Relatively high rate of quitting could be seen and the prevalence of those who smoked during the whole pregnancy was 8%. Unfortunately, within the 6 months after delivery, all former smokers started to smoke again.

The Czech cohort of ELSPAC confirms the previously published results:

- antenatal exposure to cigarette smoke is associated with fetal growth retardation

- maternal smoking during pregnancy and after delivery is associated with shorter period of breast feeding
- breast feeding had the significant protective effect on infants health
- postnatal exposure to maternal smoking is associated with significantly increased incidence of infants respiratory and gastrointestinal diseases, as well as with higher level of medical care including hospitalization
- mothers smoking is the main factor influencing the children′ exposure to ETS, also in families where with the smoking mother other smokers are living
- although older children are more exposed to ETS, the relations between the exposure and their health decreased, with an exception of wheezing
- only weak association both of antenatal and postnatal exposure to passive smoking to children′alergy were seen
- the disadvantageous antenatal developmental conditions manifested in the low birthweight are in significant relations to conduct disorders seen at the 3rd and 6th year of age.

Pregnancy is a great opportunity to smoking cessation. Nonsmoking parents behavior must be kept also after delivery and – best of all – forever. The role of physicians and other health professionals in motivating smokers to smoking cessation and in treatment of those who are dependent is crucial and essential.

INTRODUCTION

The influence of passive smoking on human health has been studied for several decades. Contemporarly wide range of damaging effects after chronical involuntary exposure of nonsmokers to secondhand smoke is commonly accepted. Infants and children are the most vulnerable target population. The specific interest is concerned on the antenatal exposure of fetuses. As smoking is associated with many other social, behavioral and habitual factors, the national studies involving different populations are needed for better understanding of the passive smoking and health problem.

The European Longitudinal Study of Pregnancy and Childhood (ELSPAC) includes 6 countries with the total cohort of 40.000 children and their parents. In the Czech Republic, all women in the urban city of Brno and the rural district Znojmo who were pregnant in the period between 1990/91 (cca 6.000 persons) were asked to participate in this study.

The data about parents′ life style, family history, education, social and living conditions, stress events and health are repeatedly collected from the second trimester (first time at 18th week of women pregnancy) through rest of pregnancy and delivery. The follow-up measurements of newborns, infants and children include the data about many conditions influencing on the child′s physical, psychical and behavioral development, skills and health. The sources of data are parents, physicians, later on also teachers and children themselves. The ongoing proces of data control and coding for PC allows the continual analysis and publishing the discovered associations.

Within the Czech cohort, about 40% of women reported the smoking history in their life, 25% of them smoked during 9 months before pregnancy. Relatively high rate of quitting could be seen and the prevalence of those who smoked during the whole pregnancy was

8,1%, most of them were light smokers (smoked less then 10 cigarettes daily). Unfortunately, within the 6 months after delivery, all former smokers started to smoke again. Although only self-reported data about smoking status were obtained, the strong agreement with other descriptive and interventional studies in the same region allows to believe they are true.

It has been mentioned, that smoking is, similarly to other form of addiction, connected with the whole complex of other characteristic factors of unhealthy life style, many of them cause significant biological effects – both direct and indirect – and potentiate deleterious influences of smoking. The complex character of smoking behaviour is both similar in its general features and has also specific particularities associated with traditions, culture and socio-economic factors in each society. In agreement with other studies (King 1997, Little et al., 1989), active smokers among ELSPAC mothers more often than non-smokers consumed alcohol and marihuana, both before and during pregnancy, and after delivery. Significantly more often the important markers of poor nutrition were seen among smokers (less fruit, vegetable and milk products consumption, abuse of sweet, fat and salty food). Smoking women were in average less educated, more often lived as single or divorced mother. In personal history, smoking women more often reported unhappy or stressful events in their childhood, adolescent and young adult period of life, they more often percieved poor health at the end of pregnancy and after delivery.

Smoking and non-smoking women had similar average gestational age and majority of the objective health problems in the current pregnancy were relatively rare and without differences in their prevalence among smokers and non-smokers. Despite of it, some pathologic outcomes have occured more often among smokers (abnormalities of placenta, placenta praevia); on the contrary, there was a significant decrease of the preeclampsia occurence in smoking women.

Those and many other results of the Czech cohort of ELSPAC confirms the previously published data (Fredricsson and Gilljam, 1992, Stillman et al., 1986, Ananth et al., 1996, Williams et al., 1991, Castles et al., 1999).

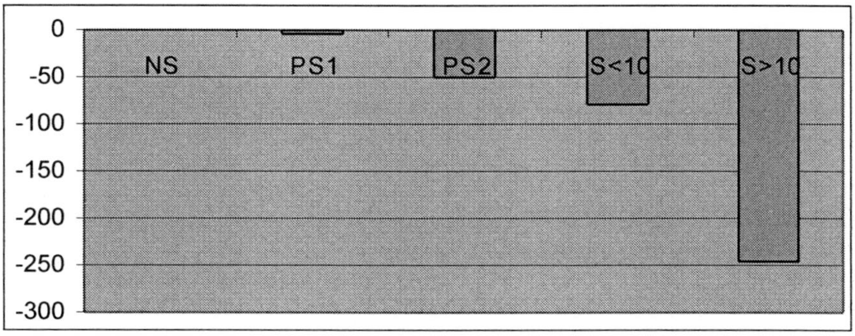

Figure 1: Average differences in birthweight (g) of babies born to women with different exposure to cigarette smoke. NS –non-smokers (average birthweight = 3322 g); PS1 – light passive smokers (spouses smoked less than 10 cig/day); PS2 – heavy passive smokers (spouses smoked more than 10 cig/day) (birthweight lower by 49g, p<0,06); S<10 – light smokers (smoke up to 10 cig/day) (birthweight lower by 79g, p<0,01); S>10- moderate smokers (smoke more than 10 cig/day) (birthweight lower by 245g, p<0,001).

PRENATAL EXPOSURE AND FETAL GROWTH RETARDATION

In the Czech ELSPAC cohort, the **clear associations between maternal exposure both to passive and active smoking and fetal growth retardation were well documented.** There were decreased average levels of birth weight, lenght and circumferences among newborns of passive and active smoking mothers; the effect was dependent on the level of exposure (Tab. 1).

Fetal growth retardation is the most common clinical consequence of antenatal tobacco smoke exposure. Many studies (for example Kramer, 1987, Wilcox 1993, Gordon et al., 1996, California EPA 1997) described the lowered birth weight of about 100 – 300 g in average; somatic retardation is proportional. Maternal smoking doubles the risk of low birthweight (<2500 g). Unfavourable effects of smoking are enhanced by the consumption of coffee and alcohol. In absence of other reasons (parental subnormal antropometric proportions, maternal poor health and/or malnutrition as the most probable conditions), and contemporal mothers′ smoking during the whole pregnancy period, the fetal growth retardation is also called fetal tobacco syndrome. There is also evidence that even involuntary pregnant women′s exposure to environmental tobacco smoke (ETS) plays a role in the reduction of fetal weight, in average about 100 g (Davis, 1991, Gordon et al. 1996, California EPA, 1997, Hruba and Kachlik, 2000, Jaakkola et al, 2001, Lindbohm et al, 2002).

Highly plausible mechanism of the influence of smoking on body growth retardation is based namely on chronic hypoxemia and hyponutrition. Nicotine induces increased production of noradrenaline, adrenaline and acetylcholine which causes vasospasm lasting approximately 40 minutes after each cigarette (during the nicotine life-time). Vasospasm in abdominal part of the maternal body lowers uteroplacental perfusion and decreases the pervasion of nutrients through the placenta to fetus. Nicotine also rapidly crosses the placenta and it is eliminated at a slower rate in the fetus than in the mothers (Spinillo 1995). Nicotine in the fetal circulation may have a direct toxic effect on the fetal cardiovascular system (Bruner and Forouzan, 1991).

Carbon monoxide (CO) inhaled by smoking women increases the content of carboxyhaemoglobin (COHb) both in maternal and fetal blood circulation. Both mothers′ and spouses′ expired air CO was significantly and dose-dependently associated with loss in birthweight, head circumference, Apgar score, increased cord blood fetal COHb and decreased number of newborns with normal fetal heart rate. Expired air CO explained alone 34% of the variance in birthweight. Carbon monoxide seems to have more deleterious effect than nicotine, as the fetus′s CO production is higher than that of a healthy man (Midwife et al, 2005).

Hydrocarbon cyanide (HCN) blocks the enzymes supporting the transfer of oxygen from erythrocytes into the tissues (Stillman, 1986).

Smoking disturbs the morphology and the function of the placenta (Schiverick and Salafia, 1999). These changes can be associated with necrotic damages caused by cumulation of cadmium; this heavy metal acts vasotoxically as it was confirmed in experimental studies (Stillman, 1986, Kuhnert et al., 1987). Maternal smoking has also been atributed to fetal zinc deficiency (Kuhnert 1987), while zinc is considered an esential trace element for many aspects of growth and development (Apgar 1985).

As the sidestream smoke contains the same compounds as mainstream smoke, it is likely that the mechanisms are similar both in active and passive smoking.

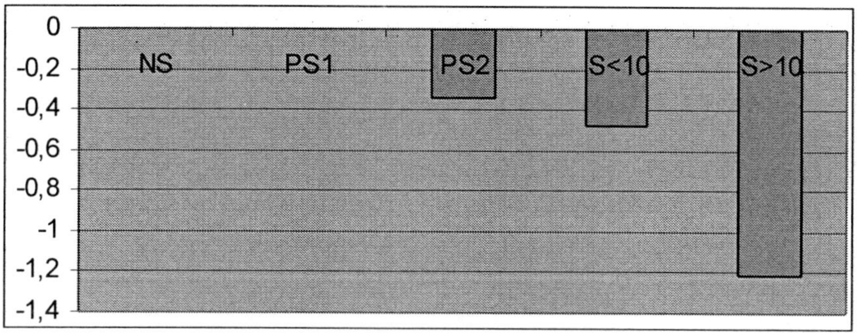

Figure 2: Average differences in body lenght (cm) of babies born to women with different exposure to cigarette smoke. NS –non-smokers (average body lenght = 50,34 cm); PS1 – light passive smokers (spouses smoked less than 10 cig/day); PS2 – heavy passive smokers (spouses smoked more than 10 cig/day) (body lenght lower by 0,34 cm, p<0,01); S<10 – light smokers (smoke up to 10 cig/day) (body lenght lower by 0,48cm, p<0,001); S>10- moderate smokers (smoke more than 10 cig/day) (body lenght lower by 1,22 cm, p<0,001).

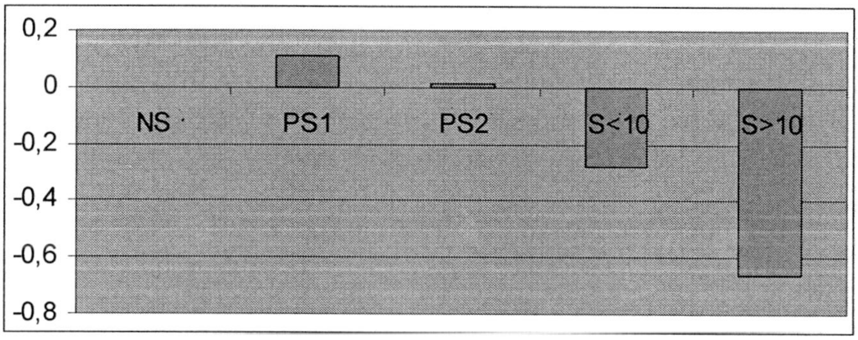

Figure 3: Average differences in head circumferences (cm) of babies born to women with different exposure to cigarette smoke. NS –non-smokers (average head circumference = 34,63 cm); PS1 – light passive smokers (spouses smoked less than 10 cig/day); PS2 – heavy passive smokers (spouses smoked more than 10 cig/day); S<10 – light smokers (smoke up to 10 cig/day) (head circumference lower by 0,28cm, p<0,001); S>10- moderate smokers (smoke more than 10 cig/day) (head circumference lower by 0,66 cm, p<0,001).

Prenatal Exposure and other Deleterious Effects on Fetus Development

According to the Meyer´s hypothesis, smoking is related to very early delivery, with a twofold increase in risk of **preterm delivery** before 32 weeks (Peacock et al, 1995).

Exposure to tobacco smoke in utero is one of the possible preventable factors influencing on **stillbirth**: smokers in several studies had about twice the risk of stillbirth and, on the other hand, the risk is comparable with that in children of non-smoking women, if smoking pregnant women stopped smoking in the first trimester (Wisborg et al., 2001, Surgeon

General 2001). Results of a study which was the first to examine the effect of smoking cessation during the first trimester, indicate that smoking exerts its influence on stillbirth at some point after the first trimester and support the causal role of fetal exposure to tobacco smoke in late pregnancy.

Smoking combined with maternal overweight were associated with dose-dependent increases in risk of stillbirth and very preterm birth (<32 weeks) (Cnattingius and Lambe, 2002). Overweight is closely associated with hyperlipidemia, which may promote vasoconstriction and platelet aggregation with consequent increasing risk of fetal asphyxia. From this point of view, smoking and overweight have synergic effects.

Smoking increased the risk of **intrauterine fetal death** by 40% during the third trimester (Cnattingius et al, 1988). The increased risk of death is due to a variety causes, which may indicate that the harmful effect of exposure to tobacco smoke is not restricted to a single organ. Some tobacco-related prenatal deaths are probably caused by the increased risk for serious malformations, including anencephaly (Fredricssom and Gilliam, 1992).

Contemporarly, there is a well documented evidence that folate levels of <900 nmol/L are associated with the lowest risk of neural tube defects (Daly et al, 1995). In the unique study, both serum folate and red blood cell folate levels were lower in pregnant women who smoked compared with non-smokers. There was also an important gene-environment interaction between methylenetetrahydrofolate reductase gene activity and tobacco exposure on serum folate levels. Deficit of folate (or vitamin B_{12}) causes hyperhomocysteinemia. Thus low levels of folate iniciated by smoking could be another contributor to poor obstetric outcomes, such as spontaneous abortion, stillbirth, abruptio placentae, intrauterine growth retardation, and fetal anomalities, all of which are associated with hyperhomocysteinemia and all of which are more often observed among smoking women (McDonald et al, 2002).

Perinatal events that modify fetal blood pressure and fetal cerebral flow could increase the possibilities of **intracranial hemorrhage** in preterm infants, which is the leading cause of neonatal death or neurologic morbidity in low birth weight infants. In the prospective case-control study (Spinillo et al, 1995), maternal smoking > 10 cig/day during the second half of pregnancy was associated with three times higher risk of intracranial hemorrhage. These associations can be explained both by hypoxia and hypertensive effect of nicotine on the fetal circulation and indirectly, as smoking may also act as a predisposing factor affecting the neonatal response to other insults (such as acidosis, respiratory distress syndrome, apnea, ventilator therapy).

Mutagenic components of tobacco smoke are likely to cause changes in the chromosomes in the DNA of germ cells or in the cells of the developing offsprings. Many chemicals in cigarette smoke have teratogenic potential in some animal tests: nicotine, pyridine, hydrazine, methylamine.

In the early 1970s, an association between maternal cigarette smoking and an increased risk of having a child with an **oral clefts** was suggested. Later on, a meta-analysis of 44 reports estimated statistically significant association between maternal smoking during the first trimester of gestation and the risk of oral clefts occurence in odds of 1,37 for each 10 cigarettes per day (Wyszynski et al, 1997). Recently, the case-control study in United Kingdom not only has confirmed the previous findings, but also described the effect of second-hand smoke: the data collected in regard to mothers′ passive smoking were comparable to those of mothers who smoked actively (Wyszynski et al, 1997).

A positive associations between maternal smoking and **limb reduction** has been also reported by some investigators (Aro 1994, Czeizel 1994).

A moderate, statistically significant association between maternal smoking and **urinary organ malformations** were found in several studies (Li et al. 1996, Kellén K, 1997) and supported by the experimental findings (Schuchardt 1996). The literature on the aetiology of urinary organ malformations is limited, alcohol could be a confounder of particular interest, as kidney dysplasia occured with fetal alcohol syndrome (Clarren and Smith 1978).

The most consistent finding was the increased risk of nervous system defects (Cal. EPA 1997). Also diaphragmatic hernia and pigmentary anomalities were found to be associated with smoking (Lindbohm, 2002).

Down syndrome is the most common identified cause of mental retardation and is predominantly caused by trisomy 21 (free- standing chromosome 21) as a result from an error in meiosis or rarely in postzygotic mitosis. Advanced maternal age has been identified as a risk factor. With the advent of DNA technology it has become possible to determine both the patternal and the time of that error during meiosis. First maternal error is initiated prenatally and continues until the egg is ovulated some 10 to 40 years later. The lenght of second maternal meiosis is only 1 to 3 days irrespective of the maternal age (Antonarakis et al., 1992).

When all Down syndrome cases were analyzed together, no evidence of an association between maternal smoking and the risk was found. When the analysis by the timing of the error separately was done, smoking has occured as significant risk increasing the cases initiated during the second meiosis. The deleterious effect of smoking was more pronounced among women younger than 35 years (OR 2,98, 95% CI 1,01-8,87) and showed clear evidence of a dose-response relationship (due to pack-years smoked). The combined use of cigarettes and oral contraceptives increased the risk further (OR 7,62, 95% CI 1,63-35,6), while oral contraceptives use alone was no risk factor (Yang et al, 1999).

The effects of smoking on meiosis is little evident, but hormonal imbalance which causes delays conception, reduced fecundity, early menopause among smoking women (Surgeon General, 1985) might also cause a less-than optimal microvasculature to develop around the maturing oocytes and consequent oxygen deficit and decreased intracellular pH in the egg. These pathways may impair the spindle and result in chromosome displacement and nondisjunction (Gaulden 1992).

The risk for severe birth defects was increased in a dose-response manner depending on the **smoking of the father**. Paternal heavy smoking (>30 cig/day) seems to be associated with an increased rate of major malformations (Lindbohm, 2002).

In the Czech ELSPAC cohort, the prevalence of congenital malformations was similar among infants born to non-smokers and smokers. However, mothers′ smoking enhanced the effect of occupational exposure to organic solvents to the higher rate of these disturbances. Compared with non-exposed non-smokers, the observed/expected ratio was higher both for smokers exposed to organic solvents before pregnancy (OR 2,08), and for smokers exposed during the first half of pregnancy (OR 2,50).

MATERNAL SMOKING INFLUENCES ON BREAST FEEDING

It was repeatedly documented in different studies that maternal smoking during pregnancy and after delivery is associated with shorter period of breast feeding (Fredricsson and Gilljam, 1992).

The same results could be seen in the Czech ELSPAC study. As soon as from the first week of newborns´ life, significant differences between prevalence of fully breast- fed and fully bottle- fed infants born to mothers with different smoking habit during pregnancy and after delivery have occured (Fig. 4a, 4b). At the end of the 6th week of infants´ age, almost 55% of babies born to non-smokers were fully breast-fed, compared with only 25% of those born to smokers. At the end of the 8th week of age, when the first control examination after delivery was performed, almost 50% of non-smokers´babies were fully breast fed and another 18% obtained the breast and bottle milk combination, in comparison with 20% plus 10% fully and combined breast feeding of smokers´ babies.

At the beginning of the 90s, the physiologic principles of breast feeding stimulation were neglected in the Czech Republic. In the desirable term, i.e. till one hour after the birth, only less than 7% of children were set to breast; only less than 60% of newborns were exclusively breast fed in the first 24 hours after the birth, and other 16% were breast fed in combination with bottle feeding.

However, the poor support of breast feeding was the common approach and so it could not explain the differences between nutrition of children born to smoking and non-smoking mothers. Although the exact mechanisms by which smoking effects on breast feeding period shortening are not known, these causes are commonly accepted:

- Chemical substances in tobacco smoke, esp. nicotine, cause hormonal dysbalance (lower prolactin levels), which projects in lower ability to produce maternal milk (Wildstrom et al, 1991)
- Chemical substances in tobacco smoke, esp. nicotine, pass into the maternal milk, where their levels exceed plasma levels up to three times (Mascola et al, 1998); these substances alters the milk´s taste and the babies refuse it
- Smoking mothers may be less motivated to breast – feeding because they suspect that the milk´s quality can be negatively influenced by smoking and taken in account the availability of bottle milk they cease to breast-feed earlier than non-smoking mothers (Haug et al, 1998)

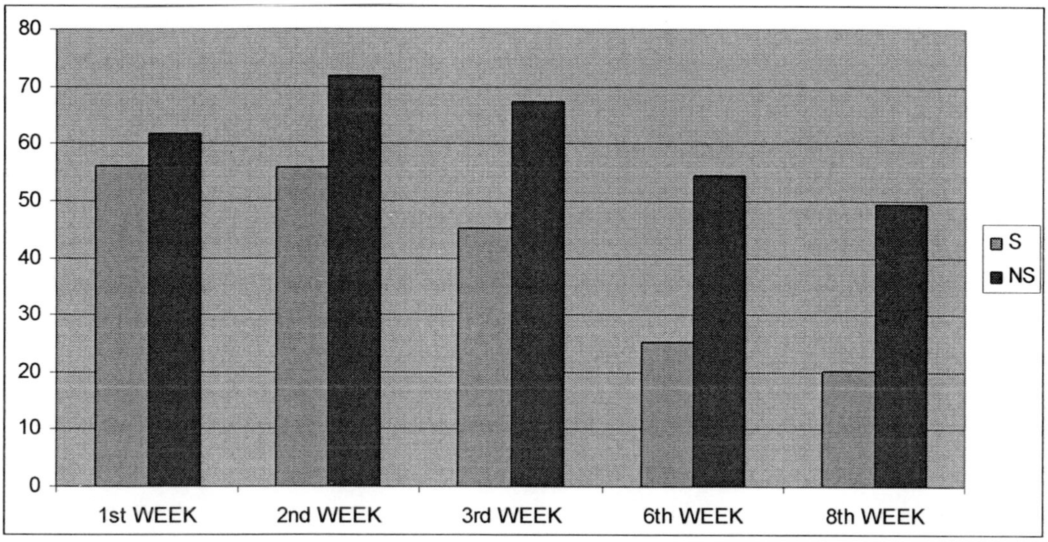

Figure 4a: The prevalence of fully breast fed infants born to smoking and non-smoking mothers during their first 8 weeks of life (%).

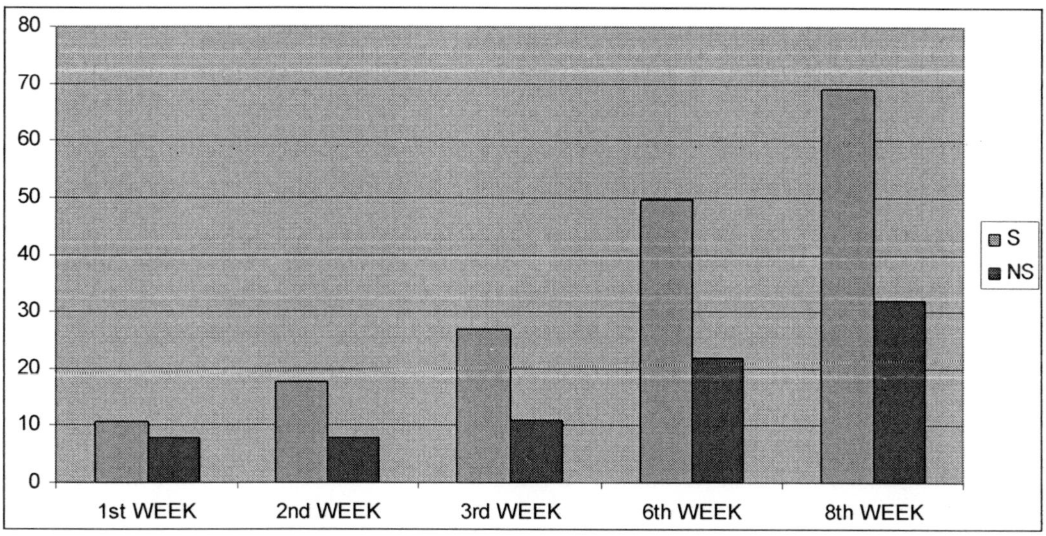

Figure 4b: The prevalence of fully bottle fed infants born to smoking and non-smoking mothers during their first 8 weeks of life (%).

Exposure to Tobacco Smoke Enhances the Risk of Sudden Infant Death Syndrome and Childhood Cancer

The **sudden infant death syndrome** (SIDS) occurs without warning to infants who are typically between 2 and 5 months of age (Golding, 1997). Observations of a relation between smoking in pregnancy and SIDS have been confirmed in several epidemiologic studies, including those of prospective. The risk for SIDS, which is the most prevalent cause of postnatal infant mortality in majority of developed countries, was found to be related to the number of cigarettes smoked per day (Pollack, 2001), and the relationship is stronger than seen with any other drugs of abuse (Haglund and Cnattingius, 1990, Golding 1997).

SIDS requires the conjunction of two developmental problems: an underlying defect in neonatal cardiovascular and respiratory control and a precipitating event (most often sleep apnea or airway obstruction) that produces hypoxia (Poets et al, 1993). Neonatal hypoxia involves unique response, the most important which is the massive release of catecholamines, which elicit the required redistribution of blood flow to the brain and heart. The adrenal catecholamine release is autonomous, independent on central reflexes, and is responsible for the neonate ability to resist hypoxia. Exposure to nicotine led to the complete loss of hypoxia-induces adrenomedullary release and to the death (in experimental animals – Slotkin et al, 1995). In addition, nicotine sensitied cardiac cells to hypoxia and, dysfunction of central respiratory control would produce fetal response patterns (respiratory arrest) as opposed to postnatal pattern (activation). Prenatal nicotine exposure results in the combined adrenomedullary, cardiac and respiratory defects which would be the mechanisms of death during neonatal apneic episodes (Slotkin et al,). Contemporarly, smoking is considered an independent risk factor for SIDS and is mainly mediated through maternal smoking during pregnancy (Alm et al, 1998).

The risk for **cancer in childhood** has been calculated to 1,3 (93% CI 0,8-2,2) for those prenataly exposed to maternal smoking during pregnancy, with the dose-dependent relationship. Smoking doubled the risk for non-Hodgkin lymphoma, acute lymphoblastic leukemia and Wilm´s tumor. Also fathers´smoking slightly increased the incidence of children´cancer, probably due to maternal passive exposure; however, damage to the male genome before conception could not be excluded (Fredricsson and Gilljam, 1992).

It was also described that natural killer-cell activity in infants may be affected by maternal active or passive smoking during pregnancy, which is in agreement with similar observations in smoking adults (Castellazzi et al, 1999). As natural killers activity represents an important immune defense mechanism against tumors, the reduction of this activity can be involved in the increased incidence of childhood cancer of tobacco smoke exposed infants.

A specific interest has been focused on brain tumors, which are the second most common cancer in childhood. Tobacco smoke contains many known human carcinogens, including N-nitroso compounds and their precursors (nitrosamines), which were recognized as animal neural carcinogens, especially when exposure is transplacental (Rice and Ward, 1982). Neither the review from 1996 (Norman et al.), nor the results of meta-analysis published 2002 (Huncharek et al.) found any clear association between maternal smoking during pregnancy and risk of childhood brain tumor development. Nevertheless, results of several studies suggest an association with paternal tobacco smoke with children brain tumors (Lindbohm et al, 2002).

PRENATAL EXPOSURE TO CIGARETTE SMOKE ENHANCES RESPIRATORY MORBIDITY DURING THE FIRST YEARS OF LIFE

Only limited information is available on normal lung growth and development during the first year of life, and there are conflicting reports on the influence of familiar and environ mental factors. Altered lung function, changes of peripheral airway and impaired imunology are the major causes of infants′ respiratory morbidity.

The evidence is sufficient to infer a causal relationship between maternal smoking during pregnancy and reduction of a lung function in infants. Prenatal exposure to tobacco smoke affects fetal intrathoracic airway development and significantly reduces airway function through the first 12 months of life (Young et al, 2000). Alhtough the mechanisms of effects are not well known, experimental and human studies have demonstrated that fetal exposure to nicotine is associated with a wide spectrum of morphological abnormalities (such as dilated bronchi, decreased fetal lung weight, reduced fetal lung volume, number of alveoli and total volume of parenchymal elastic tissue and some others. These studies also demonstrated the importance of fetal endocrine functions on the maturation of respiratory system, which can be altered by chemicals in cigarette smoke (Lieberman et al, 1992).

The alterations to the immune system have been observed in infants whose mothers smoked compared with controls: higher cords serum levels of IgG, IgA and IgM, decreased neutrophil counts in cord blood. Also natural killers activity in infants may be affected by maternal smoking during pregnancy, both active and passive, which is in agreement with previous observations in smoking adults (Castellazzi et al, 1999). Thus all these altered immune factors may be also involved in the suggestive evidence about a causal relationship between maternal smoking during pregnancy and an increase in the frequency of lower respiratory tract and other infectious illness during infancy.

Although it is difficult to distinguish between the effect of smoking during pregnancy and the infant′s exposure after delivery, prenatal exposure is considered a risk factor enhancing the morbidity, which was supported in animal models (U.S. EPA, 1992). In the Czech ELSPAC cohort, the overal morbidity of infants born to smoking mothers during their first 6 weeks of life was reported more than three times more often (2,6% vs. 0,7%).

The frequency of various respiratory symptoms or diseases was significantly higher in the Czech ELSPAC infants born to smoking mothers; breast feeding reduced the frequency of symptoms at an important level (Fig 5a, 5b).

Children′ exposure to environmental tobacco smoke (ETS) is the most ubiquitous and hazardous factor within the whole environmental exposure in childhood. Many studies have reported a dose-response relationship between degree of exposure to ETS, measured by number of cigarettes smoked by mothers or in the household, and enhanced risk of both upper and lower respiratory tract illnesses, such as cough, phlegm production, otitis media, bronchitis, bronchiolitis and pneumonia, as well as wheeze and asthma. These deleterious effects are independent of an in utero exposure to maternal smoking (U.S. EPA 1992). Odds ratios for respiratory illnesses, together with symptoms and middle ear disease range very consistently between 1,2 and 1,6 for exposed children and are usually higher in pre-school than in school children (Californian EPA, 1997, Cook and Strachan, 1999), with the peak at age of two. The effect of ETS exposure on the incidence of pneumonia and bronchiolitis seems to be the highest during the first year of life, while the cough in relation to parental smoking was described as declining after age 3 (Rylander et al, 1995). These changes in trends may be influenced by the fact that older children spend less time with their smoking parents (Li et al, 1999). Especially the increased prevalence of middle ear effusion attributable to ETS exposure is considered to be a very important public health consequence, as otitis media is a very common reason for hospitalization and operation and thus imposes children stress and a financial burden to the health care system.

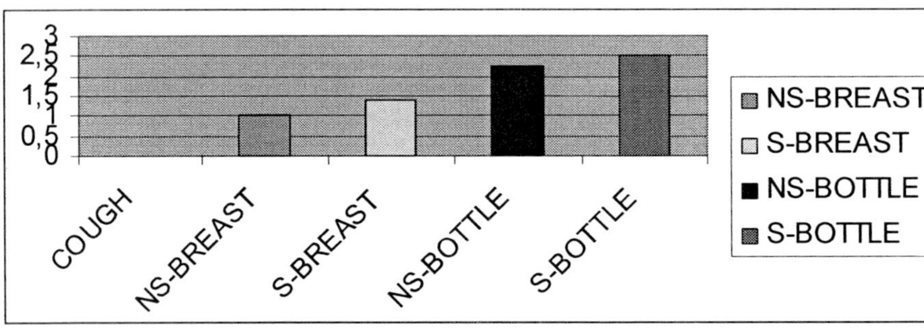

Figure 5a: The prevalence of cought in infants during their first 6 weeks of life (%). NS-BREAST – non-exposed prenataly to tobacco smoke, fully breast fed; S-BREAST – exposed prenataly to tobacco smoke, fully breast fed; NS-BOTTLE – non-exposed prenataly to tobacco smoke, fully bottle fed; S-BOTTLE – exposed prenataly to tobacco smoke, fully bottle fed.

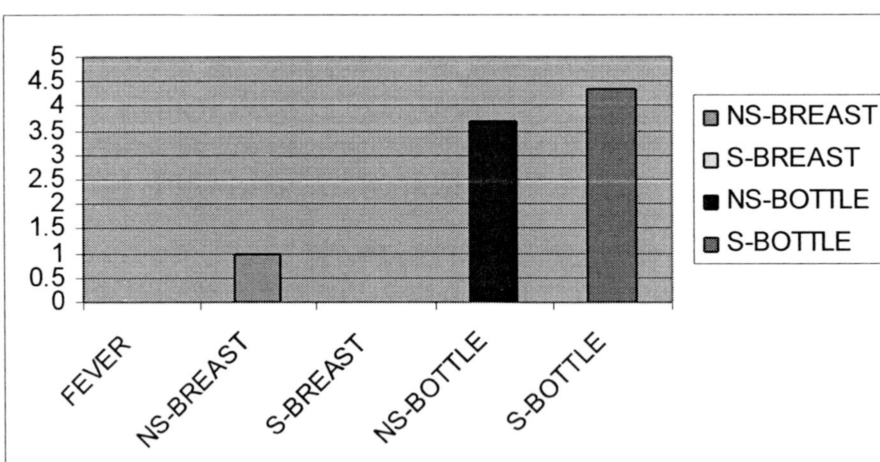

Figure 5b: The prevalence of fever in infants during their first 6 weeks of life (%). NS-BREAST – non-exposed prenataly to tobacco smoke, fully breast fed; S-BREAST – exposed prenataly to tobacco smoke, fully breast fed; NS-BOTTLE – non-exposed prenataly to tobacco smoke, fully bottle fed; S-BOTTLE – exposed prenataly to tobacco smoke, fully bottle fed.

On the other hand, the trend of development of asthmatic respiratory symptoms associated with infants′ exposure to ETS does not show similar age-related declination (Strachan and Cook, 1998); prenatal and postnatal exposure carries a substantial risk for developing asthma even in adulthood (Skorge et al, 2005). There is a corresponding increase in prevalence and exacerbation of asthma symptoms among children with raised urinary cotinine levels (Esamai, 1998). The strong support for the hypothesis about causal relationships between ETS and asthma is the report that asthma severity has improved in children after the reduction of their exposure (DiFranza et al, 2004).

Mechanisms by which exposure to ETS might cause respiratory morbidity include the decreased mucocilliary clearance and opening the respiratory ways to entry of microbes; impairing immunologic system functions; hyperplasia of adenoids (Cal EPA, 1997). To the higher risk of asthma contribute the many chemicals in cigarette smoke with their irritant effects, bronchial hyperresponsiveness to allergens, impairment of the pulmonal elasticity, decreased pulmonary function and alterations in their circadian variations (Cook and Strachan 1998, Agabiti et al, 1999).

Czech ELSPAC mothers who were smoking in the time of six months after delivery reported more often that their children were suffering from more severe health problems at their 6th month of life: 1,6% of infants exposed to ETS were sick nearly all the time compared with 0,8% of unexposed children. Infants who had smoking mothers showed significantly increased frequency of all observed signs of respiratory damages including middle ear inflammation. Almost twice as many children of heavy smokers (more than 10 cig/day) were admitted to hospital within their first half a year of life (Fig 6).

Respiratory symptomatology and morbidity has been significantly higher among children whose mothers smoked after delivery up to the 18th month of life (Fig 7). On the other hand, at the fifth year of age, the clear relationships were seen of ETS exposure to asthmatic symptomatology (wheezing) (Fig 8) and also to the more frequent alergic responses to the domestic dust (wheezing and hard breathing).

In the Czech ELSPAC cohort, mothers' smoking was the most important factor influencing the children′ exposure to ETS, as in families with smoking mother there were also other smokers and more children were exposed to ETS daily. At the age of 3 years, more children were exposed to ETS than during their first 18 months of life. At elder age (5 years), the kindergarten-visiting decreased the time of daily exposure, which was shorter on work-days than on weekends. Thus, the declining occurence of respiratory symptoms could not be explained by the lower exposure level hypothesis, except of asthmatic symptomatology.

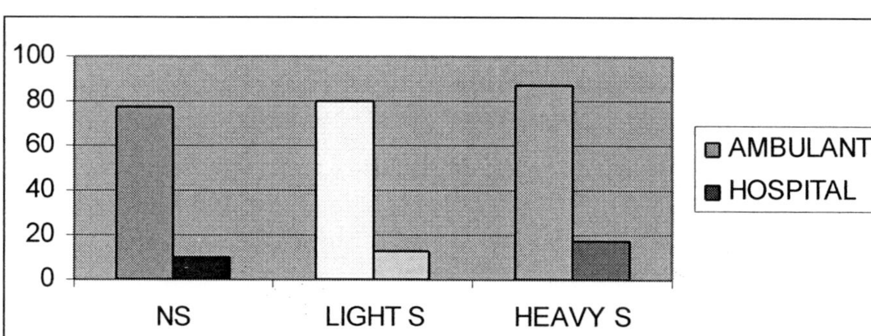

Fig. 6: The prevalence of health care during the first 6 months of life (ambulant and hospital) needed for infants of mothers with different smoking habit: non-smokers (NS), light smokers (up to 10 cig/day) and heavy smokers (more than 10 cig/day) (% of children).

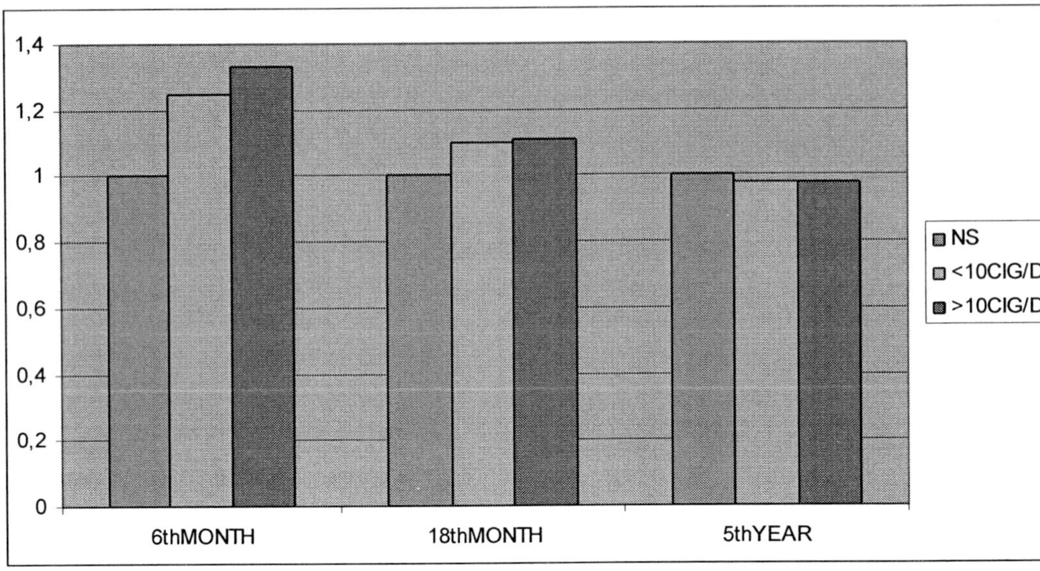

Fig 7a: The prevalence of cough in children (%) of non-smokers (NS), light smokers (<10 cig/day) and heavy smokers (> 10 cig/day) at their different age.

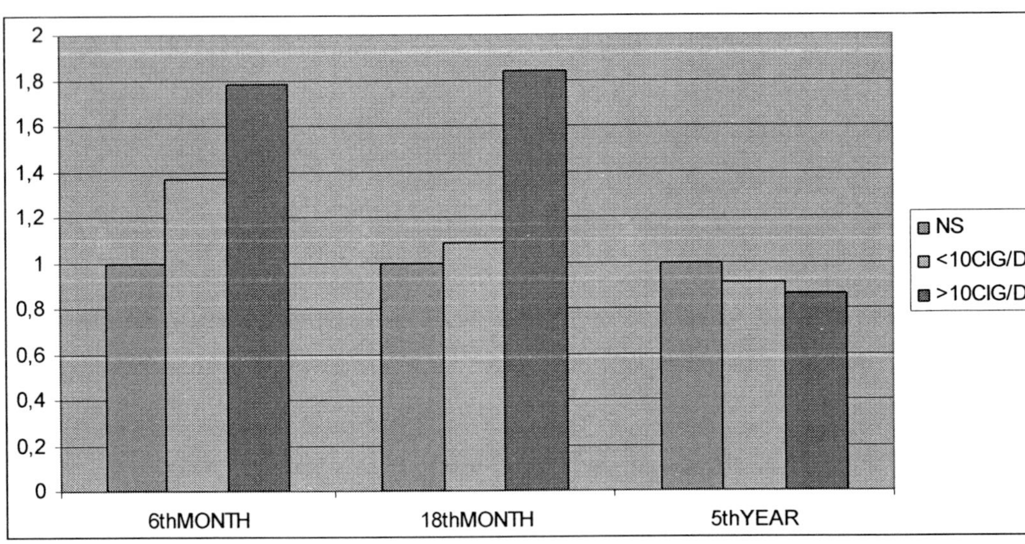

Fig 7b: The prevalence of otitis media in children (%) of non-smokers (NS), light smokers (<10 cig/day) and heavy smokers (> 10 cig/day) at their different age.

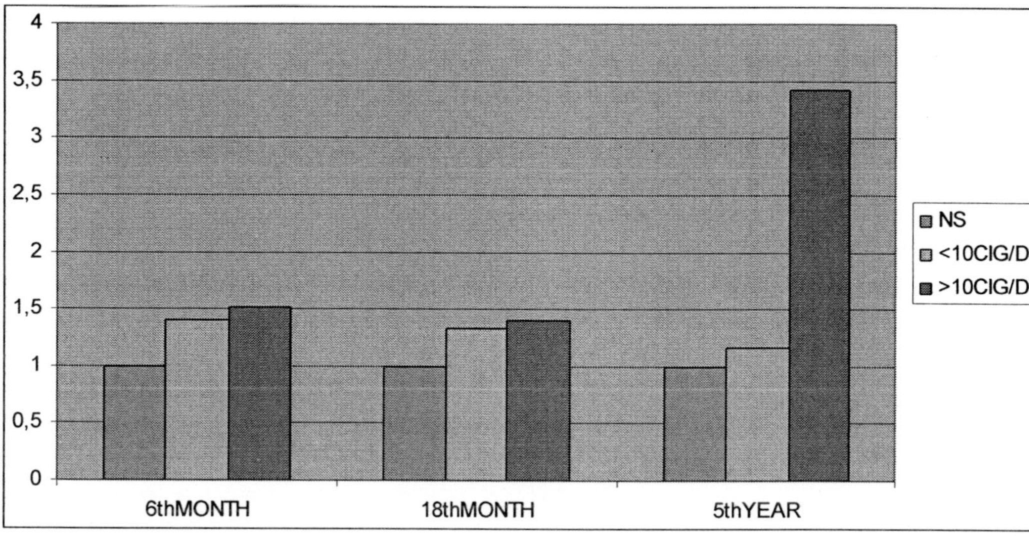

Fig 8: The prevalence of wheezing in children (%) of non-smokers (NS), light smokers (<10 cig/day) and heavy smokers (> 10 cig/day) at their different age.

PRENATAL EXPOSURE TO TOBACCO SMOKE INFLUENCES CHILDREN'S BEHAVIOR

The teratological model proposes that toxins can affect the central nervous system (CNS) of the developing fetus at levels bellow those which cause growth and morphological abnormalities (Slotkin, 1998). In animals, the CNS damage was irreversible and changes were detecable into adulthood.

In humans, an increasing number of reports describe the effect of tobacco exposure on the developing CNS. The clinical manifestations of damage are wide: impairment of auditory, language and cognitive development, decreased attention span, increased impulsivity, activity and negativity, emotional instability, oppositional behaviors and aggression among preschoolers (for example, Naeye and Peters, 1994, Olds et al 1994, Milberger et al, 1996, Orlebeke et al, 1997, Day et al. 2000). The influence of maternal smoking is greater than paternal smoking and increasing the odds of the toddler´s conduct problems is significant even after controlling for the other variables, e.g. antenatal exposure to maternal smoking is the andependent risk factor (Brook et al, 2000).

A specific interest has been focused on the attention-deficit hyperactivity disorders (ADHD), defined by the US diagnostic criteria as a separate unit. Despite the difference between US and Europen criterias, both classifications include children' inappropriate levels of inattention, hyperactivity and impulsivity that begin in childhood and cause impairment of school performance, intelectual functions, social skills, driving and occupational functions (Faraone et al, 2003). Most researchers agree that ADHD has both hereditary and environmental components. No single neuropsychological theory can explain all ADHD symptoms, but in the subcortical structures, the striatum has been of particular interest because it is rich in dopamine synapses, and is vulnerable to the perinatal hypoxic complications. Pregnancy and delivery complications which lead to chronic hypoxia and are indexed by low birthweight, are frequently associated with ADHD (Biederman and Faraone, 2005). Prenatal exposure to maternal smoking is commonly associated with lowered birthweight, so this toxaemia might be regarded as a risk factor.

Today a special attention is paid to study of these relations: existing results describe the relations of ADHD and/or conduct disorders (CD) occurence to prenatal smoking exposure even after possible bias standardization. An epidemiological study meta-analysis has confirmed that prenatal exposure to maternal smoking increases the ADHD risk more than twice (OR 2,38, 95% CI 1,61 – 3,52) (Thapar et al, 2003). Case-control studies yielded similar results (Mick et al, 2003). Low birth-weight presented even higher ADHD/CD occurence risk (OR 2,64, 95% CI 1,85-3,78) (Bhutta et al. 2002, Indredavik et al, 2004).

Several studies from different population groups confirmed the continuity of behavioral problems at ages 16 to 18 (Fergusson et al 1998), an increased risk of substance abuse in adolescence (Weissman et al, 1999), and significantly higher rate of arrests for violent and nonviolent crimes in young adulthood (Rantakallio et al, 1983, 1992, Raine et al, 1994, Brennan et al, 1999). These effects are predominantly associated with exposure in the later part of pregnancy, the time when nicotine receptors are formed (Slotkin, 1998).

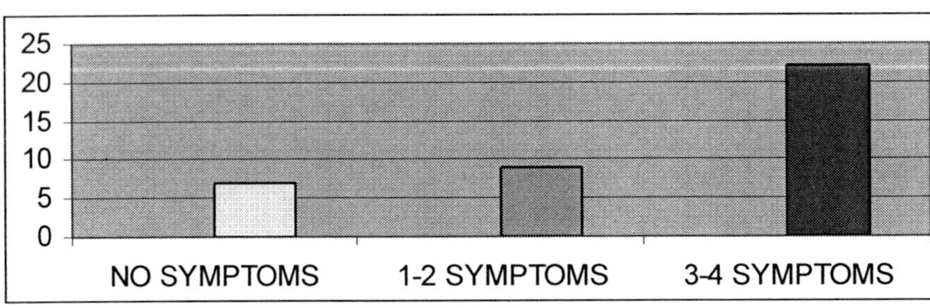

Fig 9: Prevalence of mothers of children without and with symptoms of ADHD, who smoked during the whole pregnancy ($p< 0{,}01$).

In the Czech ELSPAC cohort, the measurement of behavioral disorders was included in the period of children′ age 6 and 7 years. According to physicians′ diagnosis of symptoms of ADHD (significant and pertinacious negativity, attention deficit, aggresivity, excessive reactions) chidren were divided into 3 groups (no symptoms, 1-2 symptoms, 3-4 symptoms). The overal prevalence of ADHD was 3,5%, more frequent among boys. Mothers of children with ADHD more often smoked during pregnancy (Fig 9). The average birthweight and head circumference of children with ADHD was significantly lower (Fig. 10a, 10b). Higher prevalence of disturbances and problems of psychomotoric development at school were reported by physicians (Fig. 11) as well as by teachers for children with ADHD symptoms (Fig. 12a, 12b).

These results are not definitive. It is not possible to separate completely the effects of prenatal and postpartum exposures. It is possible that smoking mothers are more likely to be impulsive and might be modelling behaviors for the children. Women who are more impulsive or who have attention problems may have more difficulty quitting smoking than other smokers. Alternatively, women who smoke may report differently on their children′s behaviors (Williams et al, 2005).

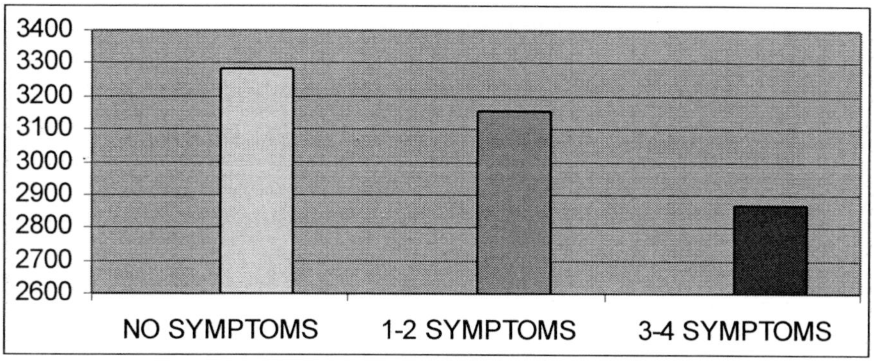

Fig.10a: An average birthweight of children without and with symptoms of ADHD (p< 0,01).

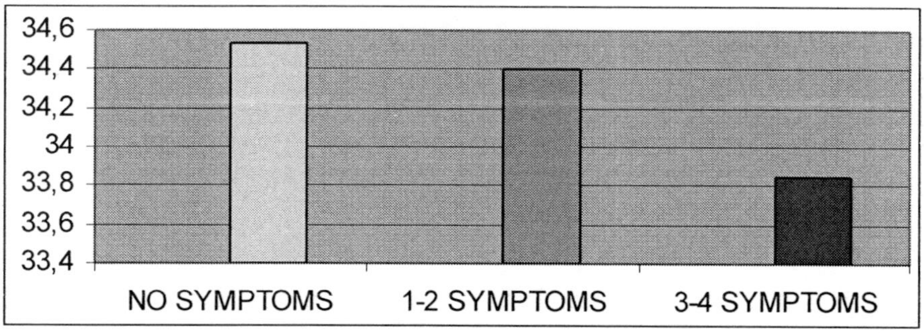

Fig.10b: An average head circumference of children without and with symptoms of ADHD (p< 0,01)

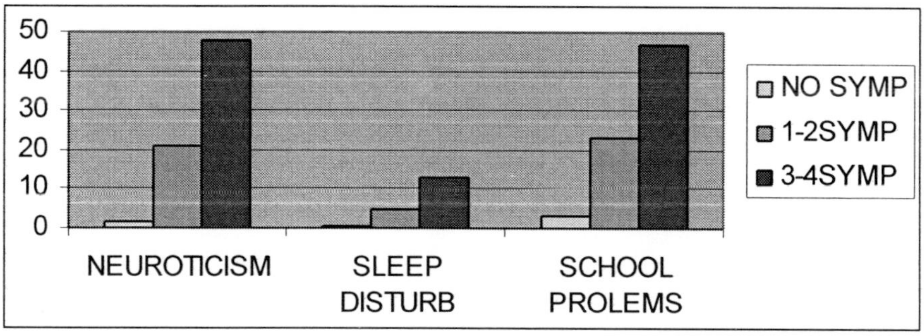

Fig. 11: Prevalence of some co-morbidity among children without and with symptoms of ADHD reported by physicians (p< 0,01).

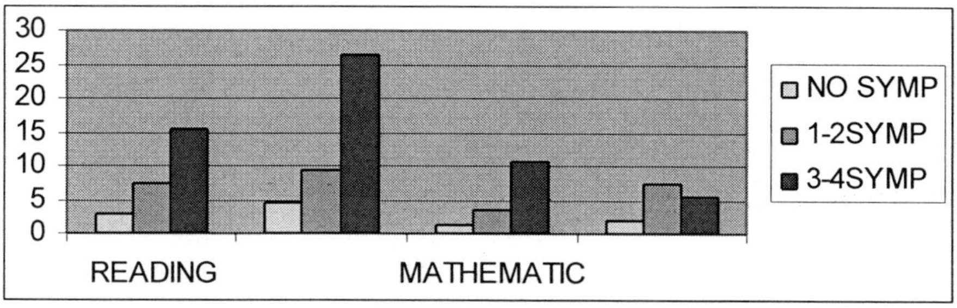

Fig. 12: Poor school performance among children without and with symptoms of ADHD reported by teachers (p< 0,01).

CONCLUSION

During the past decades, it has become increasingly clear that children born to women who smoke cigarettes during pregnancy exhibit consistent deficit in physical growth, neurologic functioning, cognitive development, school achievement, behavioral adjustment, and higher level of health problems. Although there is no doubt that women who smoke during pregnancy are much more likely to come from lower social classes and to differ from non-smokers in other health-related behaviors, personality and child rearing patterns, many studies have confirmed that prenatal exposure may be an independent risk factor for a wide range of childhood disturbances.

Pregnancy is a great opportunity to smoking cessation. Non-smoking parents′ behavior must be kept also after delivery and – best of all – forever. The role of physicians and other health professionals in motivation smokers to smoking cessation and in treatment of those who are dependent is crucial and essential.

REFERENCES

Agabiti N, Mallone S, Forastiere F et al, SIDRIA Collaborative Group: The impact of parental smoking on asthma and wheezing. *Epidemiol* 1999; 10: 692-698

Alm B, Milerad J, Wennergren G et al: A case-control study of smoking and sudden infant death syndrome in the Scandinavian countries, 1992 to 1995. *Arch Dis Child* 1998; 78: 329-334

Annanth CV, Savitz DA, Williams CV: Placental abruption and its association with hypertension and prolonged rupture of membranes: A methodological review and meta-analysis. *Obstet Gynecol* 1996; 88: 309-318

Antonarakis SE, Petersen MB, McInnis MG et al: The meiotic stage of nondisjunction in trisomy 21: Determination by using DNA polymorphisms. *Am J Hum Genet* 1992; 50: 544-550

Apgar J: Zinc and reproduction. *Ann Rew Nutr* 1985; 5: 43-48

Aro T: *Incidence, secular trend and risk indicators of reduction limb defects*. Health Services Research by the National Board of Health in Finland, 1994, Helsinki

Bhuta AT, Cleves MA, Casey PH et al: Cognitive and behavioral outcomes of school aged children who were born preterm: a meta analysis. *JAMA* 2002; 288(6): 728-737

Biederman J, Faraone SV: Attention-deficit hyperactivity disorder. *The Lancet* 2005; 366, 9482: 237-248

Brennan PA, Grekin ER, Mednick SA: Maternal smoking during pregnancy and adult male criminal outcomes. *Arch Gen Psychiatry* 1999; 56: 215-219

Brook JS, Brook DW, Whiteman M: The influence of maternal smoking during pregnancy on the toddler′s negativity. *Arch Pediatr Adolesc Med* 2000; 154: 381-385

Bruner JP, Forouzan I: Smoking and bucally administered nicotine. *J Reprod Med* 1991; 36: 435-440

California Environmental Protection Agency, Office of Environmental Health Hazard Assessment: *Health effects of exposure to environmental tobacco smoke*. Final report. Sacramento, CA, 1997

Castellazzi AM, Maccario R, Moretta A et al: Effect of active and passive smoking during pregnancy on natural killer-cell activity in infants. *J Allergy Clin Immunol* 1999; 103: 172-173

Castles A, Adams K, Melvin CL et al.: Effects of smoking during pregnancy: five meta-analysies. *Am J Prev Med* 1999; 16(3): 208-215

Clarren SK, Smith DW: The fetal alcohol syndrome. N Engl J Med 1978; 298: 1063-1067

Cnattingius S, Lambe M: Trends in smoking and overweight during pregnancy: prevalence, risks of pregnancy complications and adverse pregnancy outcomes. *Seminars in Perinatology* 2002; 26: 286-295

Cook DG, Strachan DP: Health effects of passive smoking 7: parental smoking, bronchial activity and peak flow variability in children. *Thorax* 1998; 53: 295-301

Cook DG, Strachan DP: Summary of effects of parental smoking on the respiratory health of children and implications for research. *Thorax* 1999; 54: 357-366

Cziezel A, Kodaj I, Lenz W: Smoking during pregnancy and congenital limb deficiency. *BMJ* 1994; 308: 1473-1476

Daly LE, Kirke PN, Molloy A et al: Folate levels and the risk of neural tube defects. *JAMA* 1995; 274: 1698-1702

Davis DL: Paternal smoking and fetal death. *The Lancet* 1991, 337: 123

Day NL, Richardson GA, Goldschmidt L, Cornelius MD: Effects of prenatal tobacco exposure on preschoolers′ behavior. *J Dev Behav Pediatr* 2000; 21: 180-188

DiFranza JR, Aligne AC, Weitzman M: Prenatal and postnatal environmental tobacco smoke exposure and children′s health. *Pediatrics* 2004; 113: 1007-1015

Esamai FO: Relationship between exposure to tobacco smoke and bronchial asthma in children: A review. *East African Medical J* 1998; 75: 47-50

Faraone SV, Sergeant J, Gillberg C, Biederman J.: The worldwide prevalence of ADHD: is it an American condition? *World Psychiatry* 2003; 2: 104-113

Fergusson D, Woodward L, Horwood L: Maternal smoking during pregnancy and psychiatric adjustment in late adolescence. *Arch Gen Psychiatry* 1998; 55: 721-727

Fredricsson B, Gilljam H: Smoking and reproduction. *Acta Obstet Gynecol Scand* 1992; 71: 580-592

Gaulden MR: Maternal age effect: The enigma of Down syndrome and other trisomic conditions. *Mutat. Res.* 1992; 296: 129-140

Golding J: Sudden infant death syndrome and parental smoking – a literature review. *Paediatric and Perinatal Epidemiol* 1997; 11: 67-77

Gordon AE, Johnstone FD, Prescott RJ et al.: Smoking during pregnancy: the dose dependence of birthweight deficit. *Br J Obstet Gynecol* 1996; 103: 806-813

Haglund B, Cnattingius S: Cigarette smoking as a risk factor for sudden infant death syndrome: A population-based study. *Am J Publ Health* 1990; 80: 29-32

Haug K, Irgens LM, Baste V et al.: Secular trends in breast feeding and parental smoking. *Acta Pediatr* 1998; 87: 1023-1027

Hruba D, Kachlik P: Infuence of maternal active and passive smoking during pregnancy on birthweiht in newborns. *Cent Europ J Publ Health* 2000; 8: 249-252

Huncharek M, Kupelnick B, Klassen H: Maternal smoking during pregnancy and the risk of childhood brain tumors: a meta-analysis of 6566 subjects from twelve epidemiological studies. *J Neuro-Oncology* 2002; 57: 51-57

Indredavik MS, Vik T, Heyerdal S et al: Psychiatric symptoms and disorders in adolescents with low birth weight. *Arch Dis Child Fetal Neonatal Ed* 2004; 89: F445-450

Jaakkola JK, Jaakkola N, Zahlsen K: Fetal growth and lenght of gestation in relation to prenatal exposure to environmental tobacco smoke assessed by hair nicotine concentration. *Environ Health Perspect* 2001; 109: 557-561

Kallén K: Maternal smoking and urinary organ malformations. *Int J Epidemiol* 1997; 26: 571- 574

King JC: Substane abuse in pregnancy. *Postgrad Med* 1997; 102: 135-150

Kramer MS: Determinants of low birth weight: methodological assessment and meta-analysis. *Bull WHO* 1987; 65: 663-737

Kuhnert BR, Kuhnert PM, Debanne S, Williams TG: The relationship between cadmium, zinc and birthweight in pregnant women who smoke. *Am J Obstet Gynecol* 1987; 157: 1247-1251

Li DK, Mueller BA, Hickok DE et al: Maternal smoking during pregnancy and the risk of congenital urinary tract anomalies. *Am J Publ Health* 1996; 86: 249-253

Li JS, Peat JK, Xuan W, Berry G: Meta-analysis of the association between environmental tobacco smoke (ETS) exposure and the prevalence of lower respiratory tract infection in early childhood. *Pediatr Pulmonol* 1999; 27: 5-13

Lieberman E, Torday J, Barbieri K et al.: Association of intrauterine cigarette exposure with indices of fetal lung maturation. *Obstet Gynecol* 1992; 79: 564-570

Lindbohm ML, Sallmén M, Taskinen H: Effet of exposure to environmental tobacco smoke on reproductive health. *Scand J Work Environ Health* 2002; 28 suppl 2: 84-96

Little BB, Snell LM, Klein VR et al: Coccaine abuse during pregnancy: maternal and fetal implications. *Obstet Gynecol* 1989; 73(2): 157-160

Mascola MA, Van Vunakis J, Tager IB et al: Exposure of young infants to environmental tobacco smoke: breast feeding among smoking mothers. *Am J Publ Health* 1998; 88: 893-896

McDonald SD, Perkins SL, Jodouin CA, Walker MC: Folate levels in pregnant women who smoke: An important gene/environment interaction. *Am J Obstet Gynecol* 2002; 187: 620-625

Mick E, Biederman J, Faraone SV et al: Case-control study of attention-deficit/hyperactivity disorders and maternal smoke, alcohol use, and drug use during pregnancy. *J Am Acad Child Adolesc Psychiatry* 2002; 41: 378-385

Midwife CG, Berlin I, Marquis P, Delcroix M: Expired air carbon monoxide concentration in mothers and their spouses above 5 ppm is associated with decreased fetal growth. *Prev Med* 2005; 40: 10-15

Milberger S, Biederman J, Faraone SV et al: Is maternal smoking during pregnancy a risk factor for attention deficit hyperactivity disorders in children? *Am J Psychiatry* 1996; 153: 1138-1142

Naeye R, Peters E: Mental development of children whose mothers smoked during pregnancy. *Obstet Gynecol* 1994; 64: 601-607

Norman MA, Holly EA, Preston-Martin S: Childhood brain tumors and exposure to tobacco smoke. *Cancer Epidemiol Biomarkers Prevention* 1996; 5: 85-91

Olds DL, Henderson ChR, Tatelbaum R: Intellectual impairment in children of women who smoke cigarettes during pregnancy. *Pediatrics* 1994; 93: 221-227

Orlebeke JF, Knol DL, Verhulst FC: Increase in child behavior problems resulting from maternal smoking during pregnancy. *Arch Environ Health* 1997; 52: 317-321

Peacock JL, Bland JM, Anderson HR: Preterm delivery: effects of socioeconomic factors, psychological stress, smoking, alcohol, and caffeine. *BMJ* 1995; 311: 531-536

Poets CF et al: The relationship between bradycardia, apnea and hypoxemia in preterm infants. *Pediatric Res* 1993; 34: 144-147

Pollack HA: Sudden infant death syndrome, maternal smoking during pregnancy, and the cost-effectiveness of smoking cessation intervention. *Am J Publ Health* 2001; 91: 432-436

Raine A, Brennan PA, Mednick SA: Birth complications combined with early maternal rejection at age 1 predispose to violent crime at age 18 years. *Arch Gen Psychiatry* 1994; 51: 984-988

Rantakallio P, *Laara* E, Isohanni M, Moilanen I: Maternal smoking during pregnancy and deliquency of the offspring: An association without causation. *Int J Epidemiol* 1992; 21: 1106-1113

Rantakallio P: A follow-up study up to the age of 14 of children whose mothers smoked during pregnancy. *Acta Pediatr Scand* 1983; 72: 747-753

Rice JM, Ward JM: Age dependence of susceptibility to carcinogenesis in the nervous system. *Ann NY Adac Sci* 1982;381: 274-289

Rylander E, Pershagen C, Ericksson M, Bermann G: Parental smoking, urinary cotinine, and wheezing bronchitis in children. *Epidemiology* 1995; 6: 289-293

Schiverick KT, Salafia C: Cigarette smoking and pregnancy: I. ovarian, uterine and placental effects. *Placenta* 1999; 20:265-272

Schuchardt A, Dagati V, Pachnis V, Constantini F: Renal agenesis and hypodysplasia in ret-k (-) mutant mice result from defects in uretetic bud development. *Developmen*t 1996; 122: 1919-1929

Skorge TD, Eagan TML, Eide GE et al: The adult incidence of asthma and respiratory symptoms by passive smoking in utero or in childhood. *Am J Respir Critic Care Med* 2005; 172: 61-66

Slotkin T: Fetal nicotine or coccaine exposure: Which one is worse? *J Pharmacol Exp Ther* 1998; 285: 931-945

Slotkin TA et al: Loss of neonatal hypoxia tolerance after prenatal nicotine exposure: Implications for sudden infant death syndrome. *Brain Res Bull* 1995; 38: 69-75

Smoking and orofacial clefts: A United Kingdom-based case-control study. Cleft Palate-*Craniofacial J* 2004; 41: 381-386

Spinillo A, Ornetto A, Stronati M et al.: Epidemiologic association between maternal smoking during pregnancy and intracranial hemorrhage in preterm infants. *J Pediatr* 1995; 127: 472-478

Stillman RJ, Rosenberg MJ, Sachs BP: Smoking and reproduction. *Fertil Steril* 1986; 46: 545-566

Strachan DP, Cook DG: Health effects of passive smoking 6: parental smoking and childhood asthma: longitudinal and case-control studies. *Thorax* 1998; 53: 204-212

Surgeon General 2001: Health consequences of tobacco use among women, reproductive outcomes. *Women and smoking*. Rockville, MD, U.S.Department of Health and Human Services, 2001: 272-307

Surgeon General: *The health consequences of smoking for women*. A report of the Surgeon General. Washington, DC: Government Printing Office, 1985; 189-249

Thapar A, Fowler T, Rice F et al: Maternal smoking during pregnancy and attention deficit hyperactivity disorder symptoms in offspring. *Am J Psych* 2003; 160(11): 1985-1989

U.S. Environmental Protection Agency: *Respiratory Health Effects of Passive Smoking*. U.S. EPA, Washington, D.C., 1992

Weissman M, Warner V, Wickramaratne PJ, Kandel DB: Maternal smoking during pregnancy and psychopathology in offspring followed to adulthood. *J Am Acad Child Adolesc Psychiatry* 1999; 38: 892-899

Wilcox AJ: Birth weight and perinatal mortality: the effect of maternal smoking. *Am J Epidemiol* 1993; 137: 1098-1104

Wildstrom AM, Werner S, Matthiensen AS et al: Somatostatin levels in plasma in non-smoking and smoking breast-feeding women. *Acta Paediatr Scand* 1991; 80: 13-21

Williams Cg, Wright B, Partridge I: Attention deficit hyperactivity disorder – a review. *Br J General Pract* 1999; 49: 563-571

Wisborg K, Kesmodel U, Henriksen B et al.: Exposure to tobacco smoke in utero and the risk of stillbirth and death in the first year of life. *Am J Epidemiol* 2001; 154: 322-327

Wyszynski DF, Duffy DL, Beaty TH: Maternal cigarette smoking and oral clefts: A meta-analysis. *Cleft Palate- Craniofacial J* 1997; 34: 206-210

Yang Q, Sherman SL, Hassold TJ et al: Risk factors for trisomy21: Maternal cigarette smoking and oral contraceptive use in a population-based case-control study. *Genetics in Medicine* 1999; 1(3): 80-88

Young S, Sherill DL, Arnott J et al.: Parental factors affecting respiratory function during the first year of life. *Pediatr Pulmonol* 2000; 29: 331-340

In: Smoking and Health Research Frontiers
Editor: Calvin B. Fong, pp. 119-161

ISBN 1-60021-480-0

Chapter VI

ASSESSMENT OF STEROID DISRUPTION AND METAL CONCENTRATIONS IN HUMAN PLACENTA: EFFECTS OF CIGARETTE SMOKING

Martina Piasek[1,*], Michael C. Henson[2], Maja Blanuša[1] and Krista Kostial[1]

[1]Mineral Metabolism Unit, Institute for Medical Research and Occupational Health, HR-10001 Zagreb, Croatia

[2]Department of Biological Sciences, Purdue University Calumet, Hammond, Indiana, 46323-2094, U.S.A.

ABSTRACT

Tobacco smoking is an unhealthy lifestyle linked with infertility and fetal abnormalities. Both first- and second-hand tobacco smoke can result in ill effects on female reproductive integrity and disturbances in the maternal-embryo/feto-placental functional unit. Numerous harmful substances from tobacco smoke can pass the placental barrier or accumulate in placental structures. Cigarette smoke contains several thousands of chemicals and approximately 30 metal ions, including cadmium, arsenic, lead, nickel, chromium, aluminum, antimony, copper, iron, and radioactive elements. Many metals are highly reactive and contribute to the production of oxidative stress, a starting point of toxic and carcinogenic effects of tobacco smoke. In the general population, cigarette smoke is the chief environmental source of cadmium, a confirmed human carcinogen.

By affecting woman's health and the internal environment of her descendant(s), toxic metals may cause immediate and delayed ill effects on virtually all organ systems. Women of childbearing age and growing infants are prone to deficiencies of essential elements (iron, zinc, copper, calcium) and thus are especially sensitive to toxic-essential

* Correspondence concerning this article should be addressed to Martina Piasek, Mineral Metabolism Unit, Institute for Medical Research and Occupational Health, Ksaverska cesta 2, P. O. Box 291, HR-10001 Zagreb, Croatia. Phone: +385 1 4673 188; Facsimile: +385 1 4673 303; E-mail: *mpiasek@imi.hr*

metal interactions. During pregnancy, toxic metals can compromise fetal health directly *in utero*, by passing the placental barrier, and indirectly, by accumulation in the placenta and inhibition of nutrient transfer to the fetus.

Toxic metals can interfere with principal placental functions, maintenance of pregnancy and fetal viability, by affecting the production of placental hormones. Their accumulation in the placenta may compromise prevention of placental-fetal rejection by maternal immune system and fetal response to antigen exposure *in utero*.

Only a few studies so far have validated the concept of placental steroid disruption due to metal exposure. Cadmium ions accumulate in human placental (trophoblast) cells where they suppress progesterone release without apparent inhibition of syncytial development. Increase in placental cadmium is commensurate with a decrease in placental progesterone concentrations in women exposed to cigarette smoke during pregnancy. Animal studies support the findings of cadmium-induced ovarian and placental steroid disruption during pregnancy. A concomitant low iron diet has an additive effect on cadmium-induced placental steroid disruption.

Human placenta can be used as a 'dual purpose specimen' for monitoring harmful substances in both the maternal and internal fetal environment when epidemiological variables for evaluation of exposure conditions are considered. Assessment of placental function by steroid disruption as an indicator of fetal distress *in utero* may serve as a useful noninvasive test for evaluation of risk for infant health in relation to prenatal exposure to common pollutants in environmental tobacco smoke.

> *"It is urgent that we find comprehensive solutions to the danger of tobacco use and address the epidemic among women and girls. Tobacco has been identified as a contributing factor to gender inequity and undermines the principle of women and children's right to health as a basic human right."*
>
> Kobe Declaration, WHO International Conference on Tobacco and Health, 1999 (in Ernster *et al.* 2000)

Cigarette Smoke and Maternal and Child Health: Introductory Remarks

Tobacco smoking has well known negative effects on human health. In the contemporary world, cigarette smoking is one of the most significant preventable causes of morbidity and mortality, and probably the most important preventable risk factor for delivery of low birth weight infants. This unhealthy lifestyle may place the health of future generations at risk by affecting fertility and having a strong link with fetal abnormalities.

Both first-hand, active smoking, and second-hand, passive smoking or so-called environmental tobacco smoke, pose threats for the reproductive integrity of women in childbearing age, to the normal function of the maternal-embryo/feto-placental unit during pregnancy, and to an infant's health during the perinatal period or later in life. Risks of exposure to cigarette smoke for women's health, pregnancy outcome, and developing child are summarized in Table 1.

Table 1. Health risks of cigarette smoking for woman, pregnancy outcome, and developing child.

Health risk for woman	Placental and fetal membrane disorders	Perinatal health risk for child
• primary and secondary infertility • delay in conception/impaired natural fecundity • ectopic pregnancy • uterine bleeding in pregnancy • spontaneous abortion, preterm labors and preterm delivery • cardiovascular diseases (coronary heart disese, ishaemic stroke, subarachnoid hamorrhage) • cancers (lung, oesophagus, mouth and pharynx, bladder, pancreas, kidney, cervix, uterus, breast) • chronic obstructive pulmonary disease, bronchitis and emphysema • decreased bone mineral density, bone loss, and bone fractures	• placenta previa • placental abruption • preterm rupture of membranes	• intrauterine growth retardation (IUGR) • stillborn infant • small for gestation-age infant • low birth weight infant (<2500 g) • death of infant in perinatal period • sudden infant death syndrome (SIDS) • learning and behavioral abnormalities • respiratory distress syndrome • asthma • deformities (orofacial cleft, club foot) • cancer later in life

Effects on Maternal Reproductive Health

Reproductive health risks in women related to exposure to cigarette smoke include impaired fecundity, ectopic pregnancy, improper placentation, and an increased rate of spontaneous abortion, preterm delivery and perinatal mortality.

Augood *et al.* (1998) showed in a systemic review after searching and analyzing data published in a 30-year period (1966-1997) on cigarette smoking and female fertility, a significant association with a 60% increase in the risk of infertility among cigarette smokers. Consistent results across many study populations and research designs and evidence of a dose-response relationship support a causal role of tobacco smoke in preterm birth (Lindbohm *et al.* 2002; Nishijo *et al.* 2002; Shah & Bracken 2000; Kyrklund-Blomberg & Cnattingius 1998; Peacock *et al.* 1995). Cigarette smoking may increase the incidence of spontaneous abortions, placenta previa and placental abruption, bleeding during pregnancy, premature rupture of placental membranes, perinatal mortality, and stillbirth rates (Gardella & Hill 2000; Ananth *et al.* 1996; Chelmow *et al.* 1996; Kendrick & Merritt 1996; Economides & Braithwaite 1994). Tuthill *et al.* (1999) re-evaluated, in more than 1200 cases of stillbirth or infant death, the relationship between maternal cigarette smoking and pregnancy outcome against changes in smoking habits and the causes of perinatal death by the end of 20th century and found that smoking during pregnancy continues to be strongly associated with fetal and infant mortality.

Effects on Child Health

In 1999, the World Health Organization convened an International Consultation of Environmental Tobacco Smoke and Child Health. It was concluded that environmental tobacco smoke is a real and substantial threat to child health, causing many thousands of preventable fetal and neonatal death and suffering throughout the world (ASH/WHO 1999). Disorders include lower respiratory tract infections (pneumonia, bronchitis), coughing and wheezing, worsening of asthma, tonsillitis, and middle ear disease. This association appears to be strongest during the first years of life (Forastiere *et al.* 1994).

Tobacco smoke contains numerous substances that double the risk of fetal malformations, including cleft lip or cleft palate and clubfoot, and may affect fetal growth by several mechanisms (Chung *et al.* 2000). The teratogenicity of cigarette smoke has been widely researched over the past two decades, in large part due to the percentage of pregnant women who smoke (in Mattson *et al.* 2002). Maternal smoking during pregnancy is a major cause of sudden infant death syndrome (Getahun *et al.* 2004). Another well-documented health effect is low birth weight. Smoking during pregnancy is the principal cause of low birth weight (<2500 g) in developing countries, even by exposure to passive smoke. Environmental tobacco smoke among nonsmoking pregnant women can cause decreases in birth weight and fetal biometric parameters at early gestation as well as preterm delivery (Henke *et al.* 2004; Lindbohm *et al.* 2002). Infant exposure to passive smoking may contribute to the risk of sudden infant death syndrome (ASH/WHO 1999). Babies with low birth weights face an increased risk of serious health disorders during the newborn period and chronic disabilities such as cerebral palsy, mental retardation, behavior problems, and learning abnormalities (Wasserman *et al.* 2001; Eskenazi & Castorina 1999; Rush & Callahan 1989). In a critical review on passive smoking and infants, children and adolescents, Denson (2001) pointed out that when evaluating the health impact of environmental tobacco smoke, the effects of nutritional factors and socioeconomic factors should always be taken into consideration.

Some aspects of adult health appear to be programmed *in utero*. Exposure of children to environmental tobacco smoke may contribute to chronic diseases in adulthood, such as high blood pressure and cardiovascular diseases, diabetes mellitus, infertility, neurobehavioral impairments, and cancer in later life (Milunsky *et al.* 2000; ASH/WHO 1999; Gidding *et al.* 1994).

Effects on Placenta

Child health depends upon a healthy placenta, an organ that creates a healthy internal environment for the fetus. Placenta comprises the maternal-fetal interface and has a unique structure and functions. Recent experimental studies and evidence in humans reinforces our understanding that normal structure and function of the placenta and its extraembryonic membranes, as well as proper timing of neuro-endocrine events within and between placental, fetal, and maternal compartments, are crucial for the survival and growth of the developing mammal *in utero* (Red-Horse *et al.* 2004; Mooney & Giudice 2002). Placenta is a unique organ with two separate blood sources, maternal and fetal, and a defined, limited life span. Normal placental functions include nutrient transfer, the transfer of metabolites, and the activation and deactivation of environmental chemicals. The maternal-feto-placental unit is a major site of protein and steroid hormone productions and secretion that is necessary for the maintenance of pregnancy and its termination with delivery at term (Mooney & Giudice 2002; Strauss *et al.* 1996; Solomon 1988; Pasqualini & Kincl 1985; Ferré *et al.* 1985, 1978). Placenta transfers various substances from mother to fetus, such as oxygen, nutrients, hormones, and both essential and toxic metals. Wastes and carbon dioxide are transferred from fetus to mother.

Cigarette smoking during pregnancy can decrease uterine blood flow and have an effect on placental vasculature that may consequently compromise fetal-placental blood flow and contribute to decreased birth weight (Page *et al.* 2002; Larsen al 2002; Rath *et al.* 2001; Bush *et al.* 2000a,b; Clausen *et al.* 1999; Castro *et al.* 1993). The small stem villous arteries in placentas of heavy smokers are found to be changed compared to those of nonsmokers in their mechanical properties and in vasoconstrictive response to exogenously administered endothelin-1 (Clausen *et al.* 1999). In mothers who smoke during pregnancy, reduced dimensions in fetal villous capillaries may modify placental blood flow and diminish the area for exchange of nutrients and gasses between mother and fetus. These factors may contribute to an increased risk of fetal undernourishment and reduced birth weight (Larsen al 2002; Bush *et al.* 2000b; Demir *et al.* 1994). Furthermore, there is evidence that environmental tobacco smoke can also cause the impairment of villous structure and may hinder maternal-fetal transfer, leading to adverse effects on the fetus as it was noticed in active smokers (Rath *et al.* 2001). The study of Albuquerqe *et al.* (2004) confirms that maternal cigarette smoking during pregnancy is associated with chronically increased vascular resistance in the uterine arteries with consequent reduced blood flow velocity in the umbilical-placental circulation. It gives new evidence of heavy smoking-related vascular resistance in middle cerebral arteries of the fetal brain.

Effects on Steroid Hormones

Constituents of cigarette smoke may affect or modify hormones, enzymes, and drugs in the organism (Tansavatdi *et al.* 2004; Paakki *et al.* 2000; Zevin and Benowitz 1999). Endocrine effects of tobacco smoking have also been demonstrated. The parts of the endocrine system that cigarette smoke may affect include: neuroendocrine functions and the hypothalamic-pituitary axis, function of thyroid gland, adrenal cortical hormone concentrations, glucose-ragulating hormonal function of pancreas, gastric empting, bone mass, and gonadal and reproductive functions in females, with less dramatic effects in males (Tziomalos & Cahrsoulis 2004; Shiverick & Salafia 1999).

Steroid hormones mediate a wide variety of vital physiological functions, ranging from anti-inflammatory agents to regulating events during pregnancy. They are synthesized and secreted into the bloodstream by the gonads (ovary and testis), placenta, and the adrenal cortex. Steroid sex hormones primarily affect maturation and function of secondary sex organs (estrogens and androgens), mediate the menstrual cycle, and maintain the pregnancy (progestins). These hormones are pleiotropic and act on multiple targets, in addition to their immunomodulatory role. Abnormal hormone levels may provide a mechanism (genetic, infectious) for triggering autoimmune disease (Szekeres-Bartho *et al.* 2001; Verthelyi 2001).

Estrogens

Estrogens (estrone and estradiol) are principally female steroid hormones. They are critical for the regulation of the reproductive cycle and bone remodeling and mineralization. Estrogens also affect the cardiovascular and nervous systems. Estrogens and estrogen receptors (proteins that mediate estrogen action) play major roles in the proliferation of mammary cells as well as in the origin and progression of breast cancer (Thomas *et al.* 2004).

Epidemiological studies conducted during the last two decades provide evidence that women who smoke cigarettes are relatively estrogen-deficient. Both pregnant and nonpregnant women who smoke have decreased endogenous estrogens (Shiverick & Salafia 1999; Baron *et al.* 1990; Bernstein *et al.* 1989, Baron 1984; Mochizuki *et al.* 1984; MacMahon *et al.* 1982). Barbieri *et al.* (1986) found in preparations of term placental microsomes that several nicotinic alkaloids (nicotine, cotinine and anabasine) directly inhibited aromatase and consequent conversion of testosterone (androstenedione) to estrogen. These results corroborate earlier findings of Mochizuki *et al.* (1984) of lower conversion of dehydroepiandrosterone sulphate to estradiol in pregnant women when comparing heavy smokers and nonsmokers. These results may explain, at least in part, the decreased estrogen levels observed in smoking women. Bernstein *et al.* (1989) have shown that smoking is associated with decreased concentrations of serum estradiol, human chorionic gonadotropin (hCG), and sex-hormone binding globulin in early pregnancy. The authors suggest that decreased hormone concentrations should be considered as a possible mechanism of spontaneous abortion, one of the harmful effects of smoking on pregnancy outcome.

Indirect evidence for a smoking-estrogen interaction is an elimination of the protective effect of oral estrogens on bone metabolism and an enhanced risk for hip fracture among women who smoke (Tanko & Christiansen 2004; Kiel *et al.* 1992). Smoking diminishes the beneficial effects of orally administered estrogens on osteoporosis prevention, hot flashes, urogenital symptoms, lipid metabolism, as well as positive estrogenic effects on the vasculature. The main cause seems to be a dose-dependent elevated hepatic clearance, partially in conjunction with lower estrogen levels (Mueck & Seeger 2003).

It should be also mentioned that a variety of mechanisms for potentially 'beneficial effects' of smoking have been proposed with three predominating: the anti-estrogenic effect of smoking, alterations in prostaglandin production, and stimulation of nicotinic cholinergic receptors in the central nervous system. Baron (1996) critically considered possible 'beneficial effects' and inverse associations of smoking with uterine fibroids and endometriosis, endometrial cancer, hypertensive disorders and vomiting during pregnancy, Alzheimer's dementia, and Parkinson's disease. The overall conclusion was that, although established, these inverse associations cannot provide a suitable rationale to consider cigarette smoking-related effects as 'beneficial' for estrogen-related disorders and diseases. The findings can be used only as additional evidence to clarify mechanisms and point to productive treatment or preventive options with more narrowly acting interventions of certain diseases (Tansavatdi *et al.* 2004; Mueck & Seeger 2003; Baron 1996).

Progesterone

This sex hormone is needed for preparing the uterus for implantation of the fertilized ovum (blastocyst). Progesterone originates almost entirely from the corpus luteum before six weeks' gestational age. From the 7th week of pregnancy, the placenta assumes responsibility for steroid production until the end of gestation, and beyond 12 weeks, the placenta is the major source of progesterone. It utilizes steroid precursors contributed by both maternal and fetal compartments. Maternal low-density lipoprotein (LDL)-carried cholesterol is the chief substrate for progesterone synthesis and both maternal and fetal pro-hormones are converted into active steroids in the placenta (Strauss *et al.* 2000, 1996).

Among the steroidogenic enzymes expressed by the primate placenta and involved in progesterone formation, cytochrome P-450 cholesterol side-chain cleavage (P450scc) and 3β-hydroxysteroid dehydrogenase (3β-HSD) are the key components (Miller 1988; Falcone *et al.* 1980). Steroidogenic enzyme P450scc catalyzes the conversion of cholesterol into pregnenolone, which is then converted into progesterone via 3β-HSD. Theoretically, the absence or disruption of functional enzyme(s) P450scc and/or 3β-HSD would prevent placental progesterone synthesis, as well as fetal adrenal and gonadal steroidogenesis.

It was shown that cigarette smoke-derived alkaloids inhibit cellular progesterone synthesis both by inhibiting progesterone synthesis and by causing less specific toxic effects in steroidogenic cells (cultured Leydig tumor cells) (Goecze & Freeman 2000). Cytotoxic effects of cigarette smoke-derived alkaloids and dose-related inhibition of progesterone production could be the mechanism(s) mediating reduced fertilization, implantation, and early human development, as well as impaired placental growth, disorders in the placental vasculature, and small-for-date babies. In contrast, slight stimulation or no effect on estradiol production was found. These concomitant actions of cigarette alkaloids may partly explain the higher incidence of early abortion in pregnant women who smoke (Göcze & Freeman 2000; Göcze *et al.* 1999).

In human placentas, progesterone disruption with concomitant twofold placental cadmium increase was found in urban cigarette smokers (Piasek *et al.* 2001). Evidence for the inhibitory effects of the smoke constituent cadmium on more than one site of the steroid biosynthetic pathway (prior to or after cholesterol side-chain cleavage) has been observed in male and female rat gonads (Piasek & Laskey 1999, 1994; Laskey & Phelps 1991), as well as by *in vitro* cadmium exposure in human placental (trophoblast) cells (Kawai *et al.* 2002; Jolibois *et al.* 1999a,b). Detailed results of the investigations of cadmium-induced endocrine disruption in the placenta are presented later in this chapter.

Cigarette Smoke as a Source of Exposure to Metal Ions

Tobacco smoke is a mixture of more than 4000 known components, of which about 60 are toxic and/or carcinogenic (Shiverick & Salafia 1999; Smith *et al.* 1997; Hoffman *et al.* 1997; Mulcahy 1997). It is composed of volatile and particulate phases. The gaseous portion comprises 95% of tobacco smoke by weight and about 500 gaseous compounds have been identified in this phase. The particulate phase comprises 5% of tobacco smoke and contains 3500 different compounds, of which the major one is nicotine. The particulate matter minus its alkaloid and water contents is tar, in which many carcinogens have been identified. Among their various biological effects, tobacco smoke constituents induce several drug-metabolizing enzymes that may increase the risk of cancer (Zevin and Benowitz 1999). The substances that may interact with metabolizing enzymes include polycyclic aromatic hydrocarbons, acetone, pyridine, benzene, nicotine carbon monoxide, as well as heavy metals.

Metal concentration ranges determined in smoke of various cigarettes' types are given in Table 2.

Table 2. Metal concentrations in smoke of various cigarettes' types.

Metal	Concentration in cigarette smoke [μg/cigarette]
Cadmium*	0.0-6.67[a]
Arsenic*	0.0-1.4[a]
Lead	0.017-0.98[b]
Nickel*	0.0-0.51[a,b]
Chromium*	0.0002-0.5[a]
Beryllium*	0.0-0.0005[a]
Aluminium	0.22[b]
Copper	0.19[b]
Zinc	0.12-1.21[b]
Magnesium	0.070[b]
Iron	0.042[b]
Mercury	0.004[b]
Manganese	0.003[b]
Selenium	0.001-0.063[b]

*IARC Group I Carcinogens

Sources: [a]Smith *et al.* 1997; [b]IARC 1986

Trace amounts of at least 30 elemental metals have been detected in the tobacco plant and are transferred to mainstream smoke. These are: cadmium, arsenic, lead, nickel, chromium, aluminium, antimony, copper, iron, and radioactive elements polonium-210, lead-210, potassium-40 and radium-226. Concentrations of many of them have been determined (Smith *et al.* 1997; Stohs *et al.* 1997; Chiba & Masironi 1992; Huber 1989). Most metals in tobacco smoke are present as particulate matter because of their relatively high melting point (greater than 200 °C), with the exception of mercury. The concentrations of metal ions in tobacco smoke are dependent on the soil in which tobacco was grown, fertilizers and agricultural spray used, the variety of tobacco, and how the tobacco leaves were processed. Metal ion concentrations are greater in mainstream than in sidestream smoke. Chief toxic metals present in highest concentration in cigarette smoke are cadmium, arsenic, and lead.

Much of the remainder of this chapter deals with the data on assessment of exposure to metals in cigarette smoke by using human placenta as an indicator tissue for metals, primarily cadmium, exposure. It focuses primarily on novel data that describes the relationships of cadmium accumulation and steroid hormone disruption in placental tissue that may be used as markers of cigarette smoke-related fetal distress in the assessment of perinatal health risks.

Usage of Human Placenta for Metal Biomonitoring and Steroid Disruption Evaluation: Methods and Techniques

Thirty years ago, Baglan *et al.* (1974) proposed the use of human placenta as a unique sampling tissue for the biological monitoring of metal exposure of mother and fetus. Since that time a number of papers evaluated metal exposure in different parts of the world using occasionally human placenta as an indicator organ. However, in context of health-related biomonitoring, placenta as a specimen has not received as much attention as it deserves. In a series of extensive reviews Iyengar & Rapp (2001a,b,c) recently presented advantages and examples of using human placenta as a 'dual purpose specimen' for monitoring harmful substances in both fetal and maternal environment, with the emphasis on the assessment of exposure and health risks of toxic metals for the maternal-fetal-placental unit.

Placenta could be considered an alternative to repeated maternal blood sampling for assessing exposure to metal(s) *in utero,* as well as risk for fetal distress. During pregnancy cadmium bioaccumulates in placental tissue. Under selected circumstances, placental cadmium can be used for monitoring of cadmium exposure (Lagerkvist *et al.* 1996), as well as a biomarker of exposure to cigarette smoke (Myllynen *et al.* 2005). Both human and animal data indicate that lead readily crosses the placenta and produces lead concentrations in neonates comparable to those found in maternal blood. In that capacity, placenta is not as good an indicator for lead exposure as it is for cadmium. Indeed, Lagerkvist *et al.* (1996) found that in lead-polluted areas, higher lead concentrations in both maternal and umbilical cord bloods were not commensurate with low concentation of lead in the placenta. In addition, as the concentration of lead in cigarette smoke is much lower than of cadmium (as presented in Table 2), placenta is definitely inappropriate indicator tissue for monitoring cigarette smoke-related lead exposure. Iyengar & Rapp (2001c) suggested that, if the toxic trace element concentrations in placental tissue are high (as placental cadmium is in smokers), such information could be used to diminish postnatal exposure of the fetus or maternal exposure during subsequent pregnancies.

The limited life span of the placenta presents an opportunity for evaluation of exposure to a xenobiotic and their effects during pregnancy. When using human placenta to biologically monitor metals one should keep on mind following major facts. First, a major redistribution of mineral elements occurs between the maternal and fetal body compartments, so placental metal concentrations reflect a woman's whole body burden of metals, which accumulated not only during pregnancy but also before the pregnancy. Second, usage of human placenta in assessing metal exposure and metal effects necessitates equally the proficient analytical procedures and the meticulous evaluation of specific epidemiological variables (Miller *et al.* 1988, 1983). Third, placenta is the main biosynthetic source of progesterone during pregnancy. From the luteal phase to term, maternal progesterone levels raise six- to eight-fold (Mooney & Giudice 2002). Therefore, placental tissue could be used for assessment of its function to produce progesterone, and placental progesterone concentration can serve as a biomarker of endocrine disruption in relation to toxic metal exposure.

Assessment of Epidemiological Variables

In assessing placental metal concentrations, the environment from which the placental specimen has been obtained should be carefully evaluated by collecting detailed information about each subject included in an investigation. This includes: a complete medical history; social, active smoking and eating habits (typical meals to identify source of both toxic and essential element intake); information concerning where the subject lived and worked; and information on the smoking habits of immediate family members and colleagues at work (environmental tobacco smoke data). To avoid confounding factors (major health problems during pregnancy, chronic diseases, and heterogeneity of placental samples due to relative differences in gestational lengths) otherwise healthy young women who deliver at term with no history of major health problems and with uncomplicated pregnancies should be included in an investigation.

To effectively gather relevant data on epidemiological variables, an appropriately designed questionnaire should be administered (Table 3). The questionnaire should include questions to enable collection of as much detailed data as possible for evaluation of the placental data from each parturient. Data from medical histories should be also used.

Before collecting epidemiological data and the placentas, medico-legal and ethical issues should be properly addressed. This includes obtaining informed and/or written consent from each participant and officially signed approval(s) of respective institutional Bioethical Committee(s).

Table 3. Questionnaire for collecting relevant data from a parturient whose placenta is examined that should be taken into consideration with data on placental biomarkers.

General personal data	Age Place of birth
Professional history	Education Position Current employment
Data on potential recent environmental exposure	Place of living Moving in last 24 months Vicinity of factory or smelter Vicinity of highway, street/road, big cross-roads or bus terminal with heavy traffic
General health status	Height Body weight at term Average weight before pregnancy Body weight gain during pregnancy
Data on the last pregnancy and delivery	Number of previous pregnancies (parity) Week of pregnancy when gave birth Specific health problems during pregnancy (blood pressure, peripheral edema, blood glucose) Reasons for potential sick-leaves Other health problems Previous abortions or miscarriages Twins
Data on the newborn	Sex of baby Weight and length at birth Viability score at birth in 1st and 5th minute (by Apgar)
Maternal dietary history	Self-identification of the predominate diet type: mixed, vegetarian, vegetarian plus eggs, vegetarian plus eggs plus diary products Frequency of consuming fish, shellfish, canned fish (per wk) Alcohol consumption (quantity and quality, *per die*m, per wk) Caffeine consumption (quantity and quality, *per die*m, per wk)
Smoking habit	Self-classification as active, passive or previous smoker. • For active smokers: number of cigarettes or packages *per diem*; age when started; smoking during last pregnancy. • For nonsmokers: data on potential passive smoking; data on active smokers in the family and at workplace; duration of exposure (in hours) to passive smoking *per diem*

Assessment of Cigarette Smoking as a Source of Metal (Cadmium) Exposure

Analysis of nicotine in urine or hair (Kalinić *et al.* 2003) or nicotine metabolite in biologic samples (cotinine in blood, saliva, or urine) during pregnancy and/or at term (Berny *et al.* 2002; Husgafvel-Pursiainen 2002) provides an objective and reliable assessment of perinatal exposure to cigarette smoke. Finding nicotine/cotinine at certain concentrations in persons who report nonsmoking may indicate passive smoking exposure (Henke *et al.* 2004).

Smoking life-style assessments can be based on self-reported individual active smoking habits and/or second-hand smoking exposures. Self-reporting has been widely used to document the prevalence and consequences of smoking in pregnancy when assessing metal exposure and their effects (Piasek *et al.* 2001; Kantola *et al.* 2000; Zadorozhnaja *et al.* 2000; Clausen *et al.* 1999; Demir *et al.* 1994; Miller *et al.* 1988). However, underreporting cigarette smoke exposure can decrease the likelihood of identifying differences between 'smoking' and 'nonsmoking' groups. When increased placental cadmium in the 'smoking' group is identified, it suggests that underreporting exposure has not undermined the validity of the results obtained in 'smokers' vs. group designated as 'nonsmokers' based upon self-reporting. Page *et al.* (2002) showed that self-declared smoking rate correlates with placental tissue cadmium, concentration of cotinine (nicotine metabolite) in plasma and placental enzyme ethoxyresofurin *o*-deethylase (EROD), which is dependent on cytochrome P450 and induced by cigarette smoking.

It is usually difficult to evaluate the impact of passive smoking apart from active smoking on any biomarker of effect when using either self-reported data or nicotine/cotinine concentrations as indicators of exposure to cigarette smoke. For example, for research purposes, 'smokers' could be considered persons who smoked during pregnancy (any period of time) and former smokers who stopped smoking some time within 12 months before the onset of the last pregnancy. All others are then designated as 'nonsmokers'. Our investigation (Piasek *et al.* 2001) showed that persons in the group designated as 'smokers' (according to above criteria) smoked on average 12 (3 to 20) cigarettes per day, and claimed that most of them (23 of 27) lived and/or worked with 1-2 family members who were active smokers (mostly their husbands) and spent about 9.5 h per day in environmental tobacco smoke. In the group of 'nonsmokers', less than half the women (12 of 29) claimed exposure to environmental tobacco smoke (again, mostly husbands) for about only 3.5 h per day. These findings suggest, first, that smoking habit is rather 'social' than 'individual' habit as active smokers are more frequently surrounded with other smoking persons than nonsmokers, and, second, findings in the group designated as 'smokers' are actually results of the total environmental tobacco smoke exposure and effects and not only a consequence of an active smoking.

Procedures with Placental Samples

Obtaining representative samples of placenta for element assessment is not a simple task due to placental size (a relatively large organ of around 800 g), the heterogeneity of placental cells, and the fact that decidual matter is tainted with both maternal and fetal blood. Placentas should be collected immediately after birth, preferably at term and from uncomplicated pregnancies. It is advisable to collect the entire placenta with the umbilical cord. Minimum sample manipulation rules should be followed wherever and whenever possible to avoid external metal contamination of the specimens. Further preparatory work is to be carried out in a clean analytical laboratory.

Two types of procedures with placental samples are described. They are in current use by the investigators whose results on placental metals and placental steroids are presented in detail in this chapter.

Procedures for Assessing Exposures In Vivo

To assure homogeneity for placental assay, it is advisable to either homogenize the entire placenta to obtain representative tissue samples or, as an alternative method of procuring representative samples, to randomly sample from multiple sites, pool, and homogenize. Usually, it is sufficient to take 2-3 representative full-thickness samples from the maternal part of the placenta, after trimming away the extraembryonic membranes and excluding chorionic plate and decidua basalis. One sample should be taken from a section from the midline of the placental disc, avoiding the region of umbilical cord insertion, and other (peripheral) samples from between the central region and periphery, the outermost 3 cm within the placental disc edge (Piasek *et al.* 2001; Paszkowski & Sikorski 1994; Manci & Blackburn 1987). Further procedures to be used with placental samples depend on particular analysis (of metals or steroids) and are described under respective subheadings.

Procedures for Assesing Exposures In Vitro

Placental villous tissue is enzymatically dispersed and cytotrophoblast purified via density gradient centrifugation (Henson *et al.* 1996; Kliman *et al.* 1986). Purified cytotrophoblast cells are suspended in Dulbecco Modified Eagle medium (DMEM, containing 44 mM sodium bicarbonate, 25 mM HEPES, 25 mM glucose and 4 mM glutamine plus 10% fetal bovine serum). The initial cell suspension is adjusted to a final concentration of $1x10^6$ cells/ml, containing desirable dose of metal (eg. cadmium as 0, 5, 10, or 20 mM $CdCl_2$). Cells are then cultured in 24-well culture plates (at 37 °C in a humidified atmosphere of 10% CO_2: 90% air for 96 h). In culture, cytotrophoblast differentiates into morphologically and endocrinologically active syncytiotrophoblast prior to 96 h (Henson *et al.* 1996).

To assess enzymatic (P450scc and 3β-HSD) activities, trophoblast cells are cultured under conditions (with or without pregnenolone and with or without 25-hydroxycholesterol or aminoglutethimide) designed to assess their respective steps in the progesterone biosynthetic pathway. Because 25-hydroxycholesterol (25-OHC) readily transverses the plasma and mitochondrial membranes, its conversion to progesterone provides an index of P450scc activity. Similarly, because aminoglutethimide is an inhibitor of P450scc-mediated hydroxylation, addition of this compound along with pregnenolone enables progesterone production to serve as an index of 3β -HSD activity. Therefore, trophoblast cells are cultured in DMEM plus 10% fetal bovine serum for 72 h and then incubated for 24 h with DMEM plus 10% steroid-stripped fetal bovine serum in the absence or presence of metal ions (5, 10, or 20 mM $CdCl_2$). After the incubation, trophoblast cells are incubated for 4 h (96-100 h in culture with DMEM plus 10% steroid-stripped fetal bovine serum) in the absence or presence of metal ion (20 mM $CdCl_2$, or 90 mM aminoglutethimide and 5 mg/ml pregnenolone, or 20 mg/ml 25-OHC). In some cultures, trophoblast cells are incubated in DMEM plus 10% steroid-stripped fetal bovine serum, in the absence or presence of metal ion (20 mM $CdCl_2$) between 72 and 96 h, and then 8-bromo-cAMP (1 mM) is added, in the absence or presence of metal ion (20 mM $CdCl_2$, for 48 h; 96-144 h in culture). Culture medium from all experiments is then stored at minus 20 °C until assayed for progesterone or lactate dehydrogenase (LDH) activity. Cellular protein (solubilized for 24 h in 0.1 N NaOH) is measured using bovine serum albumin as a standard (Bradford 1976).

Analysis of Trace Elements in Placental Tissue

Recommendations of tissue collection, sample preparation, and quality assurance of analytical techniques for metal analyses in human placentas should be followed (Miller *et al.* 1988, 1983; Friberg 1983; van Hattum *et al.* 1981).

Great variety of instrumental analytical methods and techniques can be applied to determine cadmium and other toxic and essential metals in clinical and biological materials. These methods include anodic stripping voltammetry (ASV), neutron activation analysis (NAA), X-ray fluorescence (XRF), inductively coupled plasma atomic emission spectrometry (ICP-AES), inductively coupled plasma mass spectrometry (ICP-MS) and atomic absoption spectrometry (Evans *et al.* 2004; Taylor *et al.* 2004). Kubala-Kukuś *et al.* (2003) successfully applied the total reflection X-ray fluorescence (TXRF) method to determine 18 elements in full-term placenta and fetal membrane samples. Most recent methods for simultaneous determination of a number of trace elements at the nanogram- and picogram-per-gram levels involve inductively coupled plasma mass spectrometry (ICP-MS). The latest method has been successfully used for determination of cadmium in placentas of nonsmokers and smokers (Page *et al.* 2002).

The most common and feasible method for quantitative determination of cadmium in the placentas is atomic absoption spectrometry (AAS). Since the ranges of cadmium and lead concentrations are at the ppb-level, electrothermal (ETAAS) method with graphite tube atomizer is considered suitable enough (Herber *et al.* 2004, 1985; Piasek *et al.* 2004, 2001). For placental iron, zinc and copper, flame AAS method can be used (Piasek *et al.* 2001; van Hattum *et al.* 1981). When using AAS methods, background correction is very important. For that purpose a deuterium continuum source or Zeeman correction is used. The latest method is more efficient in compensating interferences.

Preparation of Samples

Pretreatment of the material is of utmost importance for all the methods applied. For AAS analysis of cadmium lead, iron, zinc and copper in placentas so-called dry ashing method of organic matrix destruction is adequate. For example, representative samples for metal analyses (cubes of approximately 2 g from central and peripheral sections) are rinsed in saline, blotted on filter paper, weighed, dried to a constant weight (at 105 °C), and dry ashed at maximum temperature of 450 °C in a muffle furnace (Blanuša & Breški 1981). To avoid metal contamination, crucibles for sample ashing procedure should be made of quartz or platinum. For graphite furnace AAS measurements, ash should be dissolved in the lowest possible concentration of nitric acid (4% v/v). At higher acid concentrations the graphite tube would deteriorate prematurely. Both deionized water and acid should be of highest purity (*pro analysi; p. a.).*

Reliability of the Analytical Method

Validation of the method should be confirmed by analysis of a certified reference material to yield analytical data with sufficient reliability. The chemical composition of the standard reference material should be as close as possible to the analyzed material. Usually bovine liver from the National Institute of Standards and Technology (U.S.A.) is used for biological materials, and it is a reliable standard to validate analytical methods used for placental tissue samples (Piasek *et al.* 2004; Jureša & Blanuša 2003; Blanuša *et al.* 2002, 2001, 1999; 1985; Matek Sarić 2002; Piasek *et al.* 2001).

Analysis of Progesterone in Placental Tissue

Representative samples (cubes of approximately 1 g from central and peripheral sections) should be taken by cutting through the organ, rinsed in saline, blotted on filter paper and weighted. Samples should then be placed in test tubes, homogenized, and steroids extracted by ethanol, hexane or ether/ethyl acetate (Piasek *et al.* 2001; Ferré *et al.* 1978). Samples or supernatants with extracted steroids can be freeze-dried (lyophilized) and reconstituted in deionized water before assay. Progesterone can be measured by the usual methods for steroid assay (eg. specific radioimunnoassay, RIA). When using routine methods one should keep in mind that progesterone concentrations commonly measured in clinical practice in serum or plasma (50 to 200 ng/ml) are significantly lower than those found in full-term placentas (on average 1000 to 3000 ng/g fresh tissue weight) (Piasek *et al.* 2001; Pasqualini & Kincl 1985; Ferré *et al.* 1985; 1978).

Statistical Analysis of the Data

Data should be subjected to proper statistical evaluation. Either one-way or two-way analysis of variance (ANOVA) using the least-square means for each study group (control vs. exposed, eg. 'smokers' vs. 'nonsmokers') can be applied. Correlations between placental biomarkers (placental metals, placental steroids) and other health effect parameters (birth weight, birth length, placental weight) or toxic metal-essential element correlations can be analyzed, too.

BIOMARKERS OF METAL EXPOSURE AND STEROID DISRUPTION IN THE PLACENTA: RESULTS AND THEIR SIGNIFICANCE

Risk of Maternal and Perinatal Exposure to Metals in Tobacco Smoke

The problem of exposure to toxic heavy metals, ubiquitous inorganic xenobiotics, such as lead, cadmium, arsenic and mercury, and their biological effects have been a source of growing concern during last decades (Merian *et al.* 2004; WHO/EHC 2002, 2001, 1995,1992a,b, 1991, 1989; Zalups & Koropatnick 2000; ATSDR 2000, 1999a,b,c; Goyer 1997,1995). Exposure to metals may affect the reproductive health of women and the internal environment of their descendants causing immediate or delayed adverse health effects in virtually all organ systems.

Vulnerable population groups, such as women of childbearing age and infants, have a greater risk for toxic effects of metals as they are prone to deficiencies of essential elements iron, zinc, copper, and calcium. Female gender (including periods of gestation and lactation) and age (period of intensive growth and development) are two factors that put these groups at higher risk for increased accumulation and ill effects of toxic metals due to specific anatomical changes and physiological requirements for nutrients. These groups have increased demands for essential trace elements, particularly iron, zinc, copper, iodine, that leads to higher intestinal absorption and body burden of not only essential micronutrients, but also non-essential, toxic metals (Nishijo *et al.* 2004; Satarug *et al.* 2004; Åkesson *et al.* 2002; Laeser *et al.* 2002; Vahter *et al.* 2002; WHO/EHC 2002; Bhattacharyya *et al.* 2000; Goyer 1997; Kostial *et al.* 1991a,b).

During pregnancy a major redistribution of accumulated minerals and trace elements occurs in mothers. Some accumulate in placental tissue, and some pass the placenta more or less efficiently. If a woman had been exposed to a toxic metal that has accumulated in the body, pregnancy will increase its mobilization from the body stores. Examples of this include lead from hard tissue (skeleton and teeth) and cadmium from the kidney (Gulson *et al.* 1997; Silbergeld 1991; Carmichael *et al.* 1982). Toxic metals, such as lead, inorganic arsenic, and methylmercury, can compromise fetal health *in utero* by directly traversing the placental barrier. Indirect health effects of metals, such as cadmium, may occur due to toxicant accumulation in the placental tissue structures that affect major placental functions, transplacental nutrient passage, and steroid hormone production.

Essential trace elements together with vitamins A, C and E, and folic acid are critical for normal development and growth of the embryo and fetus *in utero*. Brain and nervous system development are particularly sensitive to zinc and folic acid deficiency. In a rapidly growing embryo, micronutrient status can dramatically affect the immune system as well. The effects may influence protective mechanisms needed for the prevention of placental-fetal rejection by the maternal immune system or may alter the fetal response to antigen exposure *in utero*. The latter can bring about allergic diseases in early childhood. Folic acid and essential elements, zinc, iron, and calcium, are of particular importance for prevention of poor pregnancy outcomes. If gestation is shortened and birth is premature, there is a failure to accumulate adequate stores of essential trace elements by the fetus, which may result in deficiencies during the postnatal period (WHO/EHC 2002; Bendich 2001). All of these ill effects can be caused by exposure to cigarette smoke.

Specific Features of Metals in Cigarette Smoke

Many of metal ions in cigarette smoke are highly reactive. They may interact with metabolising enzymes (cadmium, arsenic, nickel, lead, chromium), and some of them (nickel, chromium and cobalt) are known as antigens and/or contact allergens (Vahter *et al.* 2002; Huber 1989). Among nine agents in mainstream smoke listed as "IARC Group I human carcinogens", there are five metals: cadmium, arsenic, nickel, chromium, and beryllium (Smith *et al.* 1997).

A growing body of evidence indicates the roles of reactive oxygen species in the toxicity of transition metals. Multiple mechanisms have been proposed in the production of reactive oxygen involving these metal ions. Many highly reactive metal ions that are present in the highest concentrations in tobacco smoke are also known to actively participate in the production of oxidative stress. Mechanisms involving redox cycling with the production of superoxide anion, hydrogen peroxide, and hydroxyl radical appear to be involved for iron, copper, and chromium. Other metal ions, such as cadmium, lead, mercury, nickel, arsenic, and antimony, may deplete glutathione and protein-bound sulfhydryl groups, thus contributing to oxidative stress in this manner. Enhanced lipid peroxidation, increased DNA damage, altered calcium and sulfhydryl homeostasis, and altered redox status of NADPH may occur. As a consequence, protein damage may occur including enzyme activities with changes in membrane structure and function, cellular injury and possibly mutation. Finally, the production of toxic metabolites may be elicited (Stohs & Bagchi 1995). Metal ions can act as catalysts for the formation of reactive oxygen species and various free radicals by numerous organic, redox cycling constituents such as hydroquinone and catechol, which are present in tobacco smoke, thus greatly enhancing the potential for tissue damaging effects (eg. in lungs). In addition, radioactive elements such as polonium-210 in tobacco smoke contribute to tissue damage (Chiba & Masironi 1992). The cumulative and additive effects of metal ions are believed to play a significant role in the toxicity and carcinogenicity of tobacco smoke (Stohs *et al.* 1997).

Lead

Cigarette smoke can contribute to environmental (mainly food and air, and in some areas water) exposure to lead and its effect on all organ systems. A large body of literature clearly shows that severe lead intoxication in the past has been associated with sterility and miscarriages. Increases in neonatal mortality and morbidity along with delayed neurotoxic and behavioral effects have been reported due to high perinatal lead exposure. Lead is readily transferred to the fetus and may have direct effects even *in utero*. Human and animal studies demonstrate reproductive, perinatal and genotoxic effects of lead (ATSDR 1999b; Piasek *et al.* 1996a,b; WHO/EHC 1995).

Arsenic

Exposure to cigarette smoke may contribute to environmental (mainly dietary and in some areas water) exposure to arsenic and arsenic compounds. Inorganic arsenic is considered to be among the highest priority hazardous substances in the United States as water contaminant (WHO/EHC 2001). Epidemiological evidence in humans indicates effects on fertility and spontaneous abortion. Animal studies have showed that both inorganic forms of arsenic (arsenate and arsenite ions) are transferred to the embryo and have carcinogenic and teratogenic effects (Waalkes *et al.* 2003; Golub *et al.* 1998; Clarkson *et al.* 1985).

Cadmium

Unlike lead or arsenic, cadmium is not readily transferred to the fetus once the placenta has developed. However, it has proven carcinogenic and teratogenic potential, and cigarette smoke is considered one of the most important sources of cadmium exposure in the general non-occupationally exposed population (Herber 2004; Bhattacharyya *et al.* 2000; Järup *et al.* 1998; WHO/EHC 1992a,b; Kostial 1986). Evidence of cigarette smoke-related cadmium, lead and essential trace element concentrations and their tissue distribution in human placenta, and evidence of cadmium potential of endocrine disrupting activity in placenta is presented in detail later in this chapter.

Cadmium in Cigarette Smoke and Placenta

Cadmium is a ubiquitous pollutant in the modern environment and most of it has been released into environment (air, land and water) by human activities. High concentrations of cadmium in the soil and ground waters in certain areas in the world makes it easily detectable in the food chain, especially in seafood, grains and cereals, potatoes, fish, meat, leafy vegetables, and mushrooms (Jureša & Blanuša 2004; Blanuša *et al.* 2001; Harris & Taylor 2001; McLaughlin *et al.* 1999; Berglund *et al.* 1994; Moberg Wing *et al.* 1992). After absorption from the soil, cadmium may accumulate (up to 7 μg/g) in tobacco leaves as well (Chiba & Masioroni 1992). Single cigarettes contain approximately 1.7 μg/g cadmium, of which approximately 70% passes into the smoke. The majority of cadmium enters sidestream smoke with consequent risk to persons exposed passively (Stohs *et al.* 1997).

It has been shown in humans that about 50% of the cadmium inhaled via cigarette smoke could be absorbed (Järup *et al.* 1998; Jin *et al.* 1998). Typically, smokers have about 4 to 5 times higher blood cadmium concentrations (in nonsmokers it is$<$1.5 μg/L) (Jurasović *et al.* 2004), and twice as high concentrations in placental tissue and kidney cortex cadmium than do nonsmokers (Piasek *et al.* 2001; Blanuša *et al.* 1985). Cadmium has a long biological half-life of 15-30 years, mainly due to its slow excretion from the body. It accumulates during the entire life span in internal organs including reproductive organs, that is, ovary, testis and placenta (Chedrese *et al.* 2006; Piasek *et al.* 2001; Henson & Anderson 2000; Varga *et al.* 1993).

As early as thirty years ago, human and animal studies showed that very little cadmium crosses the placenta and that cadmium readily accumulates in placental tissue (Miller *et al.* 1988, 1983; Levin *et al.* 1983; Hanlon *et al.* 1982). In most of the studies the maternal blood cadmium concentrations were higher than the infant ones. However, data on low cadmium concentration in organs of human fetuses and infants provide evidence that placenta is not a complete barrier for fetal cadmium exposure (Lutz *et al.* 1996; Lagerkvist *et al.* 1992, Kuhnert *et al.* 1987; Carmichael *et al.* 1982; Karp & Robertson 1981; Arena 1979; Lauwerys *et al.* 1978; Chaube 1973).

Pregnant women who smoke expose themselves and their placentas to cadmium concentrations higher than those to which they would normally be exposed (Kuhnert *et al.* 1982; van Hattum *et al.* 1981). Numerous studies show higher cadmium concentrations in placentas of smoking than in nonsmoking urban parturients (Falcón *et al.* 2002; Pereg *et al.* 2001; Piasek *et al.* 2001; Osman *et al.* 2000; Reichrtova *et al.* 1998a; Loiacono *et al.* 1992). Evaluation of concentrations of cadmium, lead and several essential elements in placenta, maternal venous blood and umbilical cord blood confirms that lead, but not cadmium, easily crossed the placental barrier. Higher cadmium and lead concentrations are found in blood and in placenta of smokers than in nonsmokers. The findings are commensurate with increased concentrations of lead and only traces of cadmium in neonatal blood (Osman *et al.* 2000; Baranowska 1995).

However, some investigations failed to observe an association between placental cadmium and smoking (Odland *et al.* 2001; Zadorozhnaja *et al.* 2000). Odland *et al.* (2001) made a factor analysis of 11 essential and 5 toxic elements in human placentas from deliveries in arctic and subarctic areas of Russia and Norway. Results showed that placental concentrations of these elements depended strongly on gestational age, increasing from about week 35, and peaking near weeks 39 and 40. Elements that exhibited skewed frequency distributions and a dependence on maternal smoking were calcium, barium, magnesium and phosphorus. Associations with nickel, lead, and strontium were positive, but weaker.

Distribution of Metals and Progesterone in Placental Tissue

Some authors reported that it was important to define the location of the sampling site in studies involving elemental analysis of the placenta. Manci & Blackburn (1987) found regional variations in the concentrations of iron, copper, zinc, and calcium in human term placentas. However, it has also been suggested that placental tissue can be regarded as relatively homogenous for cadmium content (Piasek *et al.* 2001; Reichrtova *et al.* 1998a; Lagerkvist *et al.* 1996; van Hattum *et al.* 1981).

Tissue concentrations of cadmium, lead, iron, zinc, and copper in human placentas as markers of exposure to cigarette smoke are presented in Figures 1 and 2. Placental progesterone concentration as a marker of effect of cigarette smoke is given in Figure 1 (graph at the bottom). All values are given for central and peripheral sites for placental tissue sampling.

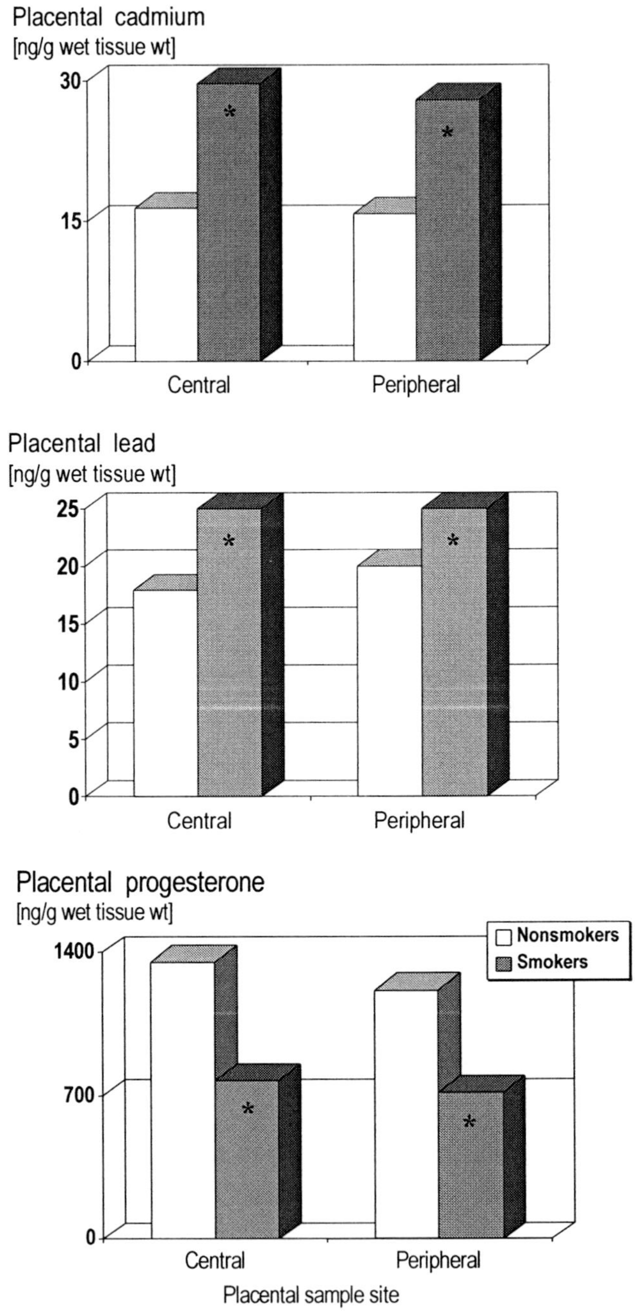

Figure 1. Average concentrations of cadmium, lead, and steroid hormone progesterone in full-term placentas of nonsmoking (N=27) and smoking parturients (N=25) at central (periumbilical) and peripheral placental sample site (within 3 cm of outer disc edge). Significant differences (at $P<0.05$) between values in smokers vs. nonsmokers are marked with asterisk.

We found no regional variation in values of either progesterone or metal concentrations. Average values of placental cadmium concentrations are significantly (two-fold) higher in smokers than in nonsmokers. Placental lead is significantly higher ($P<0.05$) in smokers than in nonsmokers. Concomitant average placental progesterone concentration is almost half of that found in nonsmokers (Figure 1). Placental concentrations of iron are significantly lower (*P<0.05*) in smokers than in nonsmokers. There is no difference in either zinc or copper concentrations in placental tissues of smokers vs. nonsmokers (Figure 2).

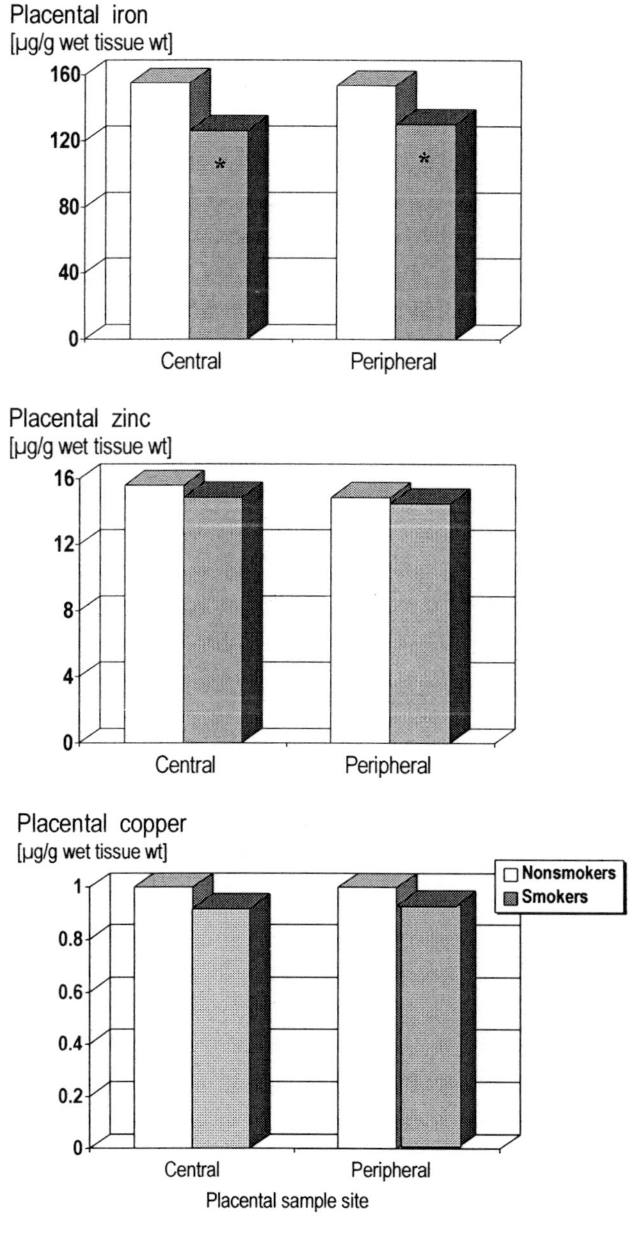

Figure 2. Average concentrations of iron, zinc and copper in full-term placentas of nonsmoking (N=27) and smoking parturients (N=25) at central (periumbilical) and peripheral placental sample site (within 3 cm of outer disc edge). Significant difference (at *P<0.05*) in placental iron between smokers vs. nonsmokers is marked with asterisk.

For determination of the exact locations of metals in the tissue, placental samples should be processed histochemically and analyzed semiquantitatively by light microscopy (Reichrtova *et al.* 1998a,b). The results show that the lead and the nickel particulates deposit in the syncytiotrophoblast, and that transport of the lead particulates from basal plate to chorionic plate occurs.

Cadmium Effects on Placental Structure

Cadmium is a highly toxic heavy metal. Beside its adverse effects on kidneys, respiratory organs, and bone, it is becoming of interest due to its effects on reproduction and placental structure and functions. There are reports of higher cadmium accumulation and concomitant histological changes in the placenta of smoking mothers (Boadi *et al.* 1991, Wier *et al.* 1990, Copius Peereboom-Stegeman 1989, Copius Peereboom-Stegeman *et al.* 1983, 1979, van der Velde *et al.* 1983, van Hattum *et al.* 1981).

After the functional placenta develops, embryo/fetal cadmium accumulation is greatly reduced. Studies in rats show that, following a single acute cadmium dose, the metal increases in placenta with advancing gestational age and maturation (Ahokas & Dilts 1979). The critical time of development when the embryo accumulates cadmium, ingested or inhaled by the mother, appears to be between implantation and development of the functional placenta, which is also a critical period of organogenesis. Cadmium administered in a single dose late in gestation can produce placental necrosis accompanied by fetal death as a direct result of the placental toxicity (Piasek *et al.* 2004, Levin *et al.* 1987, 1983; Pařízek 1983, 1964). However, no necrotic changes or effects on fetal viability are observed in rat placentas after chronic cadmium exposure during pregnancy (Piasek *et al.* 2004, 2000; Hazelhoff Roelfzema *et al.* 1988; Copius Peereboom-Stegeman *et al.* 1983). This is due to the ability of placental (trophoblast) cells to adapt to long-term cadmium exposure by synthesis and cell redistribution of placental metallothionein, a protein that binds cadmium ion and mitigates its cytotoxic effects (Breen *et al.* 1995; Torreblanca *et al.* 1992).

Cadmium and Essential Metal Interactions in the Placenta

The perinatal effects of cadmium on the fetus are indirect. Human and animal studies provide evidence that very little cadmium crosses the placenta to the fetus, as it is actually accumulated in the placental tissue (as described earlier). Cadmium in placenta may interact with essential elements that are critical for fetal growth, immune function, and development, and inhibit placental capacity to transfer nutrients to the fetus. As a result, reduced concentrations of zinc and iron in fetal tissues, fetal and neonatal iron deficiency and anemia after birth, and lower pup body weights are noted (Pillai & Gupta 2005; Piasek *et al.* 2004; Piasek *et al.* 1996b; Goyer 1995; Maitani and Suzuki 1986, Carmichael *et al.* 1982; Arizono *et al.* 1981, Webb and Samarawickrama 1981, Fox *et al.* 1980). Following acute cadmium exposure in pregnant rats, higher cadmium accumulation is found in the fetal portion than in the maternal portion of the term placenta with concurrent decreased iron concentrations (Piasek *et al.* 1994).

Less is known about interactions of toxic and essential elements in the human placenta. However, findings show a relation between maternal anemia (low serum ferritin concentrations) and placental size and birth weight (Hindmarsh *et al.* 2000). Regarding a cadmium-calcium interaction it was found that cadmium exposure significantly compromises the calcium handling ability of human placental (trophoblastic) cells (Lin *et al.* 1997). In smokers, increased placental cadmium concentrations can be accompanied by decreased placental iron concentrations (Piasek *et al.* 2001).

Reduced consumption efficiency for zinc, copper, magnesium, and selenium, which are four elements essential for life, has been indicated by the increased ratio of umbilical cord (arterial vs. venous) blood concentrations in cases of intrauterine growth retardation (Osada *et al.* 2002). The effect of maternal cadmium exposure on fetal and neonatal body weight may be due to fetal cadmium accumulation, fetal zinc deprivation, or both. Cadmium and zinc are closely associated with metallothionein, a small cysteine-rich protein that binds cadmium and may also faciliate transport of zinc and copper. Metallothionein synthesis can be induced by zinc and cadmium salts in cultured human placental (trophoblast) cells. The syncytiotrophoblast has been shown to be the site of metallothionein synthesis (Goyer 1995). It has been proposed that when trophoblast cells are exposed to cadmium, induced metallothionein facilitates zinc retention in the trophoblast, making this essential element less available to the fetal circulation (Torreblanca *et al.* 1992). Cigarette smoking increases cadmium accumulation in placental tissue and cadmium has a stimulatory effect on placental metallothionein production. Furthermore, increased metallothionein traps zinc in placental tissue (and other maternal organs) and results in a zinc-deficient fetus (Ronco *et al.* 2005; Kuhnert 1991; Kuhnert *et al.* 1988).

Placental content of essential metals in relation to exposure to cigarette smoke has been evaluated in only a few investigations. It was observed that parturients who smoke 5-20 cigarettes per day have lower placental iron concentrations than nonsmokers, with placental concentrations of other essential elements, zinc and copper being unchanged (Piasek *et al.* 2001; Paszkowski & Sikorski 1994). A negative correlation between placental concentrations of toxic metal (cadmium and lead) and birth weight and a positive correlation for the nutritionally essential element (iron, copper and zinc), with the correlation of birth weight and placental zinc being the strongest (Ward *et al.* 1990). Other investigators failed to find such relationships (Piasek *et al.* 2001; Loiacono *et al.* 1992).

Cadmium and Endocrine Disruption in the Placenta

About twenty years ago, Clarkson *et al.* (1985, 1983) proposed that there was too little information available to make a final decision on whether cadmium exerted any critical effect(s) on the placenta or not. In the interim, however, dramatic effects of cadmium on reproductive endocrine functions have been reported that may vary to some degree with respect to the experimental model employed, the tissue analyzed, and/or the dosage administered (Henson & Chedrese 2004).

Studies have reaffirmed the detrimental effects of the metal on steroidogenesis after both *in vivo* and *in vitro* exposures, in ovaries of either cycling or pregnant rats (Paksy *et al.* 1996, 1992, 1989; Piasek & Laskey 1999, 1994), and in human tissue (Paksy *et al.* 1997). In rodent and human placentas, observable symptoms of toxicity were apparent in trophoblast cells exposed to cadmium, providing an increasing body of evidence that the placenta is a site for the toxic action of cadmium (Eisenman & Miller 1995; Wier *et al.* 1990, di Sant' Agnese *et al.* 1983). These symptoms included lysosomal vesiculation, nuclear chromatin clumping, and mitochondrial calcification. In perfused human placenta, exposure to cadmium precipitated a decline in the secretion of a polypeptide product of the trophoblast, hCG (already defined in previous text) (Wier *et al.* 1990). In human placental explants, acute cadmium exposure at high concentrations caused imbalance between tromboxane A_2 and prostacyclin, a disturbance seen in late gestation in pre-eclampsia (Eisenmann & Miller 1995). The latest finding corroborated earlier observations in experimental rats following acute cadmium injection (of about 1 mg/kg b. wt) in late pregnancy who exhibited high mortality, violent convulsions, severe placental necrosis, and fetal death with pathological changes that were clinically and morphologically comparable to toxemia of pregnancy in humans (Pařízek 1983,1964).

By *in vivo* exposure before and/or during pregnancy to cadmium via cigarette smoke, concentrations of cadmium in placentas collected from urban parturients were in smokers approximately twice that of nonsmokers, with commensurate placental progesterone levels in smoking women being only one-half that of nonsmokers. Average concentrations in nonsmokers vs. smokers (mean±SEM) were for placental cadmium 15.9±1.5 vs. 28.5±2, and for progesterone 1.3±0.1 vs. 0.7±0.08 ng/g wet tissue weight (Piasek *et al.* 2002, 2001). In pregnant rats exposed to cadmium during pregnancy (at total dose 0, 3 or 5 mg/kg from day 1 through 19, that is, near term, by subcutaneosly implanted osmotic mini pumps), serum progesterone did not change, and serum estradiol concentrations were decreased (17±2, 13±3 and 9±2 pg/ml in the control, 3 and 5 mg/kg cadmium-dosed rats) and the effect was linear. Placental progesterone was reduced and this was additive and linear effect of cadmium exposure (at dose 5 mg/kg dose) and concomitant low (10 ppm) iron in diet (Piasek *et al.* 2004, 2002, 2000).

A similar pattern of increased placental cadmium accompanied by decreased placental progesterone is observed in investigations in smoking parturients and cadmium-exposed pregnant laboratory rats (Figure 3). Collectively, these results and above findings suggest a strong association between exposure to cadmium via cigarette smoking and placental endocrine disruption that could affect fetal wellbeing and pregnancy outcome.

Mechanisms of Cadmium-Mediated Disrupting Activities

The human placental syncytiotrophoblast is responsible for producing an assortment of hormones that contribute to normal embryo/fetal development and pregnancy maintenance. These hormones include progesterone, a steroid that plays a vital role by promoting uterine myometrial quiescence (Huszar 1983) and thereby preventing premature labor. In this capacity, it was demonstrated that cadmium inhibits progesterone secretion in cultured human placental cells. As indicated by assessment of lactate dehydrogenase activity, this effect was not simply the result of cadmium-induced cell death. Nor was it the result of any appreciable inhibition of syncytial maturation in culture, as immunocytochemical localization of cellular boundaries and nuclei by visualization of desmoplakin immunoflourescence (Figure 4) indicated that approximately 94% syncytial maturity was attained by both untreated and cadmium-treated cells (Jolibois *et al.* 1999a,b).

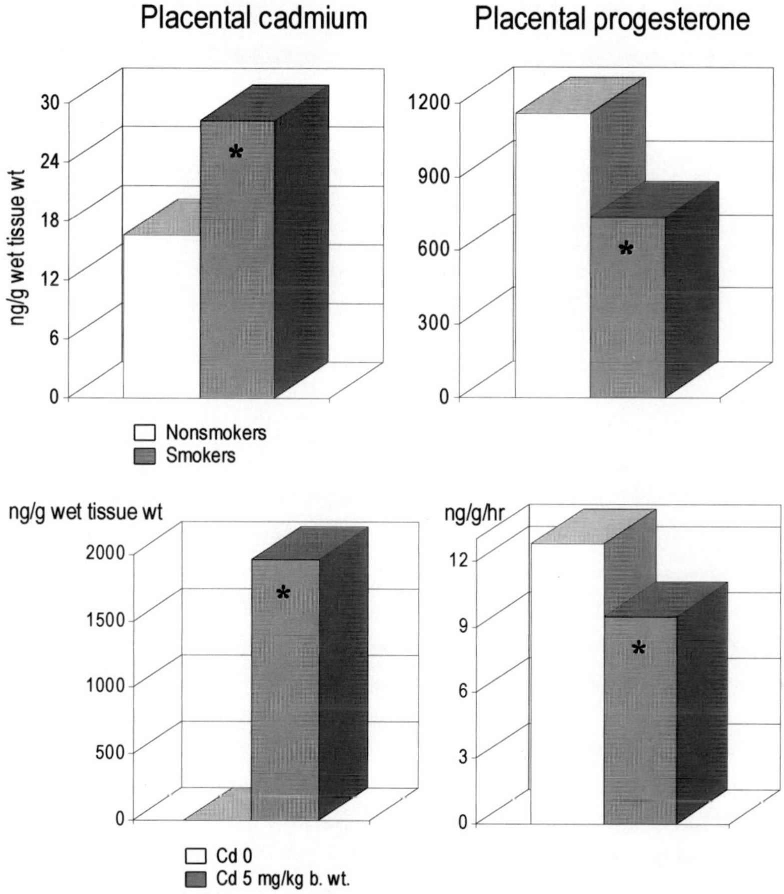

Figure 3. Comparative findings of increased cadmium concentrations in human and rat placenta and concurrent reduced progesterone concentration in human placenta (nh/g wet tissue wt) and progesterone production in culture of whole rat placentas (ng/g/h). Values in human placentas are average values irrespective of sampling site (examined subjects are described under Fig.1 and 2). Values in rat placentas were obtained after *in vivo* parenteral exposure to cadmium chloride during pregnancy (by subcutaneosly implanted osmotic mini pumps from day 1 through 19 of gestation, at total dose 5 mg Cd/kg body weight); Cd 0 - unexposed control rats (N=17); Cd 5 mg/kg b. wt. - cadmium-exposed rats (N=15).

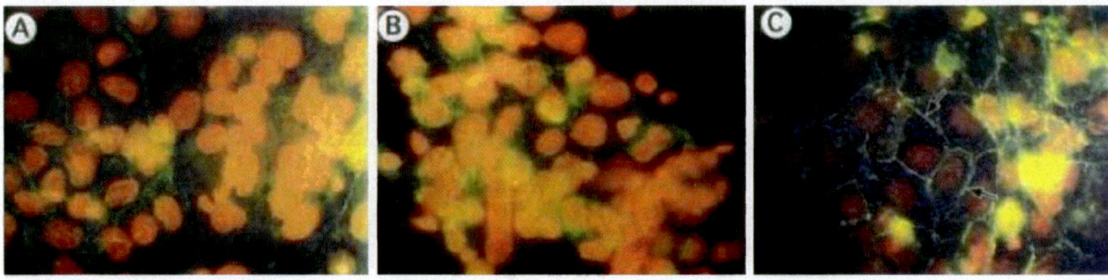

Fig. 4. Photomicrographs (x 600) demonstrating immunofluorescence of placental trophoblast cells cultured for 96 hours in different culture media: (A) dispersed in medium (Dulbecco Modified Eagle medium, DMEM) plus 10% fetal bovine serum; (B) plus 20 mM cadmium chloride; (C) plus 1% dimethyl sulfoxide (DMSO). Arrows indicate desmoplakin staining in cell juncture-associated desmosomes. Dimethyl sulfoxide is a potent inhibitor of syncytial maturation and serves as a positive control in this experiment. The lack of desmoplakin staining in both untreated and cadmium-treated cultures suggests that at the concentrations used, cadmium's inhibitory effect on progesterone synthesis is a biochemical rather than morphological one.

The above findings led to a proposal that the suppression of secretion in cultured human trophoblast cells represents a direct effect of cadmium on the progesterone biosynthetic pathway. The effect may have been attributed, at least in part, to a deleterious effect on low-density lipoprotein receptor mRNA (Jolibois *et al.* 1999b). However, because a number of steroidogenic enzymes are necessary for optimal progesterone production, the potential exists for this mechanism to be multifaceted, affecting multiple sites (Henson & Anderson 2000). As said earlier in this chapter, steroidogenic enzyme P450scc catalyzes the conversion of cholesterol into pregnenolone, which is then converted into progesterone via 3β-HSD. Syncytiotrophoblasts formed in culture (as *in vivo*) from cytotrophoblast progenitors, adapt to facilitate this transition (Henson *et al.* 1996; Ringler & Strauss 1990). Therefore, human cytotrophoblast cells were purified by density gradient centrifugation and incubated with cadmium ions (in Dulbecco Modified Eagle medium plus 10% fetal bovine serum with 0, 5, 10 or 20 μM $CdCl_2$ for 96 hours) (Kawai *et al.* 2002). Cells progressed to syncytiotrophoblastic maturity. As no differences in cell protein and lactate dehydrogenase activity were observed between untreated trophoblasts and those treated with $CdCl_2$, the metal did not impact cell viability. However, P450scc and 3β-HSD mRNA transcript levels declined in a dose-dependent manner in trophoblasts co-cultured with 5, 10 or 20 μM $CdCl_2$. Enzymatic activity of P450scc was similarly inhibited by $CdCl_2$ treatment, although activity of 3β-HSD was not affected. Co-culture with 8-bromo-cAMP enhanced progesterone secretion in untreated cultures, but did not reverse the decline in progesterone secretion induced by $CdCl_2$ treatment. $CdCl_2$ failed to influence cyclic AMP (cAMP) content in cultured cells. Taken together, results suggested that the P450scc enzyme is another site at which cadmium interferes with placental progesterone production, although it is unlikely that an inhibition of cAMP was involved. The possibility still exists, however, that the cadmium ion may interfere with the downstream cascade of the cAMP-protein kinase A-dependent pathway.

To this end, Kostrzewska *et al.* (1990) reported that higher cadmium concentrations inhibited the phosphorylation of myosin light chain kinase in the smooth muscle myosin, suggesting that cadmium interferes with the phosphorylation of protein kinases. An additional possibility is that the metal may directly affect transcription of the P450scc gene by interfering with the DNA binding zinc-finger motif through the substitution of cadmium for zinc ion (Sunderman & Barber 1988). Moreover, cations such as cadmium (Cd^{2+}) have been reported to alter the structure of nucleic acids (DNA, tRNA) and certain enzymes by reacting with their sulfydryl groups (Jacobson & Turner 1980; Vallee & Ulmer 1972). Most likely cadmium ion interferes with progesterone biosynthesis by multiple mechanisms affecting transcription of the P450scc gene (Chedrese *et al.* 2006).

It might also be postulated that cadmium could function as an endocrine disruptor by mimicking the effects of estrogens (Martin *et al.* 2003; Johnson *et al.* 2003; Safe 2003). In this regard, the effects of cadmium could be mediated by the estrogen receptor (ER)-alpha and be independent of estrogen binding (Stoica *et al.* 2000). Overall, significant evidence suggests that cadmium could function as a potent nonsteroidal estrogen *in vivo* and *in vitro*, potentially eliciting tissue-specific effects in the ovary and placenta (Chedrese *et al.* 2006; Henson & Chedrese 2004).

Further studies are called for to definitively determine the collective mechanism(s) by which cadmium interferes with steroid hormone biosynthesis *in vivo*. A better understanding of the ramifications of the mechanisms that link smoking, metal exposure, and the maintenance of pregnancy is important.

CONCLUDING REMARKS

Women are generally unaware of the adverse effects of cigarette smoke and its toxic constituents on their reproductive integrity, embryo/feto-placental function, and health of the newborn. A relatively high proportion of women worldwide, including teenage girls, are smokers, and the difference in the sex ratio of nonsmokers to smokers continues to shift toward higher female involvement. With the implementation of current public health regulations, pregnant women can no longer be occupationally exposed to toxic metals. However, other sources, which include food and water contamination, wall paint, industrial wastes, automobile exhaust fumes, pesticides, and particularly, cigarette smoking and passive environmental tobacco smoke exposure have yet to be eliminated. Pregnancy is a time when life-long smoking cessation efforts and interventions could be potentially effective due to a woman's enhanced concern at that time for her own health and that of her unborn child. This may comprise the single most important action a woman can take to improve her health, the outlook for her pregnancy, and her newborn's health and future wellbeing (Mendoza & Chaves 2003; Ebrahim *et al.* 2002).

To successfully facilitate both the primary and secondary prevention of cigarette smoking, the aggressive public health strategy directed at both parents and children should be expanded to require the strong support of physicians, with emphasis on prevention in practice, the support of public health initiatives, medical and public policy, and the funding of high-quality research (Gidding *et al.* 1994). At least two recent initiatives for cigarette smoking cessation to protect children's health are worthy to be mentioned. One involved the U. S. Environmental Agency public campaign for smoke-free homes (U. S. EPA 2004), which advised adults not to smoke indoor (in their homes and cars) in order to protect children from second-hand smoke. This is an example that will hopefully lead to the genesis of similar programs thoughout the world. The other was carried out through actions of the World Health Organization and the Fourth Ministerial Conference on Environment and Health held in Budapest, Hungary in 2004 under the motto "Children for our Future". In the Action Plan for Europe (WHO 2004) released at the Conference, an increased concern was expressed about the effects of unsafe and unhealthy environments on the health of children and developing organisms, especially during embryonic and fetal periods. It was stressed that in their early years of life children are particularly susceptible and may be exposed more often than adults to various environmental factors. Concern regarding the potential for long-term toxicity, including the carcinogenic, immunotoxic, genotoxic, neurotoxic, endocrine-disrupting and allergenic effects of many chemicals has been pointed out with the emphasis on the effects of environmental tobacco smoke and heavy metals that contaminate the environment and to which men and women of reproductive age and children may be exposed. It has been recognized that our understanding of the nature and number of health effects wrought by exposure to environmental contaminants in developing organisms, from the prenatal period to adolescence, is still incomplete. Coordinated and sustained action to protect children's health, today and in the future has been proposed. In this regard, when knowledge gaps are perceived, it should be agreed that more effort be put into research, to improve knowledge of causal links, the nature and magnitude of effects and effective interventions.

Heavy metals are mainly released into the environment by human activities that are linked to the stage of industrial development of the country. In this environment, active and passive tobacco smoke remains an important source of exposure to highly reactive, toxic and carcinogenic metals, primarily cadmium. More human and animal data are needed to elucidate association(s) between toxic metals and placental endocrine function that is essential for successful pregnancy outcome, viability of an unborn and newborn child, and the continuance of the human species in general. The biological monitoring of toxic metals and their effects in the early stages of the life cycles of all species has not received the attention it deserves so far. However, an effort has been undertaken to examine the information available and to evaluate implications for risk assessment for several well-defined areas, such as in organ systems and functions, in a workshop to identify critical windows of exposure for children's health (Selevan *et al.* 2000). The rationale for this task was that for years, although authors occasionally considered the importance of exposure timing and how it affected selected criteria, no one ever systematically compiled preconceptional, prenatal, and postnatal developmental exposure and linked them to subsequent specific outcomes. Health risk assessment of cigarette smoke exposure can be similarly applied to all defined areas to directly evaluate the reproductive system, endocrine system and general growth biomarkers. The assessment of toxicant exposures and steroid disruption using human placental tissue is just one such evaluation tool that is available today.

Human placental tissue can be used in the assessment of exposure to toxic metals, primarily cadmium, together with the assessment of other metal ions, lead, iron, zinc and copper, in relation to cigarette smoking. *In vivo* and *in vitro* investigations in laboratory animal models support the concept that cadmium, which is the most abundant, toxic, carcinogenic and teratogenic metal ion constituent of cigarette smoke, has an endocrine disrupting potential that may place female reproductive outcome and fetal viability at risk (Piasek *et al.* 2002). Appropriate biomarkers of placental toxicity are still being explored. Currently, there is no single optimal model for placental or developmental toxicology research and there is a need for new approaches, which can now include placental function, toxicity, and kinetics assessment (Myllynen *et al.* 2005). Evaluation of placental steroid disruption as an indicator of fetal distress *in utero* may serve as a useful and noninvasive test for the assessment of neonatal health risks linked to tobacco smoke exposure to metals and other common xenobiotics.

Acknowledgment

The first author (M. P.) dedicates her portion to the splendid collaboration and memory of two dear friends, coworkers, and educators: Dr John W. Laskey and the late Dr Ezra Berman of Reproductive Toxicology Branch, Developmental Toxicology Division, Health Effects Research Laboratory, United States Environmental Protection Agency, Research Triangle Park, North Carolina, for their unselfish help and sharing of experience and results to make mutual contributions to the imminent concept of cadmium as an endocrine disrupting chemical in humans in the early 1990ies.

References

Åkesson, A; Berglund, M; Schutz, A; Bjellrup, P; Bremme, K; Vahter M. Cadmium exposure in pregnancy and lactation in relation to iron status. *American Journal of Public Health*, 2002, 92, 284-287.

Albuquerque, CA; Smith, KR; Johnson, C; Chao, R; Harding R. Influence of maternal tobacco smoking during pregnancy on uterine, umbilical and fetal cerebral artery blood flows. *Early Human Development*, 2004, 80, 31-42.

Ananth, CV; Savitz, DA; Luther, ER. Maternal cigarette smoking as a risk factor for placental abruption, placenta previa, and uterine bleeding in pregnancy. *American Journal of Epidemiology*, 1996, 144, 881-889.

Arena, JM. Drug and chemical effects on mother and child. *Pediatric Annals*, 1979, 8, 690-697.

Arizono, K; Ota, Sh; Ariyoshi, T. Purification of metallothionein-like protein in rat placenta. *Bulletin of Environmental Contamination and Toxicology*, 1981, 27, 671-677.

ASH/WHO report. Action on Smoking and Health (ASH)/World Health Organization (WHO) Consultation Report WHO/NCD/TFI/ETS/99.2. International Consultation on Environmental Tobacco Smoke (ETS) and Child Health; 1999 [Available from: URL: http://ash.org/who-ets-rpt.html]

ATSDR series. Agency for Toxic Substances and Disease Registry. Atlanta, GA: U. S. Department of Health and Human Services, Public Health Service:

ATSDR Toxicological profile for arsenic; 2000;

[Available from: URL: http://www.atsdr.cdc.gov/toxprofiles/tp2.html];

ATSDR Toxicological profile for cadmium; 1999a;

[Available from: URL: http://www.atsdr.cdc.gov/tfacts5.html#bookmark01];

ATSDR Toxicological profile for lead; 1999b;

[Available from: URL: http://www.atsdr.cdc.gov/toxprofiles/tp13.html];

ATSDR Toxicological profile for mercury; 1999c;

[Available from: URL: http://www.atsdr.cdc.gov/toxprofiles/tp46.html].

Augood, C; Duckitt, K; Templeteon, AA. Smoking and female infertility: a systemic review and meta-analysis. *Human Reproduction*, 1998, 13, 1532-1539.

Baglan, RJ; Brill, AB; Schulert, A; Wilson, D; Larsen, K; Dyer, N; Schaffner, W; Hoffman, L; Davies, J. Utility of placental tissue as an indicator of trace element exposure to adult and fetus. *Environmental Research*, 1974, 8, 64-70.

Barbieri, RL; Gochberg, J; Ryan, KJ. Nicotine, cotinine, and anabasine inhibit aromatase in human trophoblast *in vitro*. *Journal of Clinical Investigation* 1986, 77, 1727–1733.

Baranowska, I. Lead and cadmium in human placentas and maternal and neonatal blood (in a heavily polluted area) measured by graphite furnace atomic absorption spectrometry. *Occupational Environmental Medicine* 1995, 52, 229–232.

Baron, JA. Smoking and estrogen-related disease. *American Journal of Epidemiology*, 1984, 19, 9-22.

Baron, JA; La Vecchia, C; Levi, F. The antiestrogenic effect of cigarette smoking in women. *American Journal of Obstetrics and Gynecology*, 1990, 162, 502-514.

Baron, JA. Beneficial effects of nicotine and cigarette smoking: the real, the possible and the spurious. *British Medical Bulletin,* 1996, 52, 58-73.

Berglund, M; Akesson, A; Nermell, B; Vahter, M. Intestinal absorption of dietary cadmium in women depends on body iron stores and fiber intake. *Environmental Health Perspectives,* 1994, 102, 1058–1066.

Berny, C; Boyer, JC; Capolaghi, B; L'Homme, GD; Desch, G; Garelik, D; Hayder, R; Houdret, N; Jacob, N; Koskas, T; Laine, G; Moel, GL; Moulsma, M; Plantin-Carrenard, E; Venembre, P. Biomarkers of tobacco smoke exposure. *Annales de Biologie Clinique (Paris)*, 2002, 60, 63-72.

Bernstein, L; Pike, MC; Lobo, RA; Depue, RH; Ross, RK; Henderson, BE. Cigarette smoking in pregnancy results in marked decrease in maternal hCG and oestradiol levels. *British Journal of Obstetrics and Gynecology*, 1989, 96, 92-96.

Bendich, A. Micronutrients in women's health and immune function. *Nutrition*, 2001, 17, 858-867.

Bhattacharyya, MH; Wilson, AK; Rajan, SS; Jonah, M. Biochemical pathways in cadmium toxicity. In: Zalups RK, Koropatnick J, editors. *Molecular biology and toxicology of metals*. London - New York: Taylor & Francis; 2000; 34-74.

Blanuša, M; Breški Dj. Comparison of dry and wet ashing procedures for cadmium and iron determination in biological material by atomic-absorption spectrophotometry. *Talanta*, 1981, 26, 681-684.

Blanuša, M; Kralj, Z; Bunarević, A. Interaction of cadmium, zinc and copper in relation to smoking habit, age and histopathological findings in human kidney cortex. *Archives of Toxicology*, 1985, 58, 115-117.

Blanuša, M; Prester, Lj; Matek, M; Kučak, A. Trace elements in soil and coniferous needles. *Bulletin of Environmental Contamination and Toxicology*, 1999, 62, 700-707.

Blanuša, M; Kučak, A; Varnai, VM; Matek Sarić, M. Uptake of cadmium, copper, iron, manganese and zinc in mushrooms (*Boletaceae*) from Croatian forest soil. *Journal of AOAC International*, 2001, 84, 1964-1971.

Blanuša, M; Mrković-Milić, R; Durbešić, P. Lead and cadmium in soil and isopoda woodlice in Croatia. *Ecotoxicology & Environmental Safety*, 2002, 52, 198-202.

Boadi, WY; Yannai, S; Urbach, J; Brandes, JM; Summer, KH. Transfer and accumulation of cadmium, and the level of metallothionein in perfused human placenta. *Archives of Toxicology*, 1991, 65, 318-323.

Bradford, MM. A rapid and sensitive method for the quantitation of microgram quantities of protein utilizing the principle of protein-dye binding. *Analytical Biochemistry,* 1976, 72, 248-254.

Breen, JG; Nelson, E; Miller, RK. Cellular adaptation to chronic cadmium exposure - intracellular localization of metallothionein protein in human trophoblast cells (JAr). *Teratology*, 1995, 51, 266-272.

Bush, PG; Mayhew, TM; Abramovich, DR; Aggett, PJ; Burke, MD; Page, KR. A quantitative study on the effects of maternal smoking on placental morphology and cadmium concentration. *Placenta* 2000a, 21, 247-256.

Bush, PG; Mayhew, TM; Abramovich, DR; Aggett, PJ; Burke, MD; Page, KR. Maternal cigarette smoking and oxygen diffusion across the placenta. *Placenta*, 2000b, 21, 824-833.

Carmichael, NG; Backhouse, BL; Winder, C; Lewis, P. Teratogenicity, toxicity and perinatal effects of cadmium. *Human Toxicology*, 1982, 1, 159-186.

Castro, LC; Allen, R; Ogunyemi, D; Roll, K; Platt, LD.Cigarette smoking during pregnancy: acute effects on uterine blood flow velocity waveforms. *Obstetrics & Gynecology*, 1993, 81, 552-555.

Chaube, Sh; Nishimura, H; Swinyard, CA. Zinc and cadmium in normal and human embryos and fetuses. *Archives of Environmental Health*, 1973, 26, 237-240.

Chedrese PJ, Piasek M, Henson MC. Cadmium as an endocrine disruptor in the reproductive system. *Immunology, Endocrine & Metabolic Agents in Medicinal Chemistry*, 2006, 1(6), 27-35.

Chelmow, D; Andrew, E; Baker, ER. Maternal cigarette smoking and placenta previa. *Obstetrics & Gynecology*, 1996, 87(5 Pt 1), 703-706.

Chiba, M; Masironi, R. Toxic and trace elements in tobacco and tobacco smoke. *Bulletin of the World Health Organization*, 1992, 70, 269-275.

Chung, KC; Kowalski, CP; Kim, HM; Buchman, SR. Maternal cigarette smoking during pregnancy and the risk of having a child with cleft lip/palate. *Plastic and Reconstructive Surgery*, 2000, 105, 485-491.

Clarkson, TW; Nordberg, GF; Sager, PR. *Reproductive and developmental toxicity of metals.* New York: Plenum Press; 1983.

Clarkson, TW; Nordberg, GF; Sager, PR. Reproductive and developmental toxicity of metals. *Scandinavian Journal of Work and Environmental Health*, 1985, 11, 145-154.

Clausen, HV; Jørgensen, JC; Ottesen, B. Stem villous arteries from the placentas of heavy smokers: Functional and mechanical properties. *American Journal of Obstetrics & Gynecology*, 1999, 180, 476-482.

Copius Peereboom, JW; de Vogt, P; van Hattum, B; van der Velde, W; Copius Peereboom-Stegeman, JHJ. The use of the human placenta as a biological indicator for cadmium exposure. In: *International Conference on Heavy Metals in the Environment, London, UK*. Edinburgh, UK: CEP Consultants Ltd.; 1979; 8-10.

Copius Peereboom-Stegeman, JHJ; van der Velde, WJ; Dessing, JWM. Influence of cadmium on placental structure. *Ecotoxicology & Environmental Safety*, 1983, 7, 79-86.

Copius Peereboom-Stegeman, JHJ. Cadmium effects on the female reproductive tract. *Toxicology & Environmental Chemistry*, 1989, 23, 91-99.

Demir, R; Demir, AY; Yinac, M. Structural changes in placental barrier of smoking mother. A quantitative and ultrastructural study. *Pathology, Research & Practice*, 1994, 190, 656-667.

Denson, KWE. Passive smoking in infants, children and adolescents. The effects of diet and socioeconomic factors. *International Archives of Occupational and Environmental Health*, 2001, 74, 525-532.

di Sant' Agnese, PA; Jensen, K; Levin, AA; Miller RK. Placental toxicity of cadmium in the rat: An ultrastructural study. *Placenta*, 1983, 4, 149-163.

Ebrahim, SH; Merrit, RK; Floyd, RL. Smoking and women's health: opportunities to reduce the burden of smoking during pregnancy. *Canadian Medical Association Journal*, 2000, 163, 281-282.

Economides, D; Braithwaite, J. Smoking, pregnancy and the fetus. *Journal of the Royal Society of Health*, 1994, 114, 198-201.

Eisenmann, CJ; Miller, RK. Cadmium and glutathione - effect on human placental thromboxane and prostacyclin production. *Reproductive Toxicology*, 1995, 9, 41-8.

Ernster, V; Kaufman, N; Nichter, M; Samet, J; Yoon, S-Y. Women and tobacco: moving from policy to action. *Bulletin of the World Health Organization*, 2000, 78, 891-901.

Eskenazi, B; Castorina, R. Association of prenatal maternal or postnatal child environmental tobacco smoke exposure and neurodevelopmental and behavioral problems in children. *Environmental Health Perspectives*, 1999, 107, 991-1000.

Evans, EH; Day, JA; Fisher, A; Price, WJ; Smith, CMM; Tyson, JF. Atomic spectrometry update. Advances in atomic emission, absorption and fluorescence spectrometry and related techniques. *Journal of Analytical Atomic Spectrometry*, 2004, 19, 775-812.

Falcón, M; Viñas, P; Osuna, E; Luna, A. Environmental exposures to lead and cadmium measured in human placenta. *Archives of Environmental Health*, 2002, 57, 598–602.

Falcone, T; Little, AB. Placental synthesis of steroid hormones. In: Tulchinsky D, Ryan KJ, editors. *Maternal-fetal endocrinology*. Philadelphia: W.B. Saunders Company; 1980; 3-16.

Ferré, F; Janssens, Y; Tanguy, G; Breuiller, M; De Pariente, D; Cedard L. Steroid concentrations in human myometrial and placental tissues at week 39 of pregnancy. *American Journal of Obstetrics & Gynecology*, 1978, 131, 500-502.

Ferré, F; Uzan, M; Jolivet, A; Janssens, Y; Tanguy, G; Sureau, C; Cedard, L. Influence of the oral administration of micronized progesterone on plasma and tissue levels of steroids in human pregnancy. *Acta Physiologica Hungarica*, 1985, 65, 443-451.

Forastiere, F; Agabiti, N; Corbo, GM; Pistelli, R; Dell'Orco, V; Ciappi, G; Perucci CA. Passive smoking as a determinant of bronchial responsiveness in children. *American Journal of Respiratory & Critical Care Medicine*, 1994, 149(2 Pt 1), 365-370.

Fox, MR; Jacobs, RM; Jones, AOL; Fry, BE Jr; Stone, CL. Effects of vitamin C and iron on cadmium metabolism. *Annals of the New York Academy of Sciences*, 1980, 355, 249-261.

Friberg, L. Quality control in laboratories testing for environmental pollution. In *Reproductive and developmental toxicity of metals*. In: Clarkson TW, Nordberg GF, Sager PR, editors. New York: Plenum Press; 1983; 811-829.

Gardela, J; Hill, JA III. Environmental toxins associated with recurrent pregnancy loss. *Seminars in Reproductive Medicine*, 2000, 18, 407-412.

Getahun, D; Amre, D; Rhoads, GG; Demissie, K. Maternal and obstetric risk factors for sudden infant death syndrome in the united States. *Obstetrics & Gynecology*, 2004, 103, 646-652.

Gidding, SS; Morgan, W; Perry, C; Isabel-Jones, J; Bricker, JT. Active and passive tobacco exposure: a serious pediatric health problem. A statement from the Committee on Atherosclerosis and Hypertension in Children, Council on Cardiovascular Disease in the Young, American Heart Association. *Circulation*, 1994, 90, 2581-2590.

Göcze, PM; Freeman, DA. Cytotoxic effects of cigarette smoke alkaloids inhibit the progesterone production and cell growth of cultured MA-10 Leydig tumor cells. *European Journal of Obstetrics, Gynecology, and Reproductive Biology*, 2000, 93, 77-83.

Göcze, PM; Szabo, I; Freeman, DA. Influence of nicotine, cotinine, anabasine and cigarette smoke extract on human granulosa cell progesterone and estradiol synthesis. *Gynecological Endocrinology*, 1999, 13, 266-272.

Golub, MS; Macintosh, MS; Baumrind, N. Developmental and reproductive toxicity of inorganic arsenic: animal studies and human concerns. *Journal of Toxicology and Environmental Health Part B*, 1998, 1, 199-241.

Goyer, RA. Transplacental transfer of lead and cadmium. In: Goyer, RA; Cherian, MG, editors. *Toxicology of metals: Biochemical aspects*. Berlin-Heidelberg, Germany: Springer-Verlag; 1995; 1-17.

Goyer, RA. Toxic and essential metal interactions. *Annual Review of Nutrition*, 1997, 17, 37-50.

Gulson, BL; Jameson, CW; Mahaffey, KR; Mizon, KJ; Korsch, MJ; Vimpani, G. Pregnancy increases mobilization of lead from maternal skeleton. *Journal of Laboratory and Clinical Medicine,* 1997, 130, 51-62.

Hanlon, DP; Specht, C; Ferm, VH. The chemical status of cadmium ion in the placenta. *Evironmental Research*, 1982, 27, 89-94.

Harris, NS; Taylor, GJ. Remobilization of cadmium in maturing shoots of near isogenic lines of durum wheat that differ in grain cadmium accumulation. *Journal of Experimental Botany*, 2001, 360, 1473-1481.

Hazelhoff Roelfzema, W; Zahn-Breidenbach, U; Copius Peereboom-Stegeman, JHJ. Light and electron microscopic investigation of the rat placenta after cadmium administration during pregnancy. *Anatomy and Embryology*, 1988, 178, 345-351.

Henke, W; Sobala, W; Kalinka, J. Environmental tobacco smoke exposure among pregnant women: impact on fetal biometry at 20-24 weeks of gestation and newborn child's birth weight. *International Archives of Occupational and Environmental Health*, 2004, 77, 47-52.

Henson, MC; Shi, W; Greene, SJ; Reggio BC. Effects of pregnant human, nonpregnant human, and fetal bovine sera on human chorionic gonadotropin, estradiol, and progesterone release by cultured human trophoblast cells. *Endocrinology*, 1996, 137, 2067-2074.

Henson, MC; Anderson, MB. The effect of cadmium on placental endocrine function. *Recent Research Developments in Endocrinology*, 2000, 1, 37-47.

Henson, MC; Chedrese, PJ. Endocrine disruption by cadmium, a common environmental toxicant with paradoxical effects on reproduction. *Experimental Biology and Medicine,* 2004, 229, 383-392.

Herber, RFM; Roelofsen, AM; Hazelhoff Roelfzema, W; Copius Peerebom-Stegeman, JHJ. Direct determination of cadmium in placenta. Comparison with a destruction atomic absorption spectrometric method. *Fresenius Journal of Analytical Chemistry*, 1985, 322, 734-746.

Herber, RFM. Cadmium. In: Merian, E; Anke, M; Ihnat, M; Stoeppler, M, editors. *Elements and their compounds in the environment: Occurrence, analysis and biological relevance. Volume 2: Metals and their compounds*. Weinheim, Germany: Wiley-VCH Verlag GmBH & Co. KgaA; 2004; 689-708.

Hindmarsh, PC; Geary, MPP; Rodeck, CH; Jackson, MR; Kingdom, JCP. Effect of early maternal iron stores on placental weight and structure. *Lancet*, 2000, 356, 719-723.

Hoffmann, D; Djordjevic, MV; Hoffmann, I. The changing cigarette. *Preventive Medicine*, 1997, 26, 427-434.

Huber, GL. Physical, chemical, and biological properties of tobacco, cigarette smoke, and other tobacco products. *Seminars in Respiratory Medicine*, 1989, 10, 297-332.

Husgafvel-Pursiainen, K. Biomarkers in the assessment of the exposure and the biological effects of environmental tobacco smoke. *Scandinavian Journal of Work and Environmental Health*, 2002, 28(Suppl 2), 21-29.

Huszar, G. Biology of the myometrium and cervix. In: Warsham J, editor. *The biological basis of reproductive and developmental medicine*. New York: Elsevier Biomedical; 1983; 85-104.

International Agency for Research on Cancer. *IARC Monographs on the Evaluation of the Carcinogenic Risk of Chemicals to Humans: Tobacco Smoking*. Volume 38. Lyon, France: IARC; 1986.

Iyengar, GV; Rapp, A. Human placenta as a 'dual' biomarker for monitoring fetal and maternal environment with special reference to potentially toxic trace elements: Part 1: Physiology, function and sampling of placenta for elemental characterization. *Science of the Total Environment*, 2001a, 280, 195-206.

Iyengar, GV; Rapp, A. Human placenta as a 'dual' biomarker for monitoring fetal and maternal environment with special reference to potentially toxic trace elements: Part 2: Essential minor, trace and other (non-essential) elements in human placenta. *Science of the Total Environment*, 2001b, 280, 207-219.

Iyengar, GV; Rapp, A. Human placenta as a 'dual' biomarker for monitoring fetal and maternal environment with special reference to potentially toxic trace elements: Toxic trace elements in placenta and placenta as a biomarker for these elements. *Science of the Total Environment*, 2001c, 280, 221-238.

Jacobson, KB; Turner, JE. The interaction of cadmium and certain other metal ions with proteins and nucleic acids. *Toxicology*, 1980, 16, 1-37.

Järup, L; Berglund, M; Elinder, CG; Nordberg, G; Vahter, M. Health effects of cadmium exposure - a review of the literature and risk estimate. *Scandinavian Journal of Work and Environmental Health*, 1998, 24 (Suppl 1), 1-52.

Jin, T; Lu, J; Nordberg, M. Toxicokinetics and biochemistry of cadmium with special emphasis on the role of metallothionein. *NeuroToxicology*, 1998, 19, 529-536.

Jolibois, LS Jr; Shi, W; George, WJ; Henson, MC; Anderson, M. Cadmium accumulation and effects on progesterone release by cultured human trophoblast cells. *Reproductive Toxicology*, 1999a; 13:215–221.

Jolibois, LS Jr; Burrow, ME; Swan, KF; George, WJ; Anderson, M; Henson, MC. Effects of cadmium on cell viability, trophoblastic development, and expression of low density lipoprotein receptor transcripts in cultured human placental cells. *Reproductive Toxicology*, 1999b, 13, 473–480.

Johnson, MD; Kenney, N; Stoica, A; Hillakivi-Clarke, L; Singh, B; Chepko, G; Clarke, R; Sholler, PF; Lirio, AA; Foss, C; Reiter, R; Trock, B; Paik, S; Martin, MB. Cadmium mimics the *in vivo* effects of estrogen in the uterus and mammary gland. *Nature Medicine*, 2003, 9, 1081-1084.

Jurasović, J; Cvitković, P; Pizent, A; Čolak, B; Telišman, S. Semen quality and reproductive endocrine function with regard to blood cadmium in Croatian male subjects. *BioMetals*, 2004, 17, 735-743.

Jureša, D; Blanuša, M. Mercury, arsenic, lead and cadmium in fish and shellfish from the Adriatic Sea. *Food Additives and Contaminants*, 2003, 20, 241-246.

Kalinić, N; Skender, Lj; Karačić, V; Brčić, I; Vadjić V. Passive exposure to tobacco smoke: Hair nicotine levels in preschool children. *Bulletin of Environmental Contamination and Toxicology*, 2003, 71, 1-5.

Kantola, M; Purkunen, R; Kroger, P; Tooming, A; Juravskaja, J; Pasanen, M; Saarikoski, S; Vartainen, T. Accumulation of cadmium, zinc, and copper in maternal blood and developmental placental tissue: differences between Finland, Estonia, and St. Petersburg. *Environmental Research*, 2000, 83, 54–66.

Karp, WB; Robertson, AF III. Cadmium, placenta, and the infant. In: Nriagu JO, editor. *Cadmium in the environment, Part II: Health effects*. Wiley & Sons: New York; 1981; 729-742.

Kawai, M; Swan, KF; Green, AE; Edwards, DE; Anderson, MB; Henson, MC. Placental endocrine disruption induced by cadmium: effects on P450 cholesterol side-chain cleavage and 3β-hydroxysteroid dehydrogenase enzymes in cultured human trophoblasts. *Biology of Reproduction,* 2002, 67, 178-183.

Kendrick, JS; Merritt, RK. Women and smoking: an update for the 1990s. *American Journal of Obstetrics and Gynecology*, 1996, 175, 528-535.

Kiel, DP; Baron, JA; Anderson, JJ; Hannan, MT; Felson, DT. Smoking eliminates the protective effect of oral estrogens on the risk for hip fracture among women. *Annals of Internal Medicine*, 1992, 116, 716-721.

Kliman, HJ; Nestler, JE; Sermasi, E; Sanger, JM; Strauss JF III. Purification, characterization and *in vitro* differentiation of cytotrophoblasts from human term placentae. *Endocrinology*, 1986; 118: 1567-1582.

Kostial, K. Cadmium. In: Merz W, editor. *Trace Elements in Human and Animal Nutrition - Fifth Edition, Volume 2.* Orlando, Florida: Academic Press, Inc.; 1986; 319-345.

Kostial, K; Blanuša, M; Kargačin, B; Piasek, M; Maljković, T; Kello, D. Sex-related differences in genetic susceptibility to toxic metals. In: Grandjean EC, editor. *Ecogenetics: Genetic predisposition to the toxic effects of chemicals.* Copenhagen, Denmark: World Health Organization, Regional Office for Europe. London: Chapman & Hall; 1991a; 111-122.

Kostial, K; Blanuša, M; Maljković, T; Kargačin, T; Piasek, M; Momčilović, B; Kello, D. Age and sex influence the metabolism and toxicity of metals. In: Momčilović B, editor. *Trace Elements in Man and Animals-7.* Zagreb, Croatia: Institute for Medical Research and Occupational Health, University of Zagreb; 1991b; 11/1-11/6.

Kostrzewska, A; Sobieszek, A. Diverse actions of cadmium on the smooth muscle myosin phosphorylation system. *FEBS Letters*, 1990, 263, 381-384.

Kubala-Kukuś, A; Banaś, A; Braziewicz, J; Majewska, U; Pajek, M. Comparative study of trace element contents in human full-term placenta and fetal membranes by total reflection X-ray fluorescence. *Spectrochimica Acta Part B*, 2003, 58, 725-734.

Kuhnert, PM; Kuhnert, BR; Bottoms, SF; Erhard, P. Cadmium levels in maternal blood, fetal cord blood, and placental tissues of pregnant women who smoke. *American Journal of Obstetrics and Gynecology*, 1982, 142, 1021-1025.

Kuhnert, PM; Kuhnert, BR; Erhard, P; Brasher, WT; Groh-Wargo, SL; Webster, S. The effect of smoking on placental and fetal zinc status. *American Journal of Obstetrics and Gynecology*, 1987, 157, 1241-1246.

Kuhnert, BR; Kuhnert, PM; Lazebnik, N; Erhard, P. The effect of maternal smoking on the relationship between maternal and fetal zinc status and infant birth weight. *Journal of the American College of Nutrition*, 1988, 7, 309-316.

Kuhnert, BR. Drug exposure to the fetus - the effect of smoking. *NIDA Research Monographs*, 1991, 114, 1-17.

Kyrklund-Blomberg, N; Cnattingius, S. Preterm birth and maternal smoking: risks related to gestational age and onset of delivery. *American Journal of Obstetrics and Gynecology*, 1998, 179, 1051-1055.

Leazer, TM; Liu, Y; Klaassen, CD. Cadmium absorption and its relationship to divalent metal transporter-1 in the pregnant rat. *Toxicology and Applied Pharmacology*, 2002, 185, 18–24.

Lagerkvist, BJ; Nordberg, GF; Söderberg, HÅ; Ekesrydh, S; Englyst, V; Gustavsson, M; Gustavsson, NO; Wiklund, DE. Placental transfer of cadmium. *IARC Scientific Publications*, 1992, 118, 287-291.

Lagerkvist, BJ; Sandberg, S; Frech, W; Jin, T; Nordberg, GF. Is placenta a good indicator of cadmium and lead exposure? *Archives of Environmental Health*, 1996, 51, 389-394.

Larsen, LG.; Clausen, HV; Jønsson, L. Stereologic examination of placentas from mothers who smoke during pregnancy. *American Journal of Obstetrics and Gynecology*, 2002, 186, 531-537.

Laskey, JW; Phelps, PV. Effect of cadmium and other metal cations on *in vitro* Leydig cell testosterone production. *Toxicology and Applied Pharmacology*, 1991, 108, 269-306.

Lauwerys, R; Buchet, J-P; Roels, H; Hubermont, G. Placental transfer of lead, mercury, cadmium, and carbon monoxide in women. I. Comparison of the frequency distributions of the biological indices in maternal and umbilical cord blood. *Environmental Research*, 1978, 15, 278-289.

Levin, AA; Miller, RK; di Sant'Agnese, PA. Heavy metal alterations of placental function: a mechanism for the induction of fetal toxicity in cadmium. In: Clarkson TW; Nordberg GF; Sager PR, editors. *Reproductive and developmental toxicity of metals.* New York: Plenum Press; 1983; 633-654.

Levin, AA; Kilpper, RW; Miller, RK. Fetal toxicity of cadmium chloride: the pharmacokinetics in the pregnant Wistar rat. *Teratology*, 1987, 36, 163-170.

Lindbohm, ML; Sallmen, M; Taskinen, H. Effects of environmental tobacco smoke on reproductive health. *Scandinavian Journal of Work and Environmental Health*, 2002, 28(Suppl 2), 84-96.

Lin, FJ; Fitzpatrick, JW; Ianotti, CA; Martin, DS; Mariani, BD; Tuan, RS. Effects of cadmium transport on trophoblast calcium transport. *Placenta*, 1997, 18, 341-356.

Loiacono, NJ; Graziano, JH; Kline, JK; Popovac, D; Ahmedi, Xh; Gashi, E; Mehmeti, A; Rajović, B. Placental cadmium and birthweight in women living near a lead smelter. *Archives of Environmental Health*, 1992, 47, 250-255.

Lutz, E; Lind, B; Herin P; Krakau, I; Bui, T-H; Vahter, M. Concentrations of mercury, cadmium and lead in brain and kidney of second trimester fetuses and infants. Journal of Trace Elements in Medicine and Biology, 1996; 10, 61-67.

MacMahon, B; Trichopoulos, D; Cole, P; Brown, J. Cigarette smoking and urinary estrogens. *New England Journal of Medicine*, 1982, 307, 1062-1065.

Maitani, T; Suzuki, KT. Effect of cadmium on essential metal concentrations in testis, liver and kidney of five inbred strains of mice. *Toxicology*, 1986, 42, 121-30.

Manci, EA; Blackburn, WR. Regional variations in the levels of zinc, iron, copper, and calcium in the term human placenta. *Placenta*, 1987, 8, 497–502.

Martin, BM; Reiter, R; Pham, T; Avellanet, YR; Camara, J; Lahm, M; Pentecost, E; Pratap, K; Gilmore, BA; Diverakar, S; Dagata, RS; Bull, JL; Stoica, A. Estrogen-like activity of metals in MCF-7 breast cancer cells. *Endocrinology*, 2003, 144, 2425-2436.

Matek Sarić. M; Blanuša, M; Piasek, M; Varnai, VM; Jureša, D; Kostial, K. Effect of dietary calcium on cadmium absorption and retention in suckling rats. *BioMetals*, 2002, 15, 175-182.

Mattson, SN; Calarco, KE; Chambers, CD; Lyons Jones, K. Interaction of maternal smoking and other in-pregnancy exposures: Analytical considerations. *Neurotoxicology and Teratology*, 2002, 24, 359-367.

McLaughlin, MJ; Parker, DR; Clarke, JM. Metals and miocronutrients - food safety issue. *Field Crops Research*, 1999, 60, 143-163.

Mendoza, ME; Chaves, FF. Helping pregnant women cope with smoking cessation. *Topics in Advanced Practice Nursing. EJournal*, 2003, 3(4). [Available from: URL: www.medscape.com/viewarticle/46298]

Merian, E; Anke, M; Ihnat, M; Stoeppler, M. *Elements and their compounds in the environment: Occurrence, analysis and biological relevance. Volume 2: Metals and their compounds.* Weinheim, Germany: Wiley-VCH Verlag GmBH & Co. KgaA; 2004.

Miller, RK; Ng, WW; Levin, AA. The placenta: the relevance to toxicology. In: Clarkson TW; Nordberg GF; Sager PR, editors. *Reproductive and developmental toxicity of metals*. New York: Plenum Press; 1983; 589-605.

Miller, RK; Mattison, DR; Plowchalk, D. Biological monitoring of the human placenta. In: Clarkson TW; Nordberg GF; Sager PR, editors. *Biological monitoring of toxic metals*. New York: Plenum Press; 1988; 567-602.

Miller, WL. Molecular biology of steroid hormone synthesis. *Endocrine Reviews*, 1988, 9, 295-318.

Milunsky, A; Carmella, SG; Ye, M; Hecht, SS. A tobacco-specific carcinogen in the fetus. *Prenatal Diagnosis*, 2000, 20, 307-310.

Moberg Wing, A; Wing, K; Tholin, K; Sjöström, R; Sandström, B; Hallmans, G. The relation of the accumulation of cadmium in human placenta to the intake of high-fibre grains and maternal iron status. *European Journal of Clinical Nutrition*, 1992, 46, 585-595.

Mochizuki, M; Maruo, T; Masuko, K; Ohtsu, T. Effects of smoking on fetoplacental-maternal system during pregnancy. *American Journal of Obstetrics and Gynecology*, 1984, 149, 413-420.

Mooney, SB; Giudice, LC. Endocrinology of Pregnancy. Chapter 13. In: Rebar RW, editor. *Female Reproductive Endocrinology. Endotext.com*; 2002 [Available from: URL: http://www.endotext.org/female/female13/femaleframe13.htm]

Mulcahy, S. The toxicology of cigarette smoke and environmental tobacco smoke. *Report Assignment - Biochemical Toxicology BC4927*; 1997 [Availabe from: URL: http://www.csn.ul.ie/~stephen/reports/bc4927.html]

Mueck, AO; Seeger, H. Smoking, estradiol metabolism and hormone replacement therapy. *Arzeneimittel-Forschung/Drug Research*, 2003, 53, 1-11.

Myllynen, P; Pasanen, M; Pelkonen, O. Human placenta: a human organ for developmental toxicology research and biomonitoring. *Placenta*, 2005, 26(5), 361-371.

Nishijo M. Nakagawa H. Honda R. Tanebe K. Saito S. Teranishi H. Tawara K. Effects of maternal exposure to cadmium on pregnancy outcome and breast milk. *Occupational & Environmental Medicine*, 2002, 59, 394-396.

Nishijo, M; Satarug, S; Honda, R; Tsuritani, I; Aoshima, K. The gender differences in health effects of environmental cadmium exposure and potential mechanisms. *Molecular & Cellular Biochemistry*, 2004, 255, 87-92.

Odland, JØ; Nieboer, E; Romanova, N; Thomassen, Y; Hofoss, D; Lund, E. Factor analysis of essential and toxic elements in human placentas from deliveries in arctic and subarctic areas of Russia and Norway. *Journal of Environmental Monitoring*, 2001, 3, 177-184.

Osada, H; Watanabe, Y; Nishimura, Y; Yukawa, M; Seki, K; Sekiya, S. Profile of trace element concentrations in the feto-placental unit in relation to fetal growth. *Acta Obstetricia Gynecologica Scandinavica*, 2002, 81, 931-937.

Osman, K; Akesson, A; Berglund, M; Bremme, K; Schűtz, A; Ask, K; Vahter, M. Toxic and essential elements in placentas of Swedish women. *Clinical Biochemistry*, 2000, 33, 131-138.

Paakki, P; Stockman, H; Kantola, M; Wagner, P; Lauper, U; Huch, R; Elovaara, E; Kirkinen, P; Pasanen, M. Maternal drug abuse and human term placental xenobiotic and steroid metabolizing enzymes *in vitro*. *Environmental Health Perspectives*, 2000, 108, 141-145.

Page, KR; Bush, PG; Abramovich, DR; Aggett, PJ; Burke, MD; Mayhew, TM. The effects of smoking on placental membranes. *Journal of Membrane Science*, 2002, 206(1-2 SI), 243-252.

Paksy, K; Varga, B; Horváth, E; Tátrai, E; Ungváry G. Acute effects of cadmium on preovulatory serum FSH, LH, and prolactin levels and on ovulation and ovarian hormone secretion in estrous rats. *Reproductive Toxicology*, 1989, 3, 241-247.

Paksy, K; Varga, B; Lázár, P. Cadmium interferes with steroid biosinthesis in rat granulosa cells *in vitro*. *BioMetals*, 1992, 5, 245-250.

Paksy, K; Varga; B, Lázár, P. Zinc protection against cadmium-induced infertility in female rats. Effect of zinc and cadmium on the progesterone production of cultured granulosa cells. *BioMetals*, 1996, 10, 27-35.

Paksy, K; Rajczy, K; Forgáscs, Z; Lázárm P; Bernard, A; Gáti, I; Kaáli, GS. Effect of cadmium on morphology and steroidogenesis of cultured human ovarian granulosa cells. *Journal of Applied Toxicology*, 1997, 17, 321-327.

Pařízek, J. Vascular changes at sites of oestrogen biosynthesis produced by parenteral injection of cadmium salts: the destruction of placenta by cadmium salts. *Journal of Reproduction and Fertility*, 1964, 7, 263-265.

Pařízek, J. Cadmium and reproduction: a perspective after 25 years. In: Clarkson TW; Nordberg GF; Sager PR, editors. *Reproductive and developmental toxicity of metals*. New York: Plenum Press; 1983; 301-313.

Paszkowski, T; Sikorski, R. Gestational smoking and placental content of essential metals. *Trace Elements in Medicine*, 1994, 11, 148-152.

Pasqualini, JR; Kincl, FA. *Hormones and the fetus. Volume I: Production, concentration and metabolism during pregnancy*. Oxford, UK: Pregamon Press; 1985.

Peacock, MJ; Bland, JM; Anderson, HR. Preterm delivery: effects of socioeconomic factors, psyhological stress, smoking, alcohol, and caffeine. *British Medical Journal*, 1995, 311, 531-535.

Pereg, D; Lagueux, J; Dewaily, É; Poirier, GG; Ayotte, P. Cigarette smoking during pregnancy: comparison of biomarkers for inclusion in epidemiological studies. *Biomarkers*, 2001, 6, 161-173.

Piasek, M; Laskey, JW. Acute cadmium exposure and ovarian steroidogenesis in cycling and pregnant rats. *Reproductive Toxicology*, 1994, 8, 495-507.

Piasek, M; Kostial, K; Laskey, JW. Experimental studies on reproductive and perinatal effects of lead and cadmium. *Environmental Management and Health*, 1996a, 7, 29-32.

Piasek, M; Schönwald, N; Blanuša, M; Kostial, K; Laskey, JW. Biomarkers of heavy metal reproductive effects and interaction with essential elements in experimental studies in female rats. *Arhiv za higijenu rada i toksikologiju*, 1996b, 47, 245–259.

Piasek, M; Laskey, JW. Effects of *in vitro* cadmium exposure on ovarian steroidogenesis in rats. *Journal of Applied Toxicology*, 1999, 19, 211-217.

Piasek, M; Laskey, JW; Blanuša, M; Kostial, K; Ferrell, JM. Low iron diet and cadmium exposure disrupt steroidogenesis in the rat. In: Roussel A-M, Anderson RA, Favier AE, editors. *Trace Elements in Man and Animals 10*. New York: Kluwer Academic/Plenum Publishers; 2000; 809-812.

Piasek, M; Blanuša, M; Kostial, K; Laskey, JW. Placental cadmium and progesterone concentrations in cigarette smokers. *Reproductive Toxicology*, 2001, 15, 673-681.

Piasek, M; Laskey, JW; Kostial, K; Blanuša, M. Assessment of steroid disruption using cultures of whole ovary and/or placenta in rat in human placental tissue. *International Archives of Occupational and Environmental Health*, 2002, 75(Suppl), S36-S44.

Piasek, M; Blanuša, M; Kostial, K; Laskey, JW. Low iron diet and parenteral cadmium exposure in pregnant rats: the effects on trace elements and fetal viability. *BioMetals*, 2004, 17, 1-14.

Pillai, A; Gupta, S. Effect of gestational and lactational exposure to lead and/or cadmium on reproductive performance and hepatic oestradiol metabolizing enzymes. *Toxicology Letters*, 2005, 155, 179-186.

Rath, G; Jain, AK; Bastia, B; Sood, M; Mukherjee, A. The effects of passive smoking on the terminal villi of human placenta. *Journal of the Anatomical Society of India*, 2001, 50, 19-23.

Red-Horse, K; Zhou, Y; Genbacev, O; Prakobphol, A; Foulf, R; McMaster, M; Fisher, SJ. Trophoblast differentiation during embryo implantation and formation of the maternal-fetal interface. *Journal of Clinical Investigation*, 2004, 114, 744-754.

Reichrtova, E; Ursinyova, M; Palkovicova, L; Wsolova, L. Contents and localization of heavy metals in human placentae. *Fresenius Journal of Analytical Chemistry*, 1998a, 361, 362–364.

Reichrtova, E; Dorociak, F; Palkovicova, L. Sites of lead and nickel accumulation in the placental tissue. *Human & Experimental Toxicology,* 1998b, 17, 176–181.

Ringler G, Strauss III JF. In vitro systems for the study of human placental endocrine function. *Endocrine Reviews*, 1990, 11, 105-123.

Ronco, AM; Arguello, G; Suazo, M; Llanos, MN. Increased levels of metallothionein in placenta of smokers. *Toxicology*, 2005, 208, 133-139.

Rush, D; Callahan, KR. Exposure to passive cigarette smoking and child development: a critical review. *Annals of the New York Academy of Sciences*, 1989, 562, 74-100.

Safe, S. Cadmium's disguise dupes the estrogen receptor. *Nature Medicine*, 2003, 9, 1000-1001.

Satarug, S; Ujjin, P; Vanavanitkun, Y; Baker, JR; Moore, MR. Influence of body iron store status and cigarette smoking on cadmium body burden of healthy Thai women and men. *Toxicology Letters*, 2004, 148, 177-185.

Selevan, SG; Kimmel, CA; Mendola, P. Identifying critical windows of exposure for children's health. *Environmental Health Perspectives*, 2000, 108(Suppl 3), 451-455.

Shah, NR; Bracken, MB. A systematic review and meta-analysis of prospective studies on the association between maternal cigarette smoking and preterm delivery. *American Journal of Obstetrics and Gynecology*, 2000, 182, 465-472.

Shiverick, KT; Salafia, C. Cigarette smoking and pregnancy - I: Ovarian, uterine and placental effects. *Placenta*, 1999, 20, 265-272.

Silbergeld, EK. Lead in bone: implications for toxicology during pregnancy and lactation. *Environmental Health Perspectives*, 1991, 91, 63-70.

Smith, CJ; Livingston, SD; Doolittle, DJ. An international literature survey of "IARC Group I carcinogens" reported in mainstream cigarette smoke. *Food and Chemical Toxicology*, 1997, 35, 1107-1130.

Solomon, S. The placenta as an endocrine organ: steroids. Chapter 51. In: Knobil E; Neill J, editors. *The physiology of reproduction*. New York, NY: Raven Press Ltd.; 1988; 2085-2091.

Stohs, SJ; Bagchi, D. Oxidative mechanism in the toxicity of metal ions. *Free Radical Biology and Medicine*, 1995, 18, 321-336.

Stohs, SJ; Bagchi, D; Bagchi, M. Toxicity of trace elements in tobacco smoke. *Inhalation Toxicology*, 1997, 9, 867-890.

Stoica A, Katzenellenbogen BS, Martin MB. Activation of estrogen receptor-alpha by the heavy metal cadmium. *Molecular Endocrinology*, 2000, 14, 545-553.

Sunderman FW Jr., Barber AM. Finger-loops, oncogenes and metals. *Annals of Clinical and Laboratory Science*, 1988, 18, 267-288.

Strauss, JF III; Martinez, F; Kiriakidou, M. Placental steroid hormone synthesis: unique featuers and unaswered questions. *Biology of Reproduction*, 1996, 54, 303-311.

Strauss, JF III; Christiansen, LK; Devoto, L; Martinez, F. Providing progesterone for pregnancy: control of cholesterol flux to the side-chain cleavage system. *Journal of Reproduction & Fertility - Supplement*, 2000, 55, 3-12.

Szekeres-Bartho, J; Barakonyi, A; Par, G; Polgar, B; Palkovics, T; Szerday, L. Progesterone as an immunomodulatory molecule. *International Immunopharmacology*, 2001, 1, 1037-1048.

Tanko, LB; Christiansen, C. An update on the antiestrogenic effect of smoking: a literature review with implications for researchers and practitioners. *Menopause*, 2004, 11, 104-109.

Tansavatdi, K; McClain, B; Herrington, DM. The effects of smoking on estradiol metabolism. *Minerva Ginecologica*, 2004, 56, 105-114.

Taylor, A; Branch, S; Halls, D; Patriarca, M; White, M. Atomic spectrometry update. Clinical and biological materials, foods and beverages. *Journal of Analytical Atomic Spectrometry*, 2004, 19, 505-556.

Thomas, T; Gallo, MA; Thomas, TJ. Estrogen receptors as targets for drug development for breast cancer, osteoporosis and cardiovascular diseases. *Current Cancer Drug Targets*, 2004, 4, 483-499.

Torreblanca, A; Del Ramo, J; Sarkar, B. Cadmium effects on zinc metabolism in human trophoblast cells: involement of cadmium-induced metallothionein. *Toxicology*, 1992, 72, 167-184.

Tuthill, DP; Stewart, JH; Coles, EC; Andrews, J; Cartlidge, PHT. Maternal cigarette smoking and pregnancy outcome. *Pediatric and Perinatal Epidemiology*, 1999, 13, 245-253.

Tziomalos, K; Charsoulis, F. Endocrine effects of tobacco smoking. *Clinical Endocrinology*, 2004, 61, 664-674.

U. S. Environmental Protection Agency (U. S. EPA). Indoor Air - Smoke-free Homes: Secondhand smoke can make children suffer serious health risks; 2004 [Available from: URL: http://www.epa.gov/smokefree/]

Vahter, M; Berglund, M; Åkesson, A; Líden, C. Metal and women's health. *Environmental Research Section A*, 2002, 88, 145-155.

Vallee, BL; Ulmer, DD. Biochemical effects of mercury, cadmium and lead. *Annual Review of Biochemistry*, 1972, 41, 91-128.

van Hattum, B; deVogt, P; Copius Peerboom, JW. An analytical procedure for the determination of cadmium in human placentae. *International Journal of Environmental Analytical Chemistry*, 1981, 10, 121-133.

van der Velde, WJ; Copius Peereboom-Stegeman, JHJ; Treffers, PE; James, J. Structural changes in the placenta of smoking mothers: a quantitative study. *Placenta*, 1983, 4, 231-240.

Varga, B; Zsolnai, B; Paksy, K; Náray, M; Ungváry, Gy. Age dependent accumulation of cadmium in the human ovary. *Reproductive Toxicology*, 1993, 7, 225-228.

Verthelyi, D. Sex hormones as immunomodulators in health and disease. *International Immunopharmacology*, 2001, 1:983-993.

Waalkes, MP; Ward, JM; Liu, J; Diwan, BA. Transplacental carcionogenicity of inorganic arsenic in the drinking water: induction of hepatic, ovarian, pulmonary, and adrenal tumors in mice. *Toxicology and Applied Pharm*acology, 2003, 186, 7-17.

Ward, NI; Durrant, S; Sankey, RJ; Bound, JP; Bryce-Smith, D. Elemental factors in human fetal development. *Journal of Nutritional Medicine*, 1990, 1, 19-26.

Wassermann, GA; Liu, X; Pine, DS; Graziano, JH. Contribution of maternal smoking during pregnancy and lead exposure to early child behavior problems. *Neurotoxicology and Teratology*, 2001, 23, 13-21.

Webb, M; Samarawickrama, GP. Placental transport and embryonic utilization of essential metabolites in the rat at the teratogenic does of cadmium. *Journal of Applied Toxicology*, 1981, 5, 270-277.

Wier, PJ; Miller, RK; Maulik, D; di Sant' Agnese, PA. Toxicology of cadmium in the perfused human placenta. *Toxicology and Applied Pharmacology*, 1990, 105, 156-171.

World Health Oganization (WHO). Children's Environment and Health Action Plan for Europe. EUR/04/5046267/7. WHO Regional Office Europe; 2004 [Available from: URL: http://www.who.dk/document/e83338.pdf].

WHO/EHC series. World Health Organization, Environmental Health Criteria. Geneva: WHO Regional Office Europe:
WHO/EHC 86 Mercury - environmental aspects; 1989;
WHO/EHC 118 Inorganic mercury; 1991;
WHO/EHC 134 Cadmium; 1992a;
WHO/EHC 135 Cadmium - environmental aspects; 1992b;
WHO/EHC 165 Inorganic lead; 1995;
WHO/EHC 224 Arsenic and arsenic compounds, 2nd Edition; 2001;
WHO/EHC 228 Principles and Methods for the Assessment of Risk from Essential Trace Elements; 2002; [Available from: URL: http://www.inchem.org/documents/ehc/ehc/ehc228.htm]

Zalups, RK; Koropatnick, J. *Molecular Biology and Toxicology of Metals*. London - New York: Taylor & Francis; 2000.

Zadorozhnaja, TD; Little, RE; Miller, RK; Mendel, NA; Taylor, RJ; Presley, BJ; Gladen, BC. Concentrations of arsenic, cadmium, copper, lead, mercury, and zinc in human placentas from two cities in Ukraine. *Journal of Toxicology and Environmental Health Part A*, 2000, 61, 255-263.

Zevin, S; Benowitz, NL. Drug interactions with tobacco smoking. An update. *Clinical Phamacokinetics*, 1999, 36, 425-438.

In: Smoking and Health Research Frontiers
Editor: Calvin B. Fong, pp. 163-182

ISBN 1-60021-480-0

Chapter VII

THE EFFECTS OF CIGARETTE SMOKING ON THE HUMAN PLASMA TOCOPHEROLS LEVELS

***Andrzej Sobczak*[1] *and Dariusz Gołka*[2]**
[1]Department of General and Analytical Chemistry, Medical University of Silesia, Sosnowiec, Poland;
[2]II Department of Pathomorphology, Medical University of Silesia, Katowice, Poland.

ABSTRACT

Free radicals levels in a healthy organism are strictly controlled by enzymatic and non-enzymatic antioxidants. In smokers, exogenous free radicals contained both in the mainstream smoke as well as in the sidestream smoke, may affect the control mechanisms involved in the oxidative balance regulation and therefore contribute to the oxidative stress, and may initiate the development of pathological changes. These processes can be followed and observed by measurements of non-enzymatic antioxidants levels. Vitamin E, being a fat-soluble antioxidant in biological membranes and plasma lipoprotein capsules, belongs to the most important non-enzymatic antioxidants. The evaluation of the actual vitamin E status in the body is very important for the estimation of vitamin E supplementation in persons showing its deficiency.

The literature review indicates that the alpha-tocopherol (the main form of vitamin E) level in plasma is in active smokers on average by 5% lower, however the data are discrepant (from –28.7% to +5.0%). Similar discrepancies are observed among reports on gamma-tocopherol metabolism. The differences in plasma levels between smokers and nonsmokers range from –3.0% to +20%. Diversity of plasma alpha- and gamma-tocopherol levels values in nonsmokers and persons exposed to environmental tobacco smoke (passive smokers) is similar to those observed among active smokers but the number of reports is minute.

Studies performed with use of deuter-labeled tocopherols unequivocally indicate a significantly faster diminishing of plasma tocopherols in smokers in comparison with nonsmokers, but this results are not confirmed in meta-analysis indicating that smoking is moderately, and frequently insignificantly associated with changes in plasma tocopherol levels. This is probably caused by physiological factors (absorption, transport, distribution) affecting vitamin E biokinetics in smokers and nonsmokers. This may also be caused by the body increased antioxidative mobilization in response to oxidative stress evoked by tobacco smoke.

This article discusses the effects of tobacco smoke on plasma alpha- and gamma-tocopherol levels in smokers and the possible causes of markedly divergent data.

Keywords: Review, Antioxidant, Alpha-tocopherol, Gamma-tocopherol, Cigarette smoking

INTRODUCTION

Free radicals, also called reactive oxygen species (ROS), have been rising particular interest in recent years due to their role in pathological processes leading to numerous disorders (Pittilo, 2000). Free radicals of the tobacco smoke origin, that enter the body cause dysfunction of the endothelial cells (Noronha-Dutra et al., 1993), are involved in oxidative streess (Epperlein et al., 1996), inactivate *α-1-antyproteinase* thus disturbing the delicate balance between proteinases and anti-proteinases which limit their activity (Evans and Pryor, 1994) finally leading to DNA damage (Liu et al., 1999), and they initiate the process of lipids peroxidation (Miller et al., 1997).

In a healthy organism, free radicals level is strictly controlled by enzymatic (superoxide dysmutase, catalase, glutathione peroxidase), and non-enzymatic (vitamin A, C, E, K, coenzyme Q, selene, thiol derivates) antioxidants. However, administration of exogenous ROSs, e.g. with tobacco smoke, may affect the control mechanisms by means of distorted oxidation-reduction balance in the body, development of oxidative stress, and initiation of free radical pathological processes that play an important role in physiological processes and pathological conditions.

Monitoring the antioxidative status in a patient, based on the measurements of the selected antioxidant levels in the body provides information regarding the need of supplementation with selected antioxidants in the person examined. Proper recognition of antioxidant vitamins storage depletion is necessary for the estimation of the appropriate dosage of supplemented substance. The purpose of the presented review is the evaluation of literature data regarding the effects of tobacco smoke on vitamin E utilization.

FREE RADICALS IN CIGARETTE SMOKE

Nearly 5000 tobacco smoke components have been identified so far (Hoffmann et al., 2001). It is estimated that the actual number of all tobacco smoke components may be even 10 to 20 times higher and constitute circa 5% of the main tobacco smoke stream (Haroun et al., 1999). The main stream of the tobacco smoke is generated at the temperature of circa 900°C and the side stream develops during slow cigarette burning at the temperature between

600°C and 700°C. Under these conditions processes of pyrolisis take place leading to formation of highly reactive molecules - free radicals (Czerwiecki, 1984).

Tobacco smoke contains 2 groups of free radicals - tarry phase radicals, and gaseous phase radicals. Most of the tarry phase radicals are semiquinone radicals $QH^\bullet$ being balanced with quinone Q and hydroquinone QH_2 (equation 1).

$$Q + QH_2 \Leftrightarrow 2QH^\bullet \tag{1}$$

Tarry phase radicals concentration is very high. It is estimated that each gram of the tarry phase contains circa 10^{17} radicals (Pryor and Stone, 1993). Zang et al. (1995) noted that tarry phase substances present in the aqueous tobacco smoke extract, after saturation with air (conditions analogous to those present in lungs) undergo the processes of autooxidation and are converted to semiquinone ($QH^\bullet$), hydroxyl ($^\bullet OH$) and peroxyl radicals ($ROO^\bullet$).

Oxygen radicals are prevalent in the gaseous phase. One 35-mililiter inhalation contains around 10^{15} radicals. They come into reaction with carbohydrates present in the tobacco smoke, e.g. isoprene and form alkyl ($R^\bullet$) and alkoxyl ($RO^\bullet$) radicals (Church and Pryor, 1985). Radicals associated with the gaseous phase are characterized by a very short lifetime, not exceeding 1 second, while particulate phase radicals and tarry phase radicals present with longer lifetime reaching up to tens of minutes (Pryor et al., 1990).

Reactive oxygen forms present in the tobacco smoke include also nitrogen oxide. Due to odd number of electrons, this compound is also considered a free radical. It easily bounds to oxygen and iron. These chemical properties are responsible for its physiological and pathophysiological role. In the tobacco smoke, they derive of amines and peroxynitrite ($O{=}N{-}OO^-$) (Shinagawa et al., 1998). Nitrogen oxide maintains high concentrations of other short-lifetime radicals for a longer time (more than 10 minutes). This process occurs through the slow oxidation of nitrogen oxide to nitrogen dioxide (equation 2), which as a more reactive one gets into reactions with unsaturated carbohydrates creating alkyl radicals (equation 3). Superoxide radicals and alkoxyle radicals are generated in following reactions (equation 4 and 5, respectively) (Church and Pryor, 1985).

$$2NO^\bullet + O_2 \rightarrow 2NO_2^\bullet \tag{2}$$

$$NO_2^\bullet + RCH{=}CH_2 \rightarrow RCH^\bullet{-}CH_2NO_2\ (R^\bullet) \tag{3}$$

$$R^\bullet + O_2 \rightarrow ROO^\bullet \tag{4}$$

$$ROO^\bullet + NO^\bullet \rightarrow RO^\bullet + NO_2^\bullet \tag{5}$$

Nitrogen oxide present in the fresh tobacco smoke under concentration of 300 ppm may also react with superoxide anion radical ($O_2^{\bullet-}$) forming peroxynitrite anion (equation 6) (Beckman et al., 1990; Pryor, 1993).

$$O_2^{\bullet-} + NO^\bullet \rightarrow ONOO^- \tag{6}$$

Peroxynitrite anion rapidly binds protone, thus forming peroxynitrous acid, which may be degraded to hydroxyl radical ($^{\bullet}OH$) and nitrogen dioxide (reaction 7 and 8):

$$ONOO^- + H^+ \rightarrow ONOOH \quad (7)$$

$$ONOOH \rightarrow NO_2^{\bullet} + {}^{\bullet}OH \quad (8)$$

Although hydroxyl radical and nitrogen dioxide may recombine to form nitric acid, the rate constant for this reaction in solution is much lower than for most of reactions involving hydroxyl radical (Beckman et al., 1990).

Also chemically stabile substances present in the tobacco smoke may be a source of free radicals. It was shown that superoxide anion radicals level in cultured pulmonary artery endothelial cells increases 3 times following the culture supplementation with tobacco smoke extract. This is due to increased nicotinamide adenine dinucleotide phosphate oxidase activity. It is believed that the main role in the increased free radical generation is played by acrolein, which is α,β-unsaturated aldehyde (Jaimes et al., 2004).

Composition, Biophysical and Antioxidant Properties of Vitamin E

Vitamin E belongs to the most important non-enzymatic antioxidants. It is the main lipophylic antioxidant of biological membranes and amphipatic capsule of the plasma lipoproteins (Thakur and Srivastava, 1996).

The term "vitamin E" encompasses 8 natural hydrophobic compounds. All of them consist of 6-chromanol ring and side chain (phytyl chain) containing 16 carbon atoms (Figure 1).

Four of the substances discussed contain saturated side chain (group of tocopherols), while the remaining four have 3 double bounds (group of tocotrienols). Both tocopherols as well as tocotrienols are designated with first four letter of the Greek alphabet α, β, γ, δ. All tocopherol molecules contain chirality centres at the positions 2, 4' and 8', which make 8 optically active stereoisomers of each tocopherol. Among them 2R,4'R,8'R-α-tocopherol (shortly, R,R,R-α-tocopherol or simply α-tocopherol) is the most common substance and also the one showing the highest biological activity. If the relative α-tocopherol antioxidative activity *in vitro* (defined on the basis of the tocopherol reaction with fatty acids peroxyl radical) expressed in percentage is regarded as 100%, then the remaining values are respectively 71% (β-tocopherol), 68% (γ-tocopherol), and 28% (δ-tocopherol) (Schneider, 2005). In the blood plasma, α-tocopherol makes circa 90% of the entire pool of substances known as vitamin E (Burton and Traber, 1990; Brigelius-Flohe and Traber, 1999). Therefore, α-tocopherol is frequently identified with vitamin E. Second most common tocopherol form in plasma is γ-tocopherol. This is why these two forms raise the most interest.

Vitmain E content in mitochondrial membranes is low, which is evidenced by the vitamin E to phospholipids molar ratio. There is one vitamin E molecule for each 1000-2000 phospholipid molecules (Sen i Packer, 2000). Incorporation of tocopherols into biological membranes and their retention is facilitated by phytyl chain attached at the position 2 of 6-hydroxychroman ring (Niki et al., 1985). Phytyl chain does not have any effect on the tocopherols' antioxidative properties (Wang and Quinn, 1999). But hydroxyl group bound to carbon '6' of the chroman ring is responsible for free radical scavenging (Figure 2).

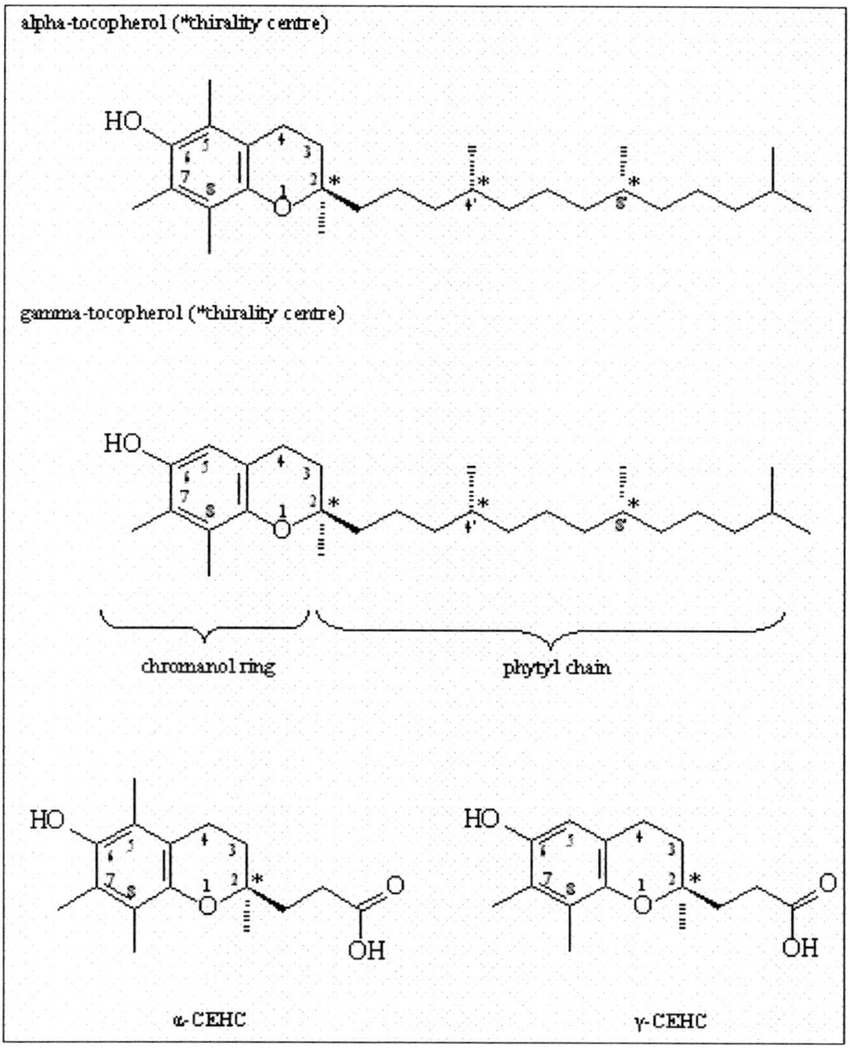

Figure 1. The structures of tocopherols and their metabolites, 2-(2'-carboxyethyl)-6-hydroxychromans (CEHC).

Such localization of the portion of tocopherol enables reactions both with lipid peroxyl radicals ($ROO^•$) as well as with aqueous phase alkoxyl radicals ($RO^•$) that frequently initiate the process lipid peroxidation chain reaction.

Antioxidant tocopherol activity is mainly based upon its involvement is the second line of defense against ROS, which is associated with scavenging of secondary organic free radicals, first of all lipid peroxyl radicals, thus terminating reactions of lipid peroxidation. Tocopherols react rapidly with organic free radicals (reaction rate constants between tocopherols and organic peroxyl radicals having different structure ranges from 10^4 to 10^9 l x mmol^{-1} x s^{-1}) (Bartosz, 2003). As a result, tocopherol transforms into free tocopheroxyl radical. The tocopheroxyl radical reactivity is relatively low, and it does not participate in the prolongation of the free radical reaction. It may, however, react with another free radical or undergo recombination with another tocopheroxyl radical. In both of these cases tocopherols lose their antioxidant properties and the developing vitamin E deficiency must be supplemented in diet. Only the tocopherol reduction by another antioxidants renders initial tocopherol structure (Figure 3).

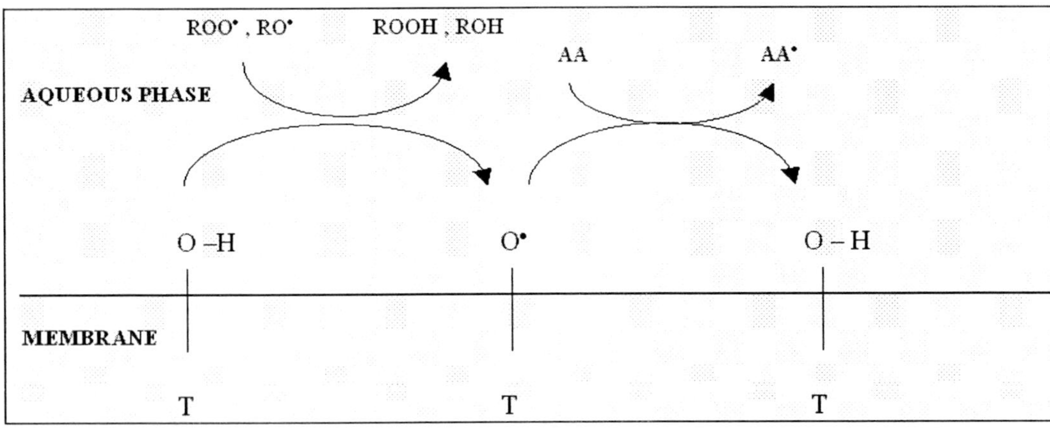

Figure 2. Tocopherol hydrophobe phytyl chain (T-OH) localized within the membrane, and the hydroxyl group bound to the carbon at the position 6 is protruding towards aqueous phase. Tocopherol reacts with lipid peroxyl radicals (ROO•) and alkoxyl radicals (RO•). Tocopheroxyl radical (T-O•) arising is then regenerated to tocopherol by ascorbic acid (AA) with simultaneous formation ascorbyl radical (AA•).

Regeneration of the tocopheroxyl radical that develops in the oxido-reductive reaction lets to maintain its amount and antioxidative potential (Sen and Packer, 2000). Radical tocopherol form is generated in its initial shape by co-antioxidants, such as glutathione, cytochrome c, ubichinol, and first of all vitamin C (Doba et al., 1985; van Acker et al., 1993; Shi et al., 1999). Ascorbyl radical that is formed in the aqueous phase may be regenerated by flavonoids (epicatechine and quercitine) present in membranes (Bandy and Bechera, 2001).

In mid eighties of the last century the main tocopherols' metabolit was identified in the urine of rats supplemented with high δ-tocopherol doses, namely 2-(2'-carboxyethyl)-6-hydroxychromans (CEHC) (Chiku et al., 1984). This compound forms due to shortening of the phytyl chain in course of the ω-oxidation reaction followed by cytochrome P-450 (CYP) mediated β-oxidation. Tocopherols are metabolized with participation of various CYP isoenzymes and to various extent, e.g. α-tocopherol is metabolized mainly by CYP3A4 (Birringer et al., 2001) and only small proportion of the administrated α-tocopherol dose (<1%) is converted to α-CEHC which is excreted with urine (Leonard et al., 2005) while γ-tocopherol is extensively metabolized by CYP4F2 to γ-CEHC (Sontag and Parker, 2002).

In course of these reactions, the chromanol ring structure remains unchanged (Lodge et al., 2001; Birringer et al. 2001; Sontag and Parker, 2002). Elimination of the hydrophobe chain makes CEHC more hydrophilic than tocopherols and tocotrienols from which they originate, but they maintain their antioxidative properties. In vitro studies showed that α-CEHC is a peroxyl radicals and peroxynitrite scavenger (Betancor-Fernandez et al., 2002). On the other hand, in rats, γ-CEHC shows protective properties. It protects from metal-induced nephrotoxicity, probably using the antioxidative mechanism (Appenroth et al. 2001). Both metabolites show similar, concentration-dependent, inhibition of the plasma and lipid LDL, but γ-CEHC is more effective perxynitrite anion ($ONOO^-$) scavenger than α-CEHC. *In vitro* they present the same antioxidative properties as tocopherols from which they are derived, but *in vivo* one should take into account different biopotentials and functions resulting from higher hydrophilic properties of metabolites (Galli et al., 2004).

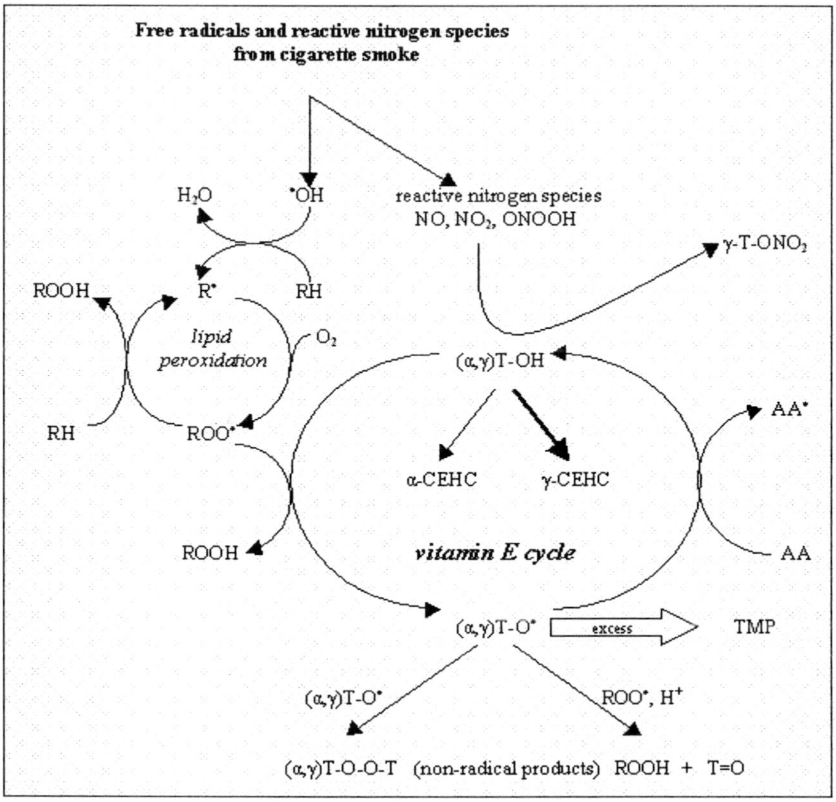

Figure 3. The effects of tobacco smoke on α- i γ-tocopherol (α,γ-T-OH) utilization. Depletion of tocopherols takes place in course of binding of reactive nitrogen forms with and reactive oxygen species leading to formation of non-radical products and their conversion to α-, γ-6-hydroxychromans (α,γ-CEHC). Tobacco smoke induces γ-tocopherol metabolism, which is evidenced by increased γ-CEHC excretion with urine in comparison with α-CEHC. At the same time, γ-tocopherol irreversibly binds with reactive nitrogen forms thus creating 5-nitro-γ-tocopferol (γ-T-ONO_2). Ascorbic acid (AA) deficiency results in restraining of the tocopherols regeneration. The excess of tocopheroxylradicals led to tocopherol-mediated peroxidation (TMP). Abbreviations: $AA^\bullet$, ascorbyl radical; $R^\bullet$, carbon-centered radical; $ROO^\bullet$, peroxyl radical; ROOH, lipid hydroperoxide; RH, polyunsaturated fatty acid; $(\alpha,\gamma)T\text{-}O^\bullet$, α,γ-tocopheroxyl radical.

Tocopherols may also act at the first line of defense against ROS, since they are effective singlet oxygen scavenger. The reaction rate constants with singlet oxygen range between 10^7 and 10^8 x mol^{-1} x s^{-1} and decrease in the following order $k_{\alpha\text{-tokoferol}} > k_{\beta\text{-tocopherol}} > k_{\gamma\text{- tocopherol}} >$

$k_{\delta\text{- tocopherol}}$. The ability to the reaction with singlet oxygen depends also on the hydroxyl group at the position '6' of the chromanol ring. Any estrification reaction of this group makes tocopherols non-reactive with singlet oxygen (Sies et al., 1992).

For a long time it was believed that γ-tocopherol, unlike its analogue α-tocopherol, does not play any important role in biochemical processes. It was because of its lower anti-oxidative activity and lower plasma concentration than α-tocopherol's. At present, more and more studies are focused on the role that γ-tocopherol plays in the pathogenesis of various disorders (Galli et al., 2003; 2004a; Hensley et al., 2004).

The difference in the molecular structure between α- and γ-tocopherol results from the lack of methyl group in the position 5 of the chromanol ring in the latter one. In healthy persons the plasma α-tocopherol / γ-tocopherol concentration ratio varies markedly according to their place of residence, and ranges from ca. 10 in women and 11 in men in Ireland to 24 and 25, respectively in Spain (Olmedilla et al., 2001). Gamma-tocopherol is a predominant dietary vitamin E form in some region of the USA (Jiang et al., 2001). Moreover, this substance may play a key role prevention of some cancers, and cardiovascular diseases (Christen et al., 1997; Jiang et al., 2000, 2001).

Besides different antioxidant potentials, α- and γ-tocopherol are characterized by different chemical properties. It is well illustrated by the inactivation of peroxynitrite anion ($O{=}N\text{-}OO^-$), which forms in the reaction of superoxide radical anion ($O_2^{\bullet -}$) and nitrogen oxide (equation 6). Peroxynitrite is not, however, a free radical but its strong oxidative properties make it react with thiol (-SH) groups of proteins and polyunsaturated fatty acids rests in lipids. The characteristic reaction for this substance is nitration of tyrozyl groups in proteins. Both α- as well as γ-tocopherol reacts promptly with peroxynitrite forming nitrogen dioxide and tocopheroxyl radical (equation 9) (Vatassery et al., 1998).

$$ONOO^- + (\alpha, \gamma)\text{-T-OH} \rightarrow NO_2^{\bullet} + (\alpha, \gamma)\text{-T-O}^{\bullet} + OH^- \qquad (9)$$

Therefore, the risk does not decrease, since instead of peroxynitrite, an active nitrogen dioxide is formed, which may nitrate proteins. However, of these two antioxidants only γ-tocopherol irreversibly binds nitrogen dioxide at the position '5' of the chromanol ring forming 5-nitro-γ-tocopherol.

This reaction is not possible in case of α-tocopherol, since all positions at the chromanol ring are already substituted. Therefore, only γ-tocopherol prevents nitration of bases in the DNA and of tyrozlyl rests in proteins, thus slowing down the development of atherosclerosis (Christen et al., 1997).

The effectiveness of γ-tocopherol in the elimination of reactive nitrogen species that enter the body with tobacco smoke was showed *in vitro* and *in vivo* studies by Leonard et al. (2003). The plasma 5-nitro-γ-tocopherol concentration in smokers is two times higher than in nonsmokers, both when comparing the crude 5-nitro-γ-tocopherol concentration as well as when adjusted to γ-tocopherol or plasma lipids levels in study persons. Moreover, a significant positive correlation ($r = 0.415$; $p = 0.015$) between the number of cigarettes smoked daily and the 5-nitro-γ-tocopherol concentration was noted. It is worth mentioning that in these studies (number of women and men, n=34), plasma α- tocopherol level in smokers and nonsmokers did not differ significantly, and the γ-tocopherol level was insignificantly lower by 4%.

Table 1. Percentage differences between serum/plasma α-tocopherol, γ-tocopherol and vitamin E levels in nonsmokers, passive smokers, and active smokers.

First author [year published]	Number of of study persons (sex)	Concentration changes in comparison with nonsmokers who are assumed as 100% [%]		
		passive smokers	active smokers	p
α-tocopherol				
Marangon [1998]	334 (M)	-	+ 5.0	< 0.006
Takatsuka [1998]	124 (F/M)	- 17.3	- 26.9	<0.05
Lykkesfeldt [2000]	75 (M)	-	- 7.4	ns
Alberg [2000]	586 (F)	- 2.8	- 1.1	ns
	560 (M)	- 5.2	+ 0.5	ns
Chopra [2000]	34 (F)	-	0.0 [1]	<0.01
Liu [2000]	59 (M)	-	- 39.6 [4]	0.001
Kim [2001]	20 (M)	-	- 20.6	<0.05
Tröbs [2002]	1077 (F/M)	0.0 [3]	- 6.7 [3]	<0.05
Daga [2003]	50 (F/M) [2]	-	- 28.7	<0.001
Dietrich [2003]	159 (F/M))	+ 1.3	- 1,0	ns
Wallström [2003]	529 (F/M)	-	-1.1	ns
Lykkesfeldt [2004]	80 (M)	-	- 2.0	ns
Lopes [2004]	133 (F)	-	- 22.1	<0.05
	49 (M)	-	- 8.2	ns
Sobczak [2004]	117 (F/M)	- 5.7	-9.2	<0.001
γ-tocopherol				
Alberg [2000]	456 (F)	+ 3.7	- 2.1	ns
	366 (M)	- 3.8	- 3.0	ns
Lykkesfeldt [2000]	75 (M)	-	+ 15.8	ns
Dietrich [2003]	159 (F/M)	+ 20.0	+ 20.0	0.032
Lykkesfeldt [2004]	80 (M)	-	-4.9	ns
Sobczak [2004]	117 (F/M)	+1.1	+3.2	ns
vitamin E				
Gökkusu [2001]	80 (F/M)	-	- 0.8	-
Wei [2001]	3901 (F)	- 3.6	- 6.1	ns
	3972 (M)	- 1.1	- 7.8	ns

F – female; M – male; p –statistical significance between smokers and nonsmokers; ns – non-significant.

[1] α-tocopherol level expressed in μmol/mmol of cholesterol;

[2] smokers with diagnosed chronic lung disease;

[3] α- and γ-tocopherol level expressed in (μmol/l) / cholesterol (mg/dl);

[4] α-tocopherol level expressed in μg/mg of the total lipids.

Cigarette Smoking and Depletion of Plasma or Serum Tocopherols

Tobacco smoke, causing oxidative stress affects also the oxidation-reduction balance and activates body protective mechanisms. As a consequence, it results in decreased concentration of some of the antioxidants.

Antioxidant vitamins concentrations are useful and frequently used indicators for the evaluation of the body oxidative-antioxidative balance. In literature, it is widely accepted that the plasma levels of ascorbic acid, α-carotene, β-carotene and kryptoxantine are more than by 25% lower in comparison with nonsmokers (Alberg, 2002). Instead, the literature data on the α-, γ-tocopherols or vitamin E in persons exposed to tobacco smoke provide divergent information. Table 1 summarizes results of the studies from 1998 -2004 on α-, γ-tocopherols plasma/blood levels changes in passive and active smokers in comparison with their levels in nonsmokers. Reports, in which authors use the term vitamin E without any additional comments are separated.

Most of the analyzed studies reported lower blood/plasma α-, γ-tocopherols or vitamin E levels in passive or active smokers then in nonsmokers. On the other hand, one should emphasize that some authors observed increased plasma levels of the substances discussed in passive and active smokers towards nonsmokers.

Dietrich et al., (2003) in their paper, report a significant, 20% increase in γ-tocopherol level both in the group of active smokers and in the group of passive ones. Margangon et al. (1998) found significantly higher plasma α-tocopherol levels (by 5.0%) in smokers vs. nonsmokers.

In a large, well-documented report, Alberg (2002) analyzed studies published in years 1986-2000 on the differences in plasma/serum antioxidants concentrations in persons exposed and non-exposed to tobacco smoke. The summary weighted average across studies for α-tocopherol (6 reports), γ-tocohperol (3 reports) and vitamin E (5 reports) was –4.2, -7.9, and –1.1, respectively. Calculations of the same parameter based on the data summarized in table 1 gave following results: – 4.8, +1.8, and – 6.9.

It is worth to notice that only in some studies, plasma tocopherols levels were evaluated in persons exposed to environmental tobacco smoke (ETS). Instead, even a short stay in the ETS environment may cause biological effect similar to those of active smoking (Baranoya and Glantz, 2005).

Sobczak at al. (2004) observed a signifficant negative correlation between plasma α-tocopherol level and urine cotinine concentration in passive smokers ($r = -0.431$, $p = 0.004$). The calculated Pearson's correlation coeficient value was similar to those of active smokers ($r=-0.534$, $p<0.001$). This suggests increased α-tocopherol disappearance with increased exposure to tobacco smoke estimated with the measurements cotinine concentration in urine. This relationship was positive in case of γ-tocopherol and it was significant only in the group of passive smokers ($r = 0.346$, $p = 0.027$).

The observed changes in plasma α- and γ-tocopherol levels in passive and active smokers in comparison with nonsmokers cannot rather be explained with differences in dietary habits. Although smokers usually consume less fruit and vegetables (Subar et al.,1990; Palaniappan et al., 2001), the amounts of vitamin E delivered with diet is similar in smokers and nonsmokers (Dietrich et al., 2003; Dyer et al., 2003). Meta-analysis of studies encompassing more than 76 thousands of people shows that the amount of vitamin E delivered with diet in smokers is only by 2.2% lesser than in nonsmokers (Alberg, 2002). There are also no significant differences in α-, γ-tocopherol, and vitamin E levels measured directly in plasma or serum from smokers and nonsmokers, and following standarization and adjustment according to the sex, age, ethnic origin, body mass index (BMI), alcohol consumption, fruit and vegetable consumption, and triacyloglyceroles concentration (Marangon et al., 1998; Wei et al., 2001; Wallström et al., 2003).

Possible Causes of Tocopherols Destruction by Cigarette Smoke

Studies on the explanation of the tobacco effects on tocopherols destruction have been intensified in recent years, mainly thanks to implementation of deuter-based methods. Unfortunately, till now only active cigarette smokers have been selected to studies, and passive smokers have been omitted.

Thanks to labeled tocopherols it was showed that one of the main causes of differences in plasma tocopherols concentration between smokers and nonsmokers is a different tobacco smoke-induced destruction rate of tocopherols.

In the study conducted by Munro et al. (1997) nosmokers and smokers were given a single dose of 50 mg deuter-labeled α-tocopherol and α-tocopherol acetate. The concentrations of both of these substances were measured after 6, 12, and 27 hours. At each of these time points, smokers revealed lower levels of both supplemented α-tocopherol forms than nonsmokers. After 12 hours the α-tocopherol to cholesterol ratio decreased markedly by 56%. The authors state that cigarette smokers are characterized either by reduced α-tocopherol absorption ability or increased α-tocopherol clearens.

Also Traber et al. (2001) indicate differences in vitamin E disintegration rate between smokers and nonsmokers as the main cause of lower plasma vitamin E level in smokers. In their experiments, authors supplemented nonsmokers (6 persons) and smokers (6 persons) daily at breakfast for seven days with a 75 mg dose of deuteric α-tocopherol and *all-rac*-α-tocopherol. The experiment was conducted on after cessation of supplementation for next 21 days in order to estimate the concentration of deuterric compounds. There was a trend toward a faster expotential disappearnce of the plasma α-tocopherol in smokers compared with nonsmokers.

After couple of years this study was repeated using a very similar study protocol, but in most of the study persons additional measurements of α-CEHC excretion in urine and plasma ascorbic acid levels were performed (Bruno et al., 2005). At baseline, no significant differences in α-tocopherol levels between smokers and nonsmokers were found. But after 17 days from the supplementation cessation, total plasma α-tocopherol (labeled and non-labeled) levels were significantly lower in smokers (by 23%, $p=0.011$). Also labeled and non-labeled urine α-CEHC concentrations were significantly lower (by 69%, $p=0.039$) in smokers than in nonsmokers. Alpha-tocopherol half-life was by 11% shorter in smokers than in nonsmokers.

A negative correlation between the fractional disappearance rates of α-tocopherol and plasma ascorbic acid concentration was found in smokers (r = - 0.713, p = 0.021), but not in nonsmokers. Authors suggest that higher fractional disappearance rates of α-tocopferol is associated with lower ascorbic acid level exclusively in the presence of an evident oxidative stress, as for example those observed in cigarette smokers. In a follow-up analysis of these same participants authors measured daily the concentrations of labeled and non-labeled α-CEHC and non-labeled γ-CEHC in order to define the pathway of α-tocopherol disappearance (Bruno et al., 2005a). The obtained results indicate that smoking does not contribute to increased α-tocopherol disappearance with participation of cytochrome P450, but rather through the antioxidant metabolism, that is in accordance with the antioxidant role of tocopherols.

Recently, a status of α- and γ-tocopherols in plasma, erytrocytes, lymphocytes, and platelets in 15 smokers and nonsmokers was compared (Jeanes et al., 2004a). No significant differences in α- and γ-tocopherols in plasma and in erytrocytes between smokers and nonsmokers were found. Instead, α-tocopherol concentration in smokers' lymphocytes (in relationship to protein) was significantly lower by 31% (p=0.001) and γ-tocopherol by 27% (p= 0.026) in comparison with the concentration in nonsmokers. Also, α-tocopherol concentration in smokers' platelets (in relationship to protein) was significantly lower (by 32%, p=0.014) as compared to nonsmokers. Gamma-tocopherol concentration in smokers' and nonsmokers' platelets was similar. Smokers presented with 53% higher γ-CEHC urinary excretion, probable as a result of cytochrom P450 induction by tobacco smoke components. This does not, however, explain the constant α-CEHC concentration in both groups. The main conclusion drawn by the authors, that is based upon the obtained results, is suggestion that the measurements of tocopherols concentration in lymphocytes and platelets is more appropriate for the evaluation of the vitamin E status under oxidative stress than their assessment in plasma or erytrocytes.

Unexpectedly, the *in vitro* results do not match the results *iv vivo*. Handelman et al. (1996) showed that in human plasma submitted to the gaseous phase of tobacco smoke, α-tocoherol level changes faster than γ-tocopherol level. Human plasma exposition to gaseous phase of tobacco smoke resulted in a significant reduction α-tocoherol level and γ-tocopherol level reduction by 70% ($p<0.001$) and 30% ($p<0.05$), respectively. These results are inconsistent with the results discussed previously, where plasma α-tocopherol level and γ-tocopherol level decreased faster in smokers than in nonsmokers.

The results of the *in vitro* studies presented above with use of labeled compounds unequivocally show the tobacco smoke-induced α-tocopherol and γ-tocopherol disappearance, however, at different rates. Should the biokinetics be the only factor influencing tocopherols disappearance, one may ask, how to explain increase in plasma tocopherols levels in smokers in comparison with nonsmokers reported in some studies (see table 1) or contradictory results obtained in *in vivo* studies?

It seems that the discrepancies result from physiological factors that come into being under *in vivo* circumstances. They may influence vitamin E absorption, transport, and distribution in humans. These processes may differ between smokers and nonsmokers. All forms of vitamin E are absorbed by enterocytes and released to circulation in chylomicrons. Most probably, at this stage different tocopherols are not distinguished. Then, they reach liver with chylomicrons remnants, where α-tocopherol transfer protein (α-TTP) isolates α-tocopherol from other tocopherols and than incorporates it into very low density lipoproteins (VLDL) (Brigelius-Flohe et al., 2002; Frank, 2005). It is possible that at this stage, mechanisms involved in the hepatic intracellular trafficking of α-tocopherol involving α-TTP are distorted in smokers. This might explain the results indicating that smokers and nonsmokers differ in their processing of natural (RRR form) and synthetic (all rac) α-tocopherol (Lodge, 2005).

Differences in tocopherols biokinetics may also result from the genetic factors. Apo E genotype effect on α-tocopherol was studied. It was showed that that apoE3 subjects take up less newly absorbed α-tocopherol into the plasma than apoE4 subjects (Lodge et al., 2004). A genetic defect in α-TTP is responsible for inducing a severe vitamin deficiency characterized by a neurodegenerative disease, ataxia with vitamin E deficiency (Stocker, 2004; Morley et al., 2004).

Vitamin E status is also influenced by dietary factors. Recently, it was found that not only the amount of fat but also the physical properties of food and food matrix have effect on vitamin E absorption (Jeanes et al., 2004).

Moreover, in response to oxidative stress caused by tobacco smoke, the body may activate protective mechanisms, including vitamin E (Elsayed, 2001). One of the theories of mechanisms of the antioxidative mobilization assumes that increased lipid peroxidation and formation of bioactive proteins molecules caused by tobacco smoke results in mobilization of vitamin E contained in membranes and its involvement in free radicals scavenging. This causes a decrease of the concentration in membranes being the oxydants' targets. This in turn, activates signal transduction pathways (Suzuki et al., 1997; Travers, 1999) stimulating the vitamin E mobilization from stores in other parts of the body and its delivery with use of very low density lipoproteins to the sites where it is supposed to "fight" free radicals (Parks et al., 2000). When the body vitamin E pool is sufficient, then the free radicals-induced damage is readily repaired. Instead, in case of vitamin E deficiency and limited antioxidant capacity, damage progression takes place. At present it is the only hypothesis that may explain higher plasma vitamin E levels in smokers in comparison with nonsmokers reported in some studies.

The body mobilization potential was confirmed in studies of Polidori et al. (2003). They found, that 4 weeks after smoking cessation plasma α- and γ-tocopherol levels were significantly higher (by 11.5% and 10%, respectively) in comparison with their levels while these persons had been smoking. This might indicate that despite the elimination of the factor that increases the use of vitamin E, the body maintains the response to oxidative stress caused by tobacco smoking and increases its plasma level.

Vitamin E is not the only antioxidant involved in scavenging of tobacco smoke-derived free radicals. The first line of defense against short living tobacco smoke-derived inhaled free radicals is the liquid coating of the pulmonary epithelium (MacNee, 2000). The main "scavenger" of the reactive oxygen spices and related forms is the intra- and extracellular glutathione (Li et al., 1996). It may react with peroxyl radicals, semiquinone radicals, organic radicals and hydroxyl radicals. The pool of free radicals migrating into the body becomes therefore markedly diminished reduced. So, this is the enzymatic activity of endothelial antioxidants that affects further antioxidant demand, including vitamin E.

Tobacco smoke is not the only external source disrupting the oxidative-reduction balance of the human body. *In vitro* studies showed that ROS might be generated by slow alternating electromagnetic fields (Kula et al., 2002). But *in vivo* studies conducted on steel plant workers operating electric ovens showed that long lasting exposure to such electromagnetic fields causes a decrease in the activity of enzymatic and non-enzymatic plasma antioxidants, including α- and γ-tocopherol (Kula et al., 2002a; Sobczak et al., 2002).

Conclusion

A range of articles reports very divergent results of plasma α- and γ-tocopherol levels in smokers and nonsmokers. This may result from various factors affecting tocopherols concentrations. Therefore, the question arises, whether plasma α- and γ-tocopherol levels reflect the actual vitamin E status? Measuring plasma tocopherols concentration one estimates exclusively their amount that is bound to circulating lipoproteins. One does not take into account the pool of tocopherols present in liver, platelets, lymphocytes and erythrocytes. One also does not measure the amount of tocopherols associated with biologic membranes, which are directly responsible for antioxidative reactions. Therefore, some authors believe that more reliable biomarker of the body vitamin E could be α-CEHC concentration in urine, which reflects the metabolism of the main form of vitamin E pool in liver (Schultz et al., 1995; Brigelius-Flohe et al., 2002; Leonard et al., 2004; Bruno and Traber, 2005). Using α-CEHC for the evaluation of the vitamin E status has some limitations. Defect of the α-tocopherol transporting protein gene may cause high α-CEHC concentrations in urine even if the plasma α-tocopherol level is very low (Schuelke et al., 2000). Moreover, in healthy subjects, α-CEHC excretion was increased only after surpassing a plasma α-tocopherol threshold of 30-40 μmol/l, which suggests that metabolism occurs when adequate or excessive hepatic α-tocopherol concentration have been achieved (Schultz et al., 1995; Bruno and Traber, 2005). Maybe an appropriate biomarker of the vitamin E status could be plasma α-tocopherol to urine α-CEHC ratio.

Most of the experiments conducted so far indicate that smoking cigarettes increases vitamin E demand in humans. However, it does not seem that this demand is very high, the observation that is supported by the results of meta-analysis of the studies conducted in recent years. Therefore, vitamin E supplementation in smokers should be very cautious in order to not evoke the effect of tocopherol-mediated peroxidation (Upston et al., 1999) and should be applied in combination with additional ascorbic acid supplementation.

References

Alberg, AJ; Chen, JC; Zhao, H; Hoffman, SC; Comstock, GW; Helzlsouer, KJ. Houshold exposure to passive cigarette smoking and serum micronutrient concentrations. *Am. J. Clin. Nutr.*, 2000, 72, 1576-1582.

Alberg, AJ. The influence of cigarette smoking on circulating concentrations of antioxidant micronutrients. *Toxicology*, 2002, 180, 121-137.

Appenroth, D; Karge, E; Kiessling, G; Wechter, WJ; Winnefeld, K; Fleck, C. LLU-alpha, an endogenous metabolite of gamma-tocopherol, is more effective against metal nephrotoxicity in rats than gamma-tocopherol. *Toxicol. Lett.*, 2001, 122, 255-265.

Bandy, B; Bechara, EJ. Bioflavonoid rescue of ascorbate at a membrane interface. J. Bioenerg. *Biomembr.*, 2001, 33, 269-277.

Barnoya, J; Glantz, SA. Cardiovascular effects of secondhand smoke. Nearly as large as smoking. *Circulation*, 2005, 111, 2684-2698.

Bartosz, G. Second face of oxygen. Free radical in nature. (in Polish). Warsaw: Polish Scientific Publishers PWN; 2003.

Beckman, JS; Beckman, TW; Chen, J; Marshall, PA; Freeman, BA. Apparent hydroxyl radical production by peroxynitrite. Implications for endothelial injury from nitric oxide and superoxide. *Proc. Natl. Acad. Sci. USA*, 1990, 87, 1620-1624.

Betancor-Fernandez, A; Sies, H; Stahl, W; Polidori, MC. In vitro antioxidant activity of 2,5,7,8-tetramethyl-2-(2'-carboxyethyl)-6-hydroxychroman (alpha-CEHC), a vitamin E metabolite. *Free Radic. Res.*, 2002, 36, 915-921.

Birringer, M; Drogan, D; Brigelius-Flohe, R. Tocopherols are metabolized in HepG2 cells by side chain omega-oxidation and consecutive beta-oxidation. *Free Radic. Biol. Med.*, 2001, 31, 226-232.

Brigelius-Flohe, R; Kelly, FJ; Salonen, JT; Neuzil, J; Zingg, JM; Azzi, A. The European perspective on vitamin E current knowledge and future research. *Am. J. Clin. Nutr.*, 2002, 76, 703-716.

Brigelius-Flohe, R; Traber, MG. Vitamin E function and metabolism. *FASEB J.*, 1999, 13, 1145-1155.

Bruno, RS; Leonard, SW; Li, J; Bray, TM; Traber, MG. Lower plasma alpha-carboxyethyl-hydroxychroman after deuterium-labeled alpha-tocopherol supplementation suggests decreased vitamin E metabolism in smokers. *Am. J. Clin. Nutr.*, 2005a, 81, 1052-1059.

Bruno, RS; Ramakrishnan, R; Montine, TJ; Bray, TM; Traber, MG. α-Tocopherol disappearance is faster in cigarette smokers and is inversely related to their ascorbic acid status. *Am. J. Clin. Nutr.*, 2005, 81, 95-103.

Bruno, RS; Traber, MG. Cigarette smoke alters human vitamin E requirements. *J.Nutr.*, 2005, 135, 671-674.

Burton, GW; Traber, MG. Vitamin E antioxidant activity, biokinetics and bioavailability. *Annu. Rev. Nutr.*, 1990, 10, 357-382.

Chiku, S; Hamamura, K; Nakamura, T. Novel urinary metabolite of d-δ-tocopherol in rats. *J. Lipid Res.*, 1984, 25, 40-48.

Chopra, M; O'Neill, ME; Keogh, N; Wortley, G; Southon, S; Thurnham, DI. Influence of increased fruit and vegetable intake on plasma and lipoprotein carotenoids and LDL oxidation in smokers and nonsmokers. *Clin. Chem.*, 2000, 46, 1818-1829.

Christen, S; Woodall, AA; Shigenaga, MK; Southwell-Keely, PT; Duncan, MW; Ames BN. γ-Tocopherol traps mutagenic electrophiles as NO_x and complements α-tocopherol. Physiological implications. *Proc. Natl. Acad. Sci. USA*, 1997, 94, 3217-3222.

Church, DF; Pryor, WA. Free-radical chemistry of cigarette smoke and its toxicological implications. Environ. *Health Perspect.*, 1985, 64, 111-126.

Czerwiecki, L. Harmful substances in cigarette smoke. (in Polish). *Roczn. PZH*, 1984, 35, 233-238.

Daga, MK; Chhabra, R; Sharma, B; Mishra, TK. Effects of exogenous vitamin E supplementation on the levels of oxidants and antioxidants in chronic obstructive pulmonary disease. *J. Biosci.*, 2003, 28, 7-11.

Dietrich, M; Block, G; Norkus, EP; Hudes, M; Traber, MG; Cross, CE; Packer, L. Smoking and exposure to environmental tobacco smoke decrease some plasma antioxidants and increase γ-tocopherol in vivo after adjustment for dietary antioxidant intakes. *Am. J. Clin. Nutr.*, 2003, 77, 160-166.

Doba, T; Burton, GW; Ingold, KU. Antioxidant and co-antioxidant activity of vitamin C. The effect of vitamin C, either alone or in the presence of vitamin E or a water-soluble vitamin E analogue, upon the peroxidation of aqueous multilamellar phospholipid liposomes. Biochim. Biophys. *Acta*, 1985, 835, 298-303.

Dyer, AR; Elliott, P; Stamler, J; Chan, Q; Ueshima, H; Zhou, BF. Dietary intake in male and female smokers, ex-smokers, and never smokers: The INTERAMP Sudy. *J. Hum. Hypertens.*, 2003, 17, 641-654.

Elsayed, NM. Antioxidant mobilization in response to oxidative stress: a dynamic environmental-nutritional interaction. *Nutrition*, 2001, 17, 828-834.

Epperlein, MM; Nourooz-Zadeh, J; Noronha-Dutra, AA; Woolf, N. Nitric oxide in cigarette smoke as a mediator of oxidative damage. *Int. J. Exp. Pathol.*, 1996, 77, 197-200.

Evans, MD; Pryor, WA. Cigarette smoking, emphysema, and damage to α_1-proteinase inhibitor. *Am. J. Physiol.*, 1994, 266, L539-L611.

Frank, J. Beyond vitamin E supplementation An alternative strategy to improve vitamin E status. *J. Plant Physiol.* 2005; 162; 834-843.

Galli, F; Lee, R; Atkinson, J; Floridi, A; Kelly, FJ. γ-Tocopherol biokinetics and transformation in humans. *Free Radic. Res.*, 2003, 37, 1225-1233.

Galli, F; Piroddi, M; Lannone, A; Pagliarani, S; Tomasi, A; Floridi, A. A comparison between the antioxidant and peroxynitrite-scavenging functions of the vitamin E matabolites alpha- and gamma-carboxyethyl-6-hydroxychromans. *Int. J. Vitam. Nutr. Res.*, 2004, 74, 362-373.

Galli, F; Stabile, AM; Betti, M; Conte, C; Pistilli, A; Rende, M; Floridi, A; Azzi, A. The effect of α- and γ-tocopherol and their carboxyethyl hydroxychroman metabolites on prostate cancer cell proliferation. Arch. Biochem. *Biophys.*, 2004a, 423, 97-102.

Gökkusu, C; Ademoglu, E; Tamer, S; Alkan, G. Oxidant-antioxidant profiles of platelet rich plasma in smokers. *Addict. Biol.*, 2001, 6, 325-330.

Handelman, GJ; Packer, L; Cross, CE. Destruction of tocopherols, carotenoids, and retinol in human plasma by cigarette smoke. *Am. J. Clin. Nutr.*, 1996, 63, 559-565.

Haroun, L; Dunn, AJ; Ting, D. Exposure Measurement and Prevalence. [In] Health effects of exposure to environmental tobacco smoke. The Report of the California Environmental Protection Agency. [Ed.] Zeise L. Bethesda: MD National Institutes of Health; 1999.

Hensley, K; Benaksas, EJ; Bolli, R; Comp, P; Grammas, P; Hamdheydari, L; Mou, S; Pye, QN; Stoddard, MF; Wallis, G; Williamson, KS; West, M; Wechter, WJ; Floyd, RA. New perspectives on vitamin E: γ-tocopherol and carboxyelthylhydroxychroman metabolites in biology and medicine. *Free Radic. Biol. Med.*, 2004, 36, 1-15.

Hoffmann, D; Hoffmann, I; El-Bayoumy, K. The less harmful cigarette: a controversial issue. A tribute to Ernst L. Wynder. *Chem. Res. Toxicol.*, 2001, 14, 767-790.

Jaimes, EA; DeMaster, EG; Tian, RX; Raij, L. Stable compounds of cigarette smoke induce endothelial superoxide anion production via NADPH oxidase activation. Arterioscler. Thromb. *Vasc. Biol.*, 2004, 24, 1031-1036.

Jeanes, YM; Hall, WL; Ellard, S; Lee, E; Lodge, JK. The absorption of vitamin E is influenced by the amount of fat in a meal and the food matrix. *Br. J. Nutr.*, 2004, 92, 575-579.

Jeanes, YM; Hall, WL; Proteggente, AR; Lodge, JK. Cigarette smokers have decreased lymphocyte and platelet alpha-tocopherol levels and increased excretion of the gamma-tocopherol metabolite gamma-carboxyethyl-hydrochroman (gamma-CEHC). *Free Radic. Res.* 2004a, 38 861-868.

Jiang, Q; Christen, S; Shigenaga, M.K; Ames, BN. γ-Tocopherol, the major form of vitamin E in the US diet, deserves more attention. *Am. J. Clin. Nutr.*, 2001, 74, 714-722.

Jiang, Q; Elson-Schwab, I; Courtemanche, C; Ames, BN. γ-Tocopherol and its major metabolite, in contrast to α-tocopherol, inhibit cyclooxygenase activity in macrophages and epithelial cells. *Proc. Natl. Acad. Sci. USA*, 2000, 97, 11494-11499.

Kim, HS; Lee, BM. Protective effects of antioxidant supplementation on plasma lipid peroxidation in smokers. *J. Toxicol. Environ. Health*, 2001, 63, 583-598.

Kula, B; Sobczak, A; Kuśka, R. A study of the effects of static and extremely low frequency magnetic fields on lipid peroxidation products in subcellular fibroblast fractions. *Electromagnet. Biol. Med.*, 2002, 21, 161-168.

Kula, B; Sobczak, A; Kuśka, R. Effects of electromagnetic field on free-radical processes in steelworkers. Part I. Magnetic field influence on the antioxidant activity in red blood cells and plasma. *J. Occup. Health*, 2002, 44, 226-229.

Leonard, SW; Bruno, RS; Paterson, E; Schock, BC; Atkinson, J; Bray, TM; Cross, CE; Traber, MG. 5-Nitro-γ-tocopherol increases in human plasma exposed to cigarette smoke in vitro and in vivo. *Free Radic. Biol. Med.*, 2003, 35, 1560-1567.

Leonard, SW; Bruno, RS; Ramakrishnan, R; Bray, TM; Traber, MG. Cigarette smoking increases human vitamin E requirements as estimated by plasma deuterium-labeled CEHC. *Ann. N. Y. Acad. Sci.*, 2004, 1031, 357-360.

Leonard, SW; Paterson, E; Atkinson, JK; Ramakrishnan, R; Cross, CE; Traber, MG. Studies in humans using deuterium-labeled α- and γ-tocopherols demonstrate faster plasma γ-tocopherol disappearance and greater γ-metabolite production. *Free Rad. Biol. Med.*, 2005, 38, 857-866.

Li, XY; Rahman, I; Donaldson, K; MacNee, W. Mechanisms of cigarette smoke induced increased airspace permeability. *Thorax*, 1996, 51, 465-471.

Liu, CS; Lii, CK; Ou, CC; Tsai, CH; Wei, YH; Chen, HW. Autoantibody against oxidized low-density lipoproteins may be enhanced by cigarette smoking. *Chem–Biol Interact.*, 2000, 127, 125-137.

Liu, X; Lu, J; Liu, S. Synergistic induction of hydroxyl radical-induced DNA single-strand breaks by chromium (VI) compound and cigarette smoke solution. *Mutat. Res.*, 1999, 440, 109-117.

Lodge, JK; Hall, WL; Jeanes, YM; Proteggente, AR. Physiological factors influencing vitamin E biokonetics. *Ann. N. Y. Acad. Sci.*, 2004, 1031, 60-73.

Lodge, JK; Ridlington, J; Leonard, S; Vaule, H; Traber, MG. Alpha- and gamma-tocotrienols are metabolized to carboxyethyl-hydroxychroman derivatives and excreted in human urine. *Lipids*, 2001, 36, 43-48.

Lodge, JK. Vitamin E bioavailabity in humans. J. Plant Physiol., 2005, 162, 790-796.

Lopes, PA; Santos, MC; Vicente, L; Viegas-Crespo, AM. Effect of cigarette smoking on serum alpha-tocopherol and the lipid profile in a Portuguese population. *Clin. Chim. Acta*, 2004, 348, 49-55.

Lykkesfeldt, J; Christen, S; Wallock, LM; Chang, HH; Jacob, RA; Ames, BN. Ascorbate is depleted by smoking and repleted by moderate supplementation: a study in male smokers and nonsmokers with matched dietary antioxidant intakes. *Am. J. Clin. Nutr.*, 2000, 71, 530-536.

Lykkesfeldt, J; Viscovich, M; Poulsen, HE. Plasma malnondialdehyde is induced by smoking: a study with balanced antioxidant profiles. Br. J. Nutr., 2004, 92, 203-206.

MacNee, W. Oxidants/antioxidants and COPD. *Chest*, 2000, 117, 303S-317S.

Marangon, K; Herbeth, B; Lecomte, E; Paul-Dauphin, A; Grolier, P; Chancerelle, Y; Artur, Y; Siest, G. Diet, antioxidant status, and smoking habits in French men. *Am. J. Clin. Nutr.*, 1998, 67, 231-239.

Miller, ER III; Appel, LJ; Jiang, L; Risby, TH. Association between cigarette smoking and lipid peroxidation in a controlled feeding study. *Circulation*, 1997, 96, 1097-1101.

Morley, S; Panagabko, C; Shineman, D; Mani, B; Stocker, A; Atkinson, J; Manor, D. Molecular determinants of heritable vitamin E deficiency. *Biochemistry*, 2004, 43, 4143-4149.

Munro, LH; Burton, G; Kelly, FJ. Plasma RRR-alpha- tocopherol concentrations are lower in smokers than in nonsmokers after ingestion of a similar oral load of this antioxidant vitamin. *Clin. Sci.* (Lond)., 1997, 92, 87-93.

Niki, E; Kawakami, A; Saito, M; Yamamoto, Y; Tsuchiya, J; Kamiya, Y. Effect of phytyl side chain of vitamin E on its antioxidant activity. *J. Biol. Chem.*, 1985, 260, 2191-2196.

Noronha-Dutra, AA; Epperlein, MM; Woolf, N. Effect of cigarette smoking on cultured human endothelial cells. *Cardiovasc. Res.*, 1993, 27, 774-778.

Olmedilla, B; Granado, F; Southon, S; Wright, AJA; Blanco, I; Gil-Martinez, E; van den Berg, H; Corridan, B; Roussel, AM; Chopra, M; Thurnham, DI. Serum concentrations of carotenoids and vitamins A, E, and C in control subjects from five European countries. *Br. J. Nutr.*, 2001, 85, 227-238.

Palaniappan, U; Starkey, LJ; O'Loughlin, J; Gray-Donald, K. Fruit and vegetable consumption is lower and saturated fat intake is higher among Canadians reporting smoking. *J. Nutr.*, 2001, 131, 1952-1958.

Parks, EJ; Dare, D; Frazier, KB; Hellerstein, MK; Neese, RA; Hughes, E; Traber, MG. Dependence of plasma alpha-tocopherol flux on very low-density triglyceride clearance in humans. *Free Radic. Biol. Med.*, 2000, 29, 1151-1159.

Pittilo, RM. Cigarette smoking, endothelial injury and cardiovascular disease. *Int. J. Exp. Path.*, 2000, 81, 219-230.

Polidori, MC; Mecocci, P; Stahl, W; Sies, H. Cigarette smoking cessation increases plasma levels of several antioxidant micronutrients and improves resistance towards oxidative challenge. *Br. J. Nutr.*, 2003, 90, 147-150.

Pryor, WA; Church, DF; Evans, MD; Rice, WY; Hayes, JR. A comparison of the free radical chemistry of tobacco-burning cigarettes and cigarettes that only heat tobacco. *Free Radic. Biol. Med.*, 1990, 8, 275-279.

Pryor, WA; Stone, K. Oxidants in cigarette smoke. Radicals, hydrogen peroxide, peroxynitrate and peroxynitrite. *Ann. N. Y. Acad. Sci.*, 1993, 686, 12-27.

Schneider, C. Chemistry and biology of vitamin E. Mol. Nutr. Food Res., 2005, 49, 7-30.

Schuelke, M; Elsner, A; Fnickh, B; Kohlschütter, A; Hübner, C; Brigelius-Flohe, R. Urinary α-tocopherol metabolites in α-tocopherol transfer protein-deficient patients. *J. Lipid Res.*, 2000, 41, 1543-1551.

Schultz, M; Leist, M; Petrzika, M; Gassmann, B; Brigelius-Flohe, R. Novel urinary metabolite of alpha-tocopherol, 2,5,7,8-tetramethyl-2(2'-carboxyethyl)-6-hydroxychroman, as an indicator of an adequate vitamin E supply? *Am. J. Clin. Nutr.*, 1995, 62(suppl), 1527S-1534S.

Sen, CK; Packer, L. Thiol homeostasis and supplements in physical exercise. *Am. J. Clin. Nutr.*, 2000, 72(suppl), 653S-669S.

Shi, H; Noguchi, N; Niki, E. Comparative study on dynamics of antioxidative action of alfa-tocopheryl hydroquinone, ubiquinol, and alfa-tocopherol against lipid peroxidation. *Free Radic. Biol. Med.*, 1999, 27, 334-346.

Shinagawa, K; Tokimoto, T; Shirane, K. Spin trapping of nitric oxide in aqueous solutions of cigarette smoke. *Biochem. Biophys. Res. Commun.*, 1998, 253, 99-103.

Sies, H; Sthal, W; Sundquist, AR. Antioxidant functions of vitamins. Vitamins E and C, beta-carotene, and other carotenoids. *Ann. N. Y. Acad. Sci.*, 1992, 669, 7-20.

Sobczak, A; Gołka, D; Szołtysek-Bołdys, I. The effects of tobacco smoke on plasma alpha- and gamma-tocopherol levels in passive and active cigarette smokers. *Toxicol. Lett.*, 2004, 151, 429-437.

Sobczak, A; Kula, B; Danch, A. Effects of electromagnetic field on free-radical processes in steelworkers. Part II. Magnetic field influence on vitamin A, E and selenium concentration in plasma. *J. Occup. Health*, 2002, 44, 230-233.

Sontag, TJ; Parker, RS. Cytochrome P450 omega-hydroxylase pathway of tocopherol catabolism. Novel mechanism of regulation of vitamin E status. *J. Biol. Chem.*, 2002, 277, 25290-25296.

Stocker, A. Molecular mechanisms of vitamin E transport. *Ann. N. Y. Acad. Sci.*, 2004, 1031, 44-59.

Subar, AF; Harlan, LC; Mattson, ME. Food and nutrient intake differences between smokers and nonsmokers in the US. *Am. J. Public Health*, 1990, 80, 1323-1329.

Suzuki, YJ; Forman, HJ; Sevanian, A. Oxidants as stimulators of signal transduction. *Free Radic. Biol. Med.*, 1997, 22, 269-285.

Takatsuka, N; Kawakami, N; Ito, Y; Kabuto, M; Shimizu, H. Effects of passive smoking on serum levels of carotenoids and α-tocopherol. *J. Epidemiol.*, 1998, 8, 146-151.

Thakur, ML; Srivastava, US. Vitamin E metabolism and its application. Nutr. Res., 1996, 16, 1767-1809.

Traber, MG; Winklhofer-Roob, BM; Robb, JM; Khoschsorur, G; Aigner, R; Cross, C; Ramakrishnan, R; Brigelius-Flohe, R. Vitamin E kinetics in smokers and nonsmokers. *Free Radic. Biol. Med.*, 2001, 31, 1368-1374.

Travers, JB. Oxidative stress can activate the epidermal platelet-activating factor receptor. *J. Invest. Dermatol.*, 1999, 112, 279-283.

Tröbs, M; Renner, T; Scherer, G; Heller, WD; Geiss, HC; Wolfram, G; Haas, GM; Schwandt, P. Nutrition, antioxidants, and risk factor profile of nonsmokers, passive smokers and smokers of the Prevention Education Program (PEP) in Nuremberg, Germany. *Prev. Med.*, 2002, 34, 600-607.

Upston, JM; Terentis, AC; Stocker, R. Tocopherol-mediated peroxidation of lipoproteins: implications for vitamin E as a potential antiatherogenic supplement. *FASEB J.*, 1999, 13, 977-994.

van Acker, SA; Koymans, LM; Bast, A. Molecular pharmacology of vitamin E structural aspects of antioxidant activity. *Free Radic. Biol. Med.*, 1993, 15, 311-328.

Vatassery, GT; Smith, WE; Quach, HT. α-Tocopherol in rat brain subcellular fractions is oxidized rapidly during incubations with low concentrations of peroxynitrite. *J. Nutr.*, 1998, 128, 152-157.

Wallström, P; Wirfält, E; Mattisson, I; Gullberg, B; Janzon, L; Berglund, G. Serum β-carotene and α-tocopherol in smokers and nonsmokers – associations with food sources and supplemental intakes. A report from the Malmö Diet and Cancer cohort. *Nutr. Res.*, 2003, 23, 163-183.

Wang, X; Quinn, PJ. Vitamin E and ist function in membranes. *Prog. Lipid Res.*, 1999, 38, 309-336.

Wei, W; Kim, Y; Boudreau, N. Association of smoking with serum and dietary levels of antioxidants in adults: NHANES III, 1988-1994. *Am. J. Public Health*, 2001, 91, 258-264.

Zang, LY; Stone, K; Pryor, WA. Detection of free radicals in aqueous extracts of cigarette tar by electron spin resonance. *Free Radic. Biol. Med.*, 1995, 19, 161-167.

In: Smoking and Health Research Frontiers
Editor: Calvin B. Fong, pp. 183-211
ISBN 1-60021-480-0

Chapter VIII

SMOKING AND ITS EFFECTS ON THE PERIODONTAL AND PERI-IMPLANT TISSUES

João B. César-Neto, Márcio Z. Casati, Enilson A. Sallum and Francisco H. Nociti Jr.
Department of Prosthodontics/Periodontics, Division of Periodontics, School of Dentistry at Piracicaba, University of Campinas, Brazil.

ABSTRACT

The impact of smoking on general health has been widely studied and is directly related to several important medical problems including cancer, low birth weight, and pulmonary and cardiovascular disease. Such a great interest is encouraged by the number of smokers in the world; more than 1,300 billion (WHO, 2005). In the past 25 years, there has also been an increasing awareness of the role of cigarette consumption in oral health problems such as periodontal disease and dental implant failures. In the field of periodontics, it has been reported that smokers have a 2.7 times greater probability of presenting periodontal disease than non-smokers, independent of age, sex and plaque index; furthermore, the disease is more severe in smokers than in former and non-smokers.

In addition, it has been reported that chronic smoking compromises periodontal health, demonstrated by an increased number of periodontally diseased sites with loss of periodontal bone height. In the field of implantology, a greater incidence of early and late implant failures has been observed for smokers when compared to non-smokers. In order to further evaluate the effect of cigarette smoke on the tissues around the tooth and dental implants, our group has been using a cigarette smoke exposure chamber and an animal model. By exposing the animals to this model of passive smoking, we have learned that ligature-induced periodontitis and the bone around titanium implants may be affected by cigarette smoke inhalation.

This chapter will then attempt to discuss recent available evidences on the impact of smoking on the periodontal and peri-implant tissues, and provide the reader with an overview of the data we have collected on the effect of cigarette smoke inhalation and its cessation on both tissues.

INTRODUCTION

Smoking has been shown to be a primary etiologic factor in many serious medical problems and has been widely investigated in these fields. However, its affect on the teeth and their surrounding tissues has been a more recent finding. One of the most investigated aspects has been the relationship between tobacco consumption and the incidence and severity of periodontal disease. The first associations were observed in the late 1940s when Pindborg (Pindborg 1947 and 1949) demonstrated that acute necrotizing ulcerative gingivitis was often observed in smokers. In the 1980s and 1990s several epidemiological studies clearly established an association between smoking and destructive periodontal disease (Bergstrom & Eliasson, 1987; Bergstrom, 1989; Goultschin et al., 1990; Haber et al., 1993; Norderyd et al., 1999). In a recent study Tomar & Asma (2000), evaluating 12,329 subjects, stated that approximately half of periodontitis cases could be attributed to smoking, and that smokers were four times more likely to have periodontitis than those who had never smoked. Evidences have also demonstrated that smoking may negatively affect periodontal therapy outcome, and that up to 90% of refractory periodontitis patients are smokers (Magnusson & Walker, 1996). With respect to titanium implants, smoking is one of the most discussed factors associated with implant failure. Clinical studies have reported that smokers present not only higher rates of early implant failure (before implant load) than non-smokers (Bain & Moy, 1993; Lambert et al., 2000; Nitzan et al., 2005; Moy et al., 2005; Moheng & Feryn, 2005), but also a greater detrimental effect around successfully integrated implants (Haas et al., 1996; Lindquist et al., 1997; Nitzan et al., 2005). In this sense, our group performed a series of studies in animal models with the objective of investigating the effect of cigarette smoke inhalation and its cessation on induced periodontitis and on bone around titanium implants. We have additionally investigated the effect of smoking on plastic periodontal procedures outcome and reported the impact of smoking on gene expression in the gingival tissues harvested from patients clinically and radiographically diagnosed with chronic periodontitis. In the present chapter we present and discuss the results of our studies, including new unpublished data, and review recent available data on the impact of smoking on the periodontal and peri-implant tissues.

SMOKING AND THE PERIODONTAL TISSUES:

The term ''periodontal disease'' in its strictest sense refers to both gingivitis and periodontitis. Gingivitis is an inflammatory condition of the soft tissues surrounding the teeth (the gingiva) and is a direct immune response to the dental microbial plaque build up on teeth. Gingivitis may be modified by several factors such as smoking, certain drugs and hormonal changes that occur in puberty and pregnancy. Periodontitis follows gingivitis and may also be influenced by the individual's immune and inflammatory response. Periodontitis is initiated by the microbial plaque, but it only occurs in a subset of the population. Periodontitis involves the destruction of the supporting structures of the teeth including the periodontal ligament, bone and soft tissues. Clearly, periodontitis is the most significant of these diseases because it causes tooth loss. Figure 1 schematically illustrates the pathogenesis of periodontal diseases.

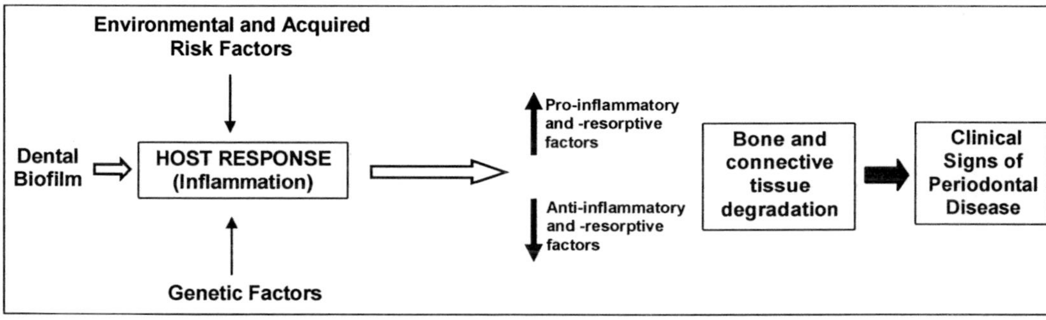

Figure 1: Schematic illustration of the pathogenesis of periodontal disease (PD): the host response to the dental biofilm may be influenced by environmental, including smoking, and genetic factors favoring disease installation and progression via their effect on pro- and anti-inflammatory [for instance, interleukin (IL)-1, IL-4, IL-6, IL-10 and TNF-α), and pro- and anti-resorptive factors [receptor activator of NF-κB ligand (RANKL) and osteoprotegerin (OPG)] involved in the host response.

Since the observation of Pindborg in the 1940s (Pindborg, 1947 and 1949), when smoking was associated with necrotizing ulcerative gingivitis, much attention has been paid to the impact of cigarette consumption on the periodontium. Nevertheless, until the 1980s there were no experimental studies, controlled for confounding factors, which provided strong evidence that smoking was a true risk factor for periodontitis. In the 1980s and 1990s, a number of epidemiological studies with well performed experimental designs and adequate statistical analysis (adjusted for confounding variables) clearly demonstrated a strong association between tobacco use and periodontal diseases (Bergstrom & Eliasson, 1987; Bergstrom, 1989; Goultschin et al., 1990; Haber et al., 1993; Norderyd et al., 1999). The effect of smoking on gingival bleeding has also been investigated. Although it has been reported that smokers may present a significantly greater plaque index, the average number of bleeding sites in smokers (27%) was smaller than in non-smokers (40%) (Preber & Bergstrom, 1985). When reviewing 369 patients with periodontitis, smokers reported fewer gingival bleeding sites (25%) than did non-smokers (51%) (Preber & Bergstrom, 1986). The influence of smoking on experimental gingivitis was evaluated in a group of dental students (Bergstrom & Preber, 1986); the subjects were free of periodontitis, not taking any medication and the group of smokers had been smoking for at least four years. This study revealed the number of gingival bleeding sites, the amount of gingival exudate and gingival sites with distinct redness to be significantly less in smokers with comparable levels of plaque indexes to non-smokers. These studies lend, therefore, support to the contention that the inflammatory gingival response could be suppressed in smokers. Another study reported that, after 28 days of plaque-induced gingivitis, the intensity of the vascular reaction was only 50% of that observed for non-smokers (Bergstrom, Person & Preber, 1988). In summary, the preponderance of evidence suggests that smoking may decrease gingival bleeding and that this may occur due to changes in the proportion of blood vessels in the periodontal tissues.

With respect to the effect of smoking on plaque-induced periodontal bone loss (e.g., periodontitis), it is now well recognized that smoking is a risk factor for periodontitis (AAP Consensus Report, 1996) and may affect not only periodontitis installation and progression, but also its treatment outcome. Risk assessment based on an increasing body of investigations over the past few years suggests that the tobacco attributable risk odds ratios (OR) range between 2.5 to 6.0 (Bergstrom & Preber, 1994, Gelskey et al., 1998, Norderyd et al., 1999, Tomar & Asma, 2000) or even more than 6.0 in heavy smokers (e.g., > 20 cigarettes/day) (Gelskey et al., 1998). One of the strongest evidences for smoking as a risk factor for periodontal diseases were the findings by Tomar & Asma (2000) based on data from the NHANES III study. In this study 12,329 subjects were evaluated and the authors observed that approximately half of the periodontitis cases in the USA could be attributed to smoking. In addition, they observed that current smokers were about 4 times more likely to be diagnosed with periodontitis than persons who had never smoked, and that there was a dose-response relationship between cigarettes smoked per day and the odds of periodontitis. Clinical studies have demonstrated that smokers have a more severe periodontal disease, showing increased bone loss (Bergstrom et al., 2000 a and b), greater periodontal attachment loss, more gingival recession as well as periodontal pocket formation (Calsina et al., 2002). Such an influence of smoking on disease severity and progression is also observed in tooth mortality (Slade et al., 1997; Krall et al., 1999; Leung et al., 2006), even in patients treated for periodontitis (Leung et al., 2006). Smoking history was associated with early attachment loss in adults (Tanner, 2005) and in a recent study; cigarette smoking was considered a strong predictor of progressive periodontitis (Heitz-Mayfield, 2005). Linden & Mullally (1994) found the odds ratio for periodontal disease to be as high as 14.1 for young smokers.

With respect to the treatment of periodontitis, it has been demonstrated that smoking has an adverse influence on all forms of periodontal therapy, and that up to 90% of refractory periodontitis patients are smokers (Magnusson & Walker, 1996). Many studies have reported that smoking is an independent risk factor for wound healing, for instance in situations where tissues are exposed to low oxygen tension, such as after lower extremity amputations (Lind et al., 1991) and mastectomies (Sorensen et al., 2002), and in tissues in direct contact with cigarette smoke during the process of wound healing such as in head and neck surgery (Kuri et al., 2005). In the periodontal field, a number of clinical studies have compared the response of smokers and non-smokers to various types of periodontal therapy, including non-surgical and surgical therapies [see Johnson and Hill (2004) for review]. Although with a lack of long-term evidence, most of the clinical trials show significantly greater reductions in probing depths and bleeding on probing, and significantly greater gain of clinical attachment following non-surgical and surgical treatments in non-smokers compared to smokers (Heasman et al., 2006). A similar scenario is observed in the treatment of furcation regions (Trombelli et al., 2003; Dannewitz et al., 2006) and after regenerative procedures (Bowers et al., 2003). Most studies on the effect of smoking on periodontal healing have in common the fact that the evaluated sites were usually contaminated by a dental biofilm. Very limited information is available from in vivo studies on whether smoking and/or nicotine may affect the self-healing capacity of periodontal tissues (periodontal ligament, bone and cementum) in the absence of dental biofilm. Our laboratory, therefore, additionally investigated the impact of cigarette smoke inhalation (CSI) or nicotine administration on the self-healing capacity of the periodontal tissues (Benatti et al., 2005). For the first time, it was demonstrated that CSI may significantly affect bone healing in artificially created fenestrations in rat alveolar bone. Both the density of newly formed bone and the extent of bone filling were less compared to the values obtained for the control and nicotine administered groups. Subcutaneous injections with nicotine had no effect on bone healing. These results indicate that cigarette smoke may have a direct impact on the self-healing capacity of the alveolar process, in the absence of a plaque biofilm. A harmful effect of smoking has also been observed when root coverage procedures are used and the outcomes of both the coronally positioned flap alone (Silva et al., 2006) and its association with connective tissue graft (Martins et al., 2004) seem to be negatively affected. Recent studies have suggested that the adjunct use of local and systemic antimicrobial therapy may improve the clinical results obtained with scaling/root planning (Mascarenhas et al., 2005; Preshaw et al., 2005) and guided tissue regeneration in smokers (Machtei el al., 2003). Data from our group (Machion et al., 2004a, 2006) are in line with these findings, showing that in the treatment of smokers with chronic periodontitis, the association of 10% doxycycline delivered locally with scaling and root planing may lead to better clinical results than the mechanical therapy alone. In Machion's studies, 48 patients (all of them smokers) with chronic periodontitis (a minimum of four pockets, > 5 mm) on anterior teeth were randomly assigned to receive, as periodontal treatment, scaling and root planing (SRP) or SRP followed by local application of doxycycline (SRP-D). Six months after active periodontal therapy it was observed that the adjunct use of doxycycline gel promoted a greater attachment gain (1.63 +/- 0.93 mm versus 1.04 +/- 0.71 mm, for SRP-D and SRP, respectively). In addition, deep periodontal pockets (>7 mm) showed a significant probing depth reduction (3.78 +/- 1.41 versus 2.60 +/- 1.28 mm, for SRP-D and SRP, respectively) and clinical attachment gain (2.54 +/- 1.27 mm versus 1.29 +/- 0.95 mm, for SRP-D and SRP, respectively) when doxycycline was applied (Machion et al., 2004a). Similar results were also observed during the 2-year follow-up of the same patients (Machion et al., 2006). In initially deep pockets (>7 mm), the SRP-D group presented a greater probing depth reduction at 6 and 18 months (mean difference between groups of 1.18 and 1.73 mm, respectively) and a greater clinical attachment gain in all periods (mean difference between groups of 1.16, 1.99, and 1.78 mm, at 6, 18, and 24 months, respectively). Microbiological examination of these patients revealed that the adjunct use of locally delivered doxycycline after scaling and root planing may favor the elimination of *T. forsythensis* and *P. gingivalis* in a greater proportion of sites than conventional mechanical therapy (Machion et al., 2004b). These studies provide valuable information for dealing with the limitations of periodontal therapy in smokers.

Animal Studies:

As an attempt to determine the mechanisms involved in smoking modulation of the periodontal tissues, in vitro and in vivo studies have investigated the impact of cigarette compounds, including nicotine and cotinine, on the periodontal tissues. In general, nicotine has been reported to adversely affect proliferation, attachment and chemotaxis of periodontal ligament cells, and induce pro-inflammatory cytokine production by human gingival fibroblasts synergically with lipopolysaccharide from Escherichia coli and P. gingivalis (Giannopoulou et al., 1999; Giannopoulou et al., 2001; Wendell & Stein, 2001). In our laboratory, we have additionally investigated, in a rat model, the impact of cigarette compounds and cigarette smoke inhalation/cessation on the periodontal tissues. In the first investigation (Nociti et al., 2000), a cotton ligature was placed in the sulcular area around one of the rat first mandibular molars in order to induce periodontitis and allow us to study the impact of nicotine on periodontitis progression. After ligature placement, the animals were randomly divided into 4 groups, the control group and three other groups that received different nicotine dosages by daily intraperitoneal injections (group A: saline solution; group B: 2 μl/g of body weight of a nicotine solution (BWNS) with a nicotine solution of 0.13 μl of nicotine/ml of saline solution; group C: 2 μl/g BWNS with a nicotine solution of 0.19 μl of nicotine/ml of saline solution; and group D: 2 μl/g BWNS with a nicotine solution of 0.26 μl of nicotine/ml of saline solution). Thirty days later, serial histological sections were obtained and the bone loss in the furcation area of the teeth was histometrically determined. The results of this initial study showed a greater bone loss in the ligated teeth of the groups that received nicotine injections (group B: 1.01 +/- 0.61 mm^2; group C: 1.14 +/- 0.72 mm^2 and group D: 1.36 +/- 0.60 mm^2) when compared to the control group (A: 0.64 +/- 0.62 mm^2), while no bone loss was observed for unligated teeth. This was the first evidence, in vivo, to suggest that nicotine alone, one of the main cigarette compounds, could affect periodontal bone loss resulting from periodontitis. However, intriguingly, contrary to findings in smokers that suggested a dose-dependent effect (Tonetti, 1998; Bergstrom et al., 2000b), different dosages of nicotine did not reproduce such an effect in rats. It was then hypothesized that higher nicotine concentrations would be required in order to reproduce the dose-dependent effect reported for smoking on the periodontium. The ligature-induced periodontitis model was used and higher nicotine concentrations applied (A - saline solution, B - 0.37 mg of nicotine per kg, C - 0.57 mg of nicotine per kg and D - 0.73 mg of nicotine per kg) (Nociti et al., 2001). Data analysis confirmed our previous findings showing a greater bone loss around the ligated teeth in which the animals were administered with nicotine than for animals that did not. As expected, this time, a dose-dependent response was observed (0.90 +/- 0.64 mm^2, 3.08 +/- 2.30 mm^2, 3.88 +/- 1.89 mm^2, 6.90 +/- 1.88 mm^2; for groups A, B, C and D, respectively). Surprisingly, a direct effect of nicotine was additionally observed in the periodontium around unligated teeth that presented a thicker periodontal ligament area, suggesting a direct effect of nicotine on the bone tissues. Although relevant and original information was gathered from these initial studies, important limitations must be highlighted. First, nicotine and cotinine serum levels were not assessed and, therefore, whether nicotine serum levels were comparable to those reported for smokers could not be determined. Secondly, the nicotine was injected once daily, while we know that smokers consume tobacco cigarettes several times a day. Thirdly, although recognized as one of the main compounds of cigarette smoke, nicotine alone may not be able to mimic the effect of cigarette smoke as a whole.

As an attempt to overcome such limitations, our group has now been using a passive smoking model aiming at further assessing the effect of passive smoking on the periodontal tissues. Pilot studies led us to determine the most appropriate experimental conditions to achieve serum nicotine and cotinine levels comparable to a moderate to heavy smoker. Ideal dimensions for the smoke exposure device and the most appropriate time line of exposures were exhaustively tested. It was found that five animals intermittently exposed three times per day for eight minutes to cigarette smoke (10 cigarettes containing 1.3 mg of nicotine, 16.5mg of tar and, 15.2mg of carbon monoxide each) would provide us with a similar scenario to that of a moderate to heavy smoker with respect to the cotinine serum levels. The exposure device ended up as being a 45 X 25 X 20 cm^3 clear acrylic chamber, an air-pump and two inflow/outflow tubes. Blood samples were taken 15 minutes after the cigarette smoke inhalation and the concentration of nicotine and cotinine was monitored by high-pressure liquid chromatography (HPLC) (César-Neto et al., 2003). Mean nicotine and cotinine serum levels were, respectively, 346.1 ng/mL +/- 114.3 and 265.4 ng/mL +/- 109.8. Taking the cotinine levels reported by Gonzalez et al. (1996) into consideration, the exposure model proposed by our group promoted levels similar to those observed in smokers that intake 10 to 20 cigarettes a day. These nicotine and cotinine serum levels were also similar to those obtained with subcutaneous injections of 3 mg/kg of nicotine (376.03 ng/mL +/- 53.85 and 294.38 ng/mL +/- 41.24, for nicotine and cotinine, respectively) (César-Neto et al., 2003). Despite being exhaustively tested and developed, some limitations may also be anticipated for this passive smoking model; smokers present several low and high peaks of nicotine during the day, a condition that is difficult to simulate experimentally. Likewise, cigarette smoke compounds are directly linked to tobacco burning temperature which differs in experimental passive smoking (a pump blowing on cigarettes) from regular smoking (an individual smoking a cigarette). Furthermore, this model does not reproduce the effect of the high temperature smoke in the airways. Although with some limitations, as discussed above, the passive smoking model is currently the only available methodology to study, in an animal model, the effects of cigarette smoke as a whole. The present model presents some advantages when compared to other passive smoking models. Its effectiveness in producing pulmonary emphysema in a short period of time has been documented (Cendon et al., 1997) and the smoking device employed is simple and inexpensive, in contrast to conventional smoking devices. By using this passive smoking model we tested the impact of cigarette smoke, as a whole, on the bone loss rate during ligature-induced periodontitis (César-Neto et al., 2004). For this investigation, twenty-seven adult male Wistar rats were used, a ligature was placed around one of the mandibular first molars of each animal and they were randomly assigned to the control or CSI (cigarette smoke inhalation) groups. Sixty days later, the animals were sacrificed, the gingival tissues harvested for MMP-2 zymography and the specimens routinely processed for decalcified sections. It was demonstrated that cigarette smoke inhalation (CSI) potentates periodontal bone destruction in ligature-induced periodontitis (0.64 +/- 0.36 mm^2 versus 1.50 +/- 0.50 mm^2, for control and CSI groups, respectively). An additional analysis of gingival tissue adjacent to periodontitis sites showed that matrix metalloproteinase (MMP)-2 levels were higher in the exposed animals when compared to the non-exposed ones, suggesting that MMP-2 may be one of the molecules responsible for the increased tissue degradation observed in periodontal tissues of smokers. The analysis of unligated teeth confirmed our previous results with nicotine injections (Nociti et al., 2001) showing, likewise, a thicker periodontal ligament area for the group which received cigarette compounds (e.g. smoke inhalation) (César-Neto et al., 2004). In general, our results with the passive smoking model corroborate with the ones obtained with nicotine injections, suggesting that nicotine seems to be a key molecule for the intensified periodontal destruction observed in smokers and may contribute, at least partially, to the negative impact of cigarette smoke as a whole. With most of the available evidence to indicate smoking as a risk factor for periodontal destruction, in a subsequent study we evaluated whether the interruption of smoke exposure would reverse the negative impact of CSI on periodontitis-related bone loss (César-Neto et al., 2005a). Additionally, we radiographically investigated the effect of CSI on mandibular bone quality (César-Neto et al., 2005a). Fifty-three Wistar rats were randomly assigned to group 1: control; group 2: 83 days of CSI prior to ligature placement; or group 3: 90 days of CSI before and 60 days after ligature placement. The animals were sacrificed 60 days after ligature placement for histometric and photodensitometric analyses. The results revealed similar levels of bone loss for both the control and cessation groups, while the group continuously exposed to CSI presented a significantly increased periodontal destruction (0.90 +/- 0.33 mm^2; 0.96 +/- 0.32 mm^2; 1.64 +/- 0.65 mm^2; for groups 1, 2 and 3, respectively). Radiographically, continuous exposure to cigarette smoke promoted a significantly reduced bone density in the basal manibular bone (1.74 +/- 0.38 aluminum equivalence [Al eq]; 1.74 +/- 0.14 Al eq; and 0.68 +/- 0.10 Al eq for groups 1, 2, and 3, respectively). In line with previous findings (Tomar & Asma, 2000), these data strongly suggest that the effect of smoking on periodontium may be reversible, which may be of great clinical significance when dealing with smokers in clinical practice. Moreover, the radiographic findings regarding bone quality may be of particular relevance in the field of clinical implantology, since bone quality and smoking are well recognized factors associated with clinical implant failures. In order to confirm the radiographic findings and to investigate whether the figure observed for the basal mandibular bone would also occur in the tooth supporting alveolar bone, a complementary study was performed (César-Neto et al., 2006). Sixty male Wistar rats were randomly assigned to: group 1 - control, group 2 - 2 months of CSI, group 3 - 3 months of CSI and 2 months without exposure to CSI and group 4 - 5 months of CSI. Five months after beginning the cigarette smoke inhalation regime (2 months for group 2), the animals were killed and the mandibles removed and routinely prepared for histological sections. The proportion of mineralized tissue in the inter-radicular area (e.g. a 1,000-micrometer zone under the furcation and between the roots) was obtained for the first mandibular molar. Data analysis showed that the animals continuously exposed to cigarette smoke inhalation presented a decreased proportion of mineralized tissue (groups 2 and 4) when compared to the control and cessation groups (groups 1 and 3), while both control and cessation groups presented similar results. These findings confirm the previous data for the mandibular basal bone showing a beneficial effect of smoking cessation on mandibular bone tissue. However, it remains to be investigated whether the decreased mineral density in the tooth supporting alveolar bone would favor periodontitis progression and/or have any effect on tooth function. In summary, this series of studies shows that the scenario observed clinically in smokers was reproducible in laboratory animals and confirmed, in a controlled environment with a highly reliable methodology of measurement (histometrical analysis), the events observed in clinical epidemiological studies. Such findings reinforce tobacco consumption as a risk factor for periodontal disease and provide an important methodological tool for the study of smoking related subjects that may not be clinically evaluated due to ethical and methodological limitations. Table 1 summarizes the data with respect to the impact of nicotine alone and cigarette smoke on both the ligature-induced periodontitis and the fenestration model.

Effect of Smoking on Cytokine Expression in the Periodontium:

Although a number of studies have established smoking as a true risk factor for periodontitis onset and progression, as previously discussed in this chapter, the mechanisms involved are still not clear. Cytokine profiles are of considerable value when studying periodontal tissue destruction. It has been proposed that bacteria proliferation and/or its products in periodontal pockets results in the recruitment and activation of the monocyte/T-lymphocyte axis. This, in turn, leads to the enhanced release of inflammatory cytokines, including interleukin (IL)-1β, IL-6 and tumor necrosis factor (TNF)-α, associated with periodontal tissue destruction. IL-8, secreted by monocytic cells but also from fibroblasts and endothelial cells, induces release of matrix metalloproteinases (MMPs) by neutrophils. Tobacco smoking, mostly in the form of cigarette smoking, is recognized as the most important environmental risk factor in periodontitis, and as a major risk factor that contributes to the pathogenesis of periodontal disease. It would seem logical to expect that factors that are associated with tissue destruction should be higher in smokers than in non-smokers. In agreement with this assumption, there are some data showing that cytokine expression may in fact be up-regulated by smoking and/or its compounds. In an in vitro study, nicotine, in association or not with lipopolysaccharide (LPS) from periodontopathogenic bacteria, was shown to increase IL-6 and IL-8 protein production by human gingival fibroblasts (Wendell & Stein, 2001). In a recent study, a microarray analysis demonstrated that peripheral blood mononuclear cells exposed for 5 minutes to tobacco smoke presented elevated expression of 20 genes previously reported to be associated with periodontal pathogenesis (Ryder et al., 2004). Higher levels of TNF-α and IL-8 in the gingival crevicular fluid in smokers have additionally been reported compared to non-smokers (Giannopoulou et al., 2003, Bostrom et al., 1999). In contrast, pro- and anti-inflammatory cytokines have been reported to be lower in association with smoking and its compounds. It seems that cigarette smoke contains potent inhibitors of both gene expression and protein production, at least for IL-1β, IL-8, IL-2 and TNF-α (Morozumi et al., 2004, Ouyang et al., 2000). Corroborating the data from in vitro studies, productions of IL-1β, IL-1ra, IL-1α and IL-4 have been reported to be significantly lower in the gingival crevicular fluid of smokers from periodontally diseased sites compared with non-smokers (Giannopoulou et al., 2003, Petropoulos et al., 2004). In addition, although not statistically significant, other studies have shown a tendency towards reduced levels of IL-1β and TNF-α in the gingival crevicular fluid of smoker subjects with moderate to severe periodontal disease (Bostrom et al., 2000, Erdemir et al., 2004).

Table 1- Summary of the studies evaluating the impact of nicotine alone and cigarette smoke on both the ligature-induced periodontitis and the fenestration models.

Author (year)	Model (experimental period)	Animal	Exposure regimen	Experimental Groups	Mean bone loss in the ligated teeth (mm^2)		Mean periodontal ligament area in the unligated teeth (mm^2)		General findings
Nociti et al. (2000)	Ligature-induced periodontitis (30 days)	rat	Nicotine administration after ligature placement	Control (n=5) Group 1[*] (n=5) Group 2[&] (n=5) Group 3[#] (n=5)	0.64 +/- 0.62 1.01 +/- 0.61 1.14 +/- 0.72 1.36 +/- 0.60	S	0.25 +/- 0.05 0.28 +/- 0.05 0.28 +/- 0.09 0.23 +/- 0.09	NS	Nicotine enhanced periodontitis related bone loss, but a dose-dependent effect was not observed.
Nociti et al. (2001)	Ligature-induced periodontitis (30 days)	rat	Nicotine administration after ligature placement	Control (n=5) 0.37mg/Kg (n=5) 0.57mg/Kg (n=5) 0.73mg/Kg (n=5)	0.90 +/- 0.64 3.08 +/- 2.30 3.88 +/- 1.89 6.90 +/- 1.88	S	0.25 +/- 0.04 0.72 +/- 0.05 0.81 +/- 0.08 0.83 +/- 0.11	S	Nicotine enhanced bone loss in a dose-dependent fashion and promoted a wider periodontal ligament area.
César-Neto et al. (2004)	Ligature-induced periodontitis (60 days)	rat	60 days of CSI after ligature placement	Control (n=13) CSI (n=14)	0.64 +/- 0.36 1.50 +/- 0.50	S	0.16 +/- 0.03 0.24 +/- 0.09	S	CSI enhanced bone loss and promoted a wider periodontal ligament area.
César-Neto et al. (2005a)	Ligature-induced periodontitis (60 days)	rat	83 days of CSI prior or 90 prior and 60 after ligature	Control (n=16) CSI prior to ligature (n=17) CSI prior and after ligature (n=20)	0.90 +/- 0.33 0.96 +/- 0.32 1.64 +/- 0.65	S	0.15 +/- 0.06 0.15 +/- 0.04 0.18 +/- 0.06	S	CSI before ligature placement did not affect ligature-induced periodontitis progression
					Bone Filling (%)		Bone Density (%)		
Benatti et al. (2005)	Fenestration defects (4x3mm) created buccally to the distal root of the first mandibular molar (21 days of healing)	rat	30 days of CSI or nicotine administration prior and 21 after defect creation	Control (n=14) 3mg/Kg (n=14) CSI (n=14)	95.97 +/- 4.64 90.62 +/- 4.64 85.34 +/- 7.70	S	80.07 +/- 3.45 76.37 +/- 5.27 72.74 +/- 6.24	S	No new cementum was formed along the root surface in any of the three groups.

CSI – Cigarette smoke inhalation, S - Statistically different, NS - Non-statistically different.

[*] 2 µl/g of body weight of a nicotine solution (BWNS) with a nicotine solution of 0.13 µl of nicotine/ml of saline solution; [&] 2 µl/g of BWNS with a nicotine solution of 0.19 µl of nicotine/ml of saline solution; [#] 2 µl/g of BWNS with a nicotine solution of 0.26 µl of nicotine/ml of saline solution.

Although significant, these studies collectively do not provide an accurate description of the underlying mechanisms by which smoking affects the periodontium since contradictory findings have been reported. In order to further investigate possible mechanisms involved in the smoking modulation of periodontal bone loss, we have simultaneously assessed the profile of a number of pro- and anti-inflammatory cytokines plus pro- and anti-resorptive agents in the gingival tissues of smokers versus non-smokers with moderate to severe chronic periodontitis, including IL-1β, IL-1ra, IL-6, IL-8, IL-10, interferon (INF)-γ, TNF-α, MMP-2 and -8, receptor activator of NF-κB ligand (RANKL) and osteoprotegerin (OPG) (César-Neto et al., 2006 a and b – in press). Gingival biopsies were divided into 3 groups: Healthy group: periodontally healthy subjects; Periodontitis group: subjects who had never smoked with severe chronic periodontitis (probing depth >7mm) and Smoking group: subjects diagnosed with severe chronic periodontitis who smoked >1 pack/day for at least 10 years. Gene and protein expressions were quantitatively assessed. In general, data analysis confirmed a number of previous reports which indicated that elevated levels of pro-inflammatory cytokines, such as IL-1β, IL-6, IL-8, INF-γ and TNF-α, plus the pro-resorptive factor RANKL, and low levels of the anti-resorptive factor OPG, are associated with sites showing periodontal destruction. In addition, as also previously reported, higher mRNA levels for MMP-2, a potent collagenase that plays a critical role in depredating connective tissue, were found in inflamed versus non-inflamed sites. With respect to smoking modulation on gene expression, it was found that IL-1β, IL-8, IL-10, TNF-α, MMP-8 and OPG were lower in smokers than non-smokers with comparable types of periodontitis, while IL-6, INF-γ and IL-1ra were higher. Increased RANKL:OPG and IL-6:IL-10 ratios were found in sites with periodontitis in smokers versus non-smokers, whereas in smokers the 1β:IL-1ra ratio was similar to the healthy group. It was then concluded that smoking modulation of bone destruction in periodontal disease may involve reduced levels of anti-inflammatory and anti-resorptive factors such as IL-10 and OPG, respectively, and may also involve high levels of pro-inflammatory cytokines such as IL-6 and INF-γ. A list of the main findings on the effect of smoking on gene expression in the periodontal tissues is shown in Table 2.

In summary, passive or active tobacco smoking presents widespread systemic effects, many of which may provide mechanisms for the increased susceptibility to periodontal diseases and the poorer response to treatment. As we get closer to elucidating mechanisms, we have accepted that smoking is a significant factor in the development and progression of periodontal diseases and that gingival inflammation (bleeding on probing) is decreased in these patients. Treatment in smokers appears not to be as effective as in non-smokers and the microbial role is still being clarified. A number of studies have also suggested that genetic variations may also play a role in susceptibility to the disease, disease severity and patients' response to therapy.

Table 2- Main findings on the effect of smoking on gene expression of pro- and anti-inflammatory and pro- and anti-resorptive factors in the periodontium.

.Author (year)	Disease type	Method	Substract	Factors										
César-Neto et al. (2006a,b) *in press*	Chronic Periodontitis	Real-Time PCR (mRNA)	Extract of gingival tissue	IL-1β ↓	IL-1ra ↑	IL-6 ↑	IL-8 ↓	IL-10 ↓	TNF-α ↓	IFN-γ ↑	MMP-2 ↓	MMP-8 ↓	RANKL -	OPG ↓
Bostrom et al. (1999)	Chronic Periodontitis	ELISA (protein)	GCF			-			↑					
Bostrom et al. (2000)	Chronic Periodontitis	ELISA (protein)	GCF	-	-									
Rawlinson et al. (2003)	Chronic Periodontitis	ELISA (protein)	GCF	↓	↓									
Erdemir et al. (2004)	Chronic Periodontitis	ELISA (protein)	GCF			-			-					
Gianno-poulou et al. (2003)	Experimental Gingivitis	ELISA (protein)	GCF	-	IL-4 ↓		↑							
Kamma et al. (2004)	Aggressive Periodontitis	ELISA (protein)	GCF		IL-4 ↑	-	-							

- no effect, ↑ increase, ↓ decrease, GCF: gingival crevicular fluid

SMOKING AND OSSEOINTEGRATED IMPLANTS:

The functional and aesthetic damage caused by tooth loss has long been a concern. With the development of prosthetic dentistry, many alternatives have been proposed, such as removable partial and complete dentures and crown and bridge prosthesis. Although widely used, these kinds of oral rehabilitation have important limitations, such as decreased chewing efficiency, loss of healthy dental tissue and, in some cases, difficult oral hygiene care and functional overload. In 1952, Professor Per-Ingvar Brånemark found that titanium is a biocompatible metal that can establish a firm union with bone tissue, termed osseointegration. This finding revolutionized the technique of implantology with the emergence of a new and promising method of oral rehabilitation, and in 1965 the first patient was treated by this principle. The original protocol consisted of five to seven titanium screws that were inserted in the mandible and, after a bone healing period of 4 to 6 months, an implant-supported overdenture was built. Longitudinal studies have documented the long-term success of the osseointegrated implants (Adell et al., 1990), and the promising discovery became a real alternative for tooth replacement. Since this time, a great number of studies, focusing on titanium implant development, have been performed and a number of different implant systems have been created, with high success rates also being reported for single (Bahat, 2000; Sullivan et al., 2001; Romeo et al., 2002; Lambrecht et al., 2003) and partial implant-supported prostheses (Bahat, 2000; Sullivan et al., 2001; Romeo et al., 2004). At this time, the long-term success of implant supported prostheses, with success rates in excess of 95%

up to 15 years, has been reported (Adell et al., 1990). In addition, quality of life assessments comparing implant supported prostheses with removable partial and complete dentures have shown implant retained prosthesis to be a highly satisfactory method of tooth replacement (Adell et al., 1990; Lindquist et al., 1997). However, some patients loose a disproportionately high number of implants. This clustering of failure has been a limitation of implantology and several studies have investigated the factors that may favor such a phenomenon (Esposito et al., 1998; Lemmerman & Lemmerman, 2005). Some local, behavioral and systemic conditions have been correlated with higher rates of failure and, similarly to the scenario observed for the periodontal tissues, smoking has been one of the most widely discussed factors. Jones & Triplett (1992), evaluating fifteen patients who underwent intraoral bone grafting with simultaneous implant placement, were the first to suggest an association between tobacco use and higher rates of implant failures. Five of 15 patients showed impaired healing (defined as loss of bone or implants) and four of these five patients admitted to smoking in the peri-operative period. The first strong evidence of smoking as a risk factor for osseointegrated implants failure was provided by Bain & Moy (1993) one year later. They retrospectively evaluated 2,194 implants placed by the same operator over a 6-year period. It was observed that the overall failure rate was 5.92%, however, when smokers and non-smokers were separately evaluated it was evident that tobacco use exerted a negative impact on titanium implants survival with a failure rate of 11.3% for smokers and 4.76% for non-smokers. The harmful effect was still more evident when the maxilla alone was considered, with failure rates of 17.9% and 7.3% for smokers and non-smokers, respectively. Gorman et al. (1994) analyzed more than 2,000 implants regarding their survival at the second stage surgery, when the implants were exposed to allow prosthetic rehabilitation, and concluded that smoking is detrimental to implant success. In one of the few prospective studies, Moheng and Feryn (2005) evaluated during a 2-year period, 266 titanium implants placed in 93 patients. In addition to the implant survival analysis they investigated the urinary biomarkers of bone formation and resorption (i.e. osteocalcin, pyridinoline and deoxypyridinoline) as predictive factors for oral implant failure. Whilst the biomarkers investigated were not considered predictors for failure, smoking was identified as a major risk factor of implant failure. In another prospective study (Ortorp & Jemt, 2002), the influence of the prosthesis framework type on implant failures was evaluated in 126 edentulous patients. The patients were provided, by random distribution, with 67 prostheses with CNC (computer numeric controlled)-milled titanium frameworks in 23 upper and 44 lower jaws and 62 conventional prostheses with gold-alloy castings in 31 upper and 31 lower jaws. The results revealed that while the framework type did not affect the implant survival in a 3-year follow-up period; patients with smoking habits experienced significantly more implant failures than non-smokers. Considering the already osseointegrated implants, Lindquist et al. (1997) and Hass et al (1996) reported that smoking was the most important factor correlated with peri-implant bone loss. These reports are in line with a recent study by Roos-Jansaker et al. (2006) that examined 1,057 implants in 218 patients for biological complications in existing implants 9-14 years after initial therapy. The effects of several potentially explanatory variables, both on the patient and implant levels, were assessed. On the patient level, smoking was associated with mucositis (inflammation of the peri-implant tissues), low bone level and peri-implantitis (inflammation of the peri-implant tissues associated with bone loss around the implant). In a

3-year follow-up study, Lambert et al. (2000) reported that although success may be achieved for both smokers and non-smokers, titanium implants placement in smokers may be almost 1.5 times more likely to fail than in non-smokers (2.9% difference). De Bruyn & Collaert (1994) verified that cigarette consumption also enhanced early implant failures (i.e. before functional loading) in maxillae, demonstrating 9% of failure for smokers and 1% for non-smokers. The negative impact of smoking on titanium implants survival was confirmed by several authors, using different implant systems in distinct populations (Kourtis et al., 2004; Levin & Schwartz-Arad, 2005; Hinode et al., 2006), and currently is considered one of the main risk factors for implant failure. The preponderance of evidence suggests that smoking may decrease titanium implant success rates (before and after functional loading) and may potentate the bone loss around successfully integrated implants. In a recent study, Saldanha et al. (2006) reported that the effect of smoking on bone healing may precede implant placement. Twenty-one individuals (11 non-smokers and 10 smokers) requiring a non-molar extraction in the upper jaw were selected for the study. Periapical radiographs and linear tomographies were taken 7 and 180 days after tooth extraction, and the following parameters obtained: alveolar process height, alveolar process width, radiographic bone density in the post-extraction socket, and in the pre-existing bone apical to the tooth root. Data analysis demonstrated that smokers presented lower values than non-smokers with regard to the radiographic density in the pre-existing bone apical to the post-extraction socket. Six months after tooth extraction, smoking was found to lead to a more significant dimensional reduction of the residual alveolar ridge and postpone post-extraction socket healing.

The biological basis of the effect of smoking on titanium implants survival and its correlation with bone healing and metabolism is still poorly understood. Although the influence of hormones on bone density has been discussed, it seems that there are no differences between smokers and non-smokers concerning hormonal profile (Law et al., 1997; Fung et al., 1999; Payne et al., 2000; Ward & Klesgues, 2001). It was recently proposed that genetic factors may be important for the incidence of implant failures and complications. Gruica et al. (2004) retrospectively evaluated the charts of 180 patients that had received one or more titanium implants (total of 292 implants), which had been in function for at least 8 (range: 8-15) years. From these, 51 implants in 34 patients showed late (infectious) biological complications. Of the 180 patients, 53 were smokers; these smokers were subdivided in a series of classes according to their intensity of smoking, and 127 had never been smokers. Sixty-four of 180 (36%) patients tested positive for the interleukin (IL)-1 genotype polymorphism. The results of the heavy smokers group (more than 20 cigarettes/day) showed that there was a clear association between a positive IL-1 genotype and implant complications in smokers. Half of the heavy smokers and IL-1 genotype-positive patients (6 of 12) had either loss of implant or a biological complication during the follow-up period.

In vitro studies have shown that cigarette smoke compounds have cytotoxic effects on the cells responsible for bone formation and remodeling. Nicotine has shown a biphasic effect on osteoblast cultures, with an anti-proliferative effect at high levels and stimulatory effects at very low levels (Walker et al., 2001). Henemyre et al. (2003) observed that, at clinically relevant levels, nicotine is not toxic to osteoclasts. It appears to stimulate osteoclast differentiation and resorption of calcium phosphate, the major component of bone. The influence of a cigarette smoke extract (CSE) was evaluated on human osteoprogenitor cells and osteoblast-like cells. CSE inhibited the proliferation of osteoprogenitor cells and the differentiation of osteoprogenitor cells toward osteoblast-like cells (Liu et al., 2001). The chemotactic response of both cell types to fibronectin and platelet-derived growth factor (PDGF)-BB, important molecules for bone repair and remodeling, was inhibited by CSE (Liu et al., 2003). CSE additionally suppressed the production of fibronectin by both cell types (Liu et al., 2003). These studies suggest that tobacco compounds may alter the metabolism of the cells related to bone formation and remodeling and such interference may be one of the mechanisms responsible for the delayed bone healing and poor bone quality observed in smokers. Such a hypothesis was further investigated by Theiss et al. (2001) who evaluated the influence of nicotine (delivered by an osmotic minipump) on gene expression of bone morphogens and related proteins expressed during surgical spine fusion in rabbits. Data analysis demonstrated that nicotine inhibited the expression of both type I and II collagen, bone morphogenic protein-2, -4, and -6, basic fibroblast growth factor (bFGF) and vascular endothelial growth factor (VEGF). Despite the above mentioned studies it is still not known whether different genes to those previously studied may take part in this regulation, and whether cigarette smoke may cause a different overall effect to that of nicotine alone. Thus, further studies are necessary in the near future to elucidate these intriguing questions.

Animal Studies:

As an attempt to further address the impact of cigarette smoke on the behavior of the bone tissue around titanium implants, our group has pioneered the use of animal models to perform histological analysis. We first found that nicotine alone may not affect bone healing around titanium implants placed in rabbits (Stefani et al., 2002; Nociti et al., 2002b). However, in these preliminary studies, nicotine and/or cotinine serum levels were not assessed and, therefore, caution should be used with respect to these initial observations. In order to further investigate the contribution of nicotine to the already reported effect of cigarette smoke on bone healing around titanium implants, we used the same smoke exposure device used to assess the effect of passive smoking on the periodontal tissues (César-Neto et al., 2003). Forty-five rats that received one screw-shaped titanium implant in each tibia were randomly assigned to: Group 1: control; Group 2: intermittent cigarette smoke inhalation; and Group 3: subcutaneous administration of nicotine (3 mg/kg) twice daily. We first determined by HPLC analysis that the nicotine dosage used in this study promoted cotinine serum levels similar to those of the 8-minute smoke exposure used in our passive smoking model. The results demonstrated that, in the cortical bone, cigarette smoke presented a significant negative influence on the bone-to-implant contact and on the amount of new formed bone within the limits of the implant threads, while no effect was found when nicotine alone was administered. In the cancellous bone, cigarette smoke inhalation also resulted in a decreased percentage of bone-to-implant contact when compared to the control group. In addition, the bone filling of the threads was significantly decreased by both cigarette smoke and nicotine. It was concluded that the negative impact of smoking on implant outcomes may be related to more than one molecule present in the cigarette smoke and nicotine seems to partially contribute, especially in the cancellous bone. These findings were later confirmed by studies that evaluated the effect of nicotine administration on bone regeneration in dogs (Saldanha et al., 2004 a and b). For these studies, 16 mongrel dogs were used. One defect was surgically created bilaterally and randomly assigned as an expanded polytetrafluoroethylene (ePTFE) membrane site or a non-membrane control site. The animals randomly received, or not, subcutaneous administration of nicotine (2 mg/kg) twice daily. In general, data analysis demonstrated that at least part of the negative influence of smoking on the bone tissue seems to be caused by nicotine. A relevant issue that still remained to be further investigated was whether the effect of cigarette smoke was limited to the newly formed bone closely associated to the implant surface or if the pre-existing bone would also be affected. By using the already validated passive smoking device, it was further investigated whether cigarette smoke would alter the pre-existing bone in a region adjacent to titanium implants inserted in the tibiae of rats (Nociti et al., 2002a). Thirty-two animals that received a screw-shaped titanium implant (4.0 mm in length and 2.2 mm in diameter) in each tibia were used. After the surgical placement of the implants, the animals were randomly assigned to either the control (non-exposed animals) or test (intermittent cigarette smoke exposure) groups. Sixty days later, the animals were sacrificed and the bone density (i.e. the proportion of mineralized bone in a 500-micrometers-wide zone lateral to the implant) was separately determined in the cortical and cancellous bone areas. Data collected from the cortical and cancellous bone areas were evaluated separately because of the anatomic and metabolic differences between these areas, and also because previous studies reported that the bone in the cancellous compartment may be more susceptible to systemic factors (Motohashi et al., 1999; Pan et al., 2000). It was found that cigarette smoke inhalation was able to affect bone quality in the pre-existing cancellous bone, while the cortical bone seemed to be less sensitive. Thus, although the local effect of tobacco on oral cavity, e.g. heating and local presence of the cigarette smoke compounds, may be involved in the effect of smoking on titanium implant outcome, we clearly demonstrated that the systemic presence of cigarette compounds in blood flow may also play an important role, resulting in a poorer bone quality around titanium implants.

Despite medical studies have suggested a synergic effect of smoking and estrogen deficiency on bone tissue (Fujiwara, 2005), since the former is considered a risk factor for osteoporosis and the latter is the main cause of mineral content loss, an intriguing scenario has recently been brought up suggesting that cigarette smoke inhalation may act synergistically with hormone deficiency on the bone around titanium implants (Carvalho et al., 2006). In order to investigate the effect of cigarette smoke inhalation associated with estrogen deficiency, 45 female Wistar rats that had received one titanium implant in one of the tibiae were randomly assigned to the following groups: OVX (ovariectomized rats), SHAM (sham-operated rats), and CSI + OVX (4 months of intermittent cigarette smoke inhalation, starting 2 months before implant placement in ovariectomized rats). The implants were placed at the time of OVX or SHAM surgery. Sixty days after implant placement it was observed that the CSI + OVX group presented the lowest degree of bone-to-implant and bone density (a 500 μm zone lateral to the implant surface) in both cortical and cancellous bone. The results of this study demonstrated that cigarette smoke inhalation may amplify the deleterious effects of estrogen deficiency on the bone tissue and that such an effect may extend to the bone around titanium implants. With this series of studies we provided important information that i) at least partially document why titanium implants fail more frequently in smokers, ii) establishes a model that allows for the observation of the smoking effects on bone tissue around titanium implants, iii) confirms the interaction between cigarette smoke inhalation and other systemic factors such as hormone deficiency, and iv) provides us with a model to search for alternatives that may be adopted to attenuate the negative influence of tobacco use on bone tissue around titanium implants. Tables 3 and 4 summarize the data in animal models and humans with respect to the impact of cigarette smoke and its compounds (nicotine) on the bone with and without the presence of titanium implants.

Table 3- Summary of histological studies evaluating the effect of nicotine and cigarette smoke on bone around titanium implants inserted in the tibiae of animals.

Author (year)	**Animal**	**Exposure regimen**	**Experimental Groups**	**Histometric Parameters**				**General findings**
				BIC		**BF**		
				Cortical	**Cancellous**	**Cortical**	**Cancellous**	
Stefani et al. (2000)	rabbit	Nicotine administration after implant placement	Control (n=8) 0.37 mg/kg (n=8) 0.57 mg/kg (n=8) 0.93 mg/kg (n=8)	34.98 +/- 7.52 33.58 +/- 6.40 30.13 +/- 4.97 27.79 +/- 3.93 **NS**	-	75.45 +/- 4.61 72.19 +/- 5.82 74.72 +/- 5.3 71.09 +/- 6.8 **NS**	-	Nicotine did not affect bone healing around implants. **Obs. Data from machined implants**
César-Neto et al. (2003)	rat	Nicotine administration and CSI after implant placement	Control (n=19) CSI (n=15) 3 mg/kg (n=11)	55.60 +/- 11.00 41.39 +/- 15.64 45.54 +/- 3.06 S	36.67 +/- 7.11 25.55 +/- 13.34 27.95 +/- 11.93 S	86.47 +/- 4.80 79.85 +/- 6.17 81.54 +/- 5.06 S	32.01 +/- 6.62 20.71 +/- 8.57 21.91 +/- 6.48 S	The impact of smoking on implant outcomes may be related to more than one molecule. Nicotine seems to contribute, especially in the cancellous bone.
César-Neto et al. (2005c)	rat	CSI before and after implant placement	Control CSI Definitive Cessation Temporary Cessation	55.34 +/- 14.57 47.84 +/- 11.36 51.09 +/- 11.97 47.77 +/- 12.43 **NS**	42.70 +/- 10.78 33.21 +/- 12.51 39.67 +/- 11.96 37.46 +/- 10.28 **NS**	88.91 +/- 4.29 80.66 +/- 6.55 84.27 +/- 6.96 85.71 +/- 4.7 S	51.28 +/- 6.49 38.69 +/- 10.78 48.87 +/- 8.47 49.47 +/- 8.04 S	Temporary and complete CSI cessation reversed the effect of smoke exposure on bone healing around titanium implants
				BD				
Nociti et al. (2002)	rat	CSI after implant placement	Control (n=18) CSI (n=14)	96.18 +/- 1.08 95.38 +/- 1.17 **NS**	17.57 +/- 6.45 11.30 +/- 6.81 **S**	-	-	Although CSI may not seriously affect cortical bone density, it may jeopardize bone quality around implants in the cancellous area

Table 3- Summary of histological studies evaluating the effect of nicotine and cigarette smoke on bone around titanium implants inserted in the tibiae of animals. (Continued)

Author (year)	Animal	Exposure regimen	Experimental Groups	Histometric Parameters				General findings
				BIC		BF		
				Cortical	Cancellous	Cortical	Cancellous	
César-Neto et al. (2005b)	rat	CSI before and after implant placement	Control CSI Definitive Cessation Temporary Cessation	BD 97.66 +/- 3.69 98.30 +/- 0.95 98.83 +/- 0.73 98.11 +/- 1.14 **NS**	25.69 +/- 9.41 18.08 +/- 6.0 25.46 +/- 5.42 26.20 +/- 6.77 **S**	-	-	Smoking affected bone quality around implants in cancellous area, and cessation resulted in a return toward to the levels of the control group

CSI – Cigarette smoke inhalation, **S** - Statistically different, **NS** - Non-statistically different, **BIC** – Bone-to-implant contact, **BF** – Bone filling within the limits of the threads, **BD** – Bone Density (proportion of mineralized tissue).

Table 4- Summary of key and recent articles comparing implant outcome in smokers and non-smokers.

Author (year)	Type of study	Evaluation Period	# Patients			# Implants			% of Failures		Type of Implant	General comments
			Total	NSm	Sm	Total	NSm	Sm	NSm	Sm		
Bain & Moy (1993)	Retrospective; 1 center	0 to 6 years	540	nd	nd	2,194	1804	390	4.8	11.3	Brane-mark machined	Include post-loading data
De Bruin & Collaert (1994)	Retrospective; 1 center	6 months	61	45	16	244	166	78	1	9	Brane-mark machined	Data from maxilla; Only pre-loading data
Kan et al. (1999)	Retrospective; 1 center	0-60 months	60	44	16	228	158	70	**Cumulative success rate** 82.7	65.2	nd	Implants placed in grafted maxillary sinus
Wallace (2000)	Retrospective; 1 center	0 to 4 years	56	nd	nd	187	nd	nd	6.9	16.6	nd	Include post-loading data
Schwartz-Arad et al. (2002)	Retrospective; 1 center	At least 6 months	261	172	89	959	579	380	2	4	nd	Include data from immediate implants with high and flat cover screws

Table 4- Summary of key and recent articles comparing implant outcome in smokers and non-smokers. (Continued)

Author (year)	Type of study	Evaluation Period	# Patients			# Implants			% of Failures		Type of Implant	General comments
Bain et al. (2002)	Prospective; 25 centers	3 years	778	637	141	2,274	1877	397	1.6	1.3	**3i Osseotite acid etched**	Include post-loading data
			1013	821	192	2609	2117	492	7.2	6.5	**3i machined**	Include post-loading data
Kourtis et al. (2004)	Retrospective; 4 centers	1 to 12 years (mean 4.6)	405	205	200	1692	839	853	**Survival rate probability (6 years)** 97.1	93.7	Frialit-2, IMZ, Free-Hex and Frialoc	Include data from immediate implants
Moheng & Feryn (2005)	Prospective; 1 center	2 years	93	78	15	266	nd	nd	Risk of implant failure (Sm vs. NSm) **14.4**		Frialit-2 (73% of the cases) or IMZ Twin Plus	Include post-loading data
Hinode et al. (2006)	Meta-analysis; 19 studies								Odds ratio of implant failures (Sm vs. NSm) **2.17**			Include post-loading data

nd - non-described, Sm – smokers, NSm - non-smokers

Overcoming the Effect of Cigarette smoking and/or its Compounds on Implant Outcome

Once established that smoking, isolated or in association with another systemic condition, may significantly affect the success rates reported for osseointegrated implants, a natural goal is to search for alternative approaches to clinically overcome such a problem. It has been shown that the effect of smoking on most living tissues may be transient, and reversion of such effects is seen once cigarette consumption is interrupted (Fielding, 1985; Tomar & Asma, 2000; Ward & Klesges, 2001; Smith et al., 2003). Therefore, it seems logical that definitively interrupting cigarette consumption is the ideal strategy to avoid its consequences. However, it is known that the adherence to quit-smoking programs is low, and individuals often return to their smoking status. In the face of this reality, Bain (1996) was the first to purpose a temporary smoking cessation protocol to deal with implant failure in smokers. Bain suggested a program that consisted of a cessation perioperative period in which potential implant patients who smoked were encouraged to stop for 1 week before and 8 weeks after implant placement. Based on a prospective study of 223 consecutive titanium implants placed in 78 patients, the authors found no difference in failure rate between non-smoking controls and the smokers who quit, whereas a significant difference was noted between the continuing smokers and smokers who followed the cessation protocol. In order to further document the beneficial effect of smoking cessation on bone around titanium implants, a protocol based on Bain's proposal was adapted to the passive smoking model used in rats (Cesar-Neto et al., 2005 b and c). Sixty-six rats were randomly assigned to one of four groups: Control; CSI - intermittent cigarette smoke inhalation (C-CSI) throughout the entire 150-day experiment; P-CSI - CSI for 83 days prior to implant placement; or R-CSI - CSI for 83 days, cessation 7 days before and 21 weeks after implant placement, and return to CSI for 39 days. The animals were sacrificed sixty days after the surgeries and the degree of bone-to-implant contact, the bone area within the limits of the implant threads and the proportion of mineralized tissue lateral to the implants were obtained. Data analyses confirmed that the cortical bone seems to be less sensitive to the influence of smoking than the cancellous bone. Furthermore, it was observed that both temporary and complete CSI cessation reversed the effect of smoke exposure on bone healing around titanium implants in both areas.

Despite the promising results attributed to smoking cessation, we have to take into account that quitting smoking is not an easy task. Nicotine is a drug with a high addiction potential and most patients have difficulties in interrupting its intake, even temporarily. Data from Bain's study (1996) (where all patients were advised to stop smoking) showed that 51 patients started on the cessation protocol and, one year later just 23 patients remained without smoking. In a recent study (Killen et al., 2006) testing bupropion (the most effective non-nicotine based cessation drug) as adjunct therapy for smoking cessation, it was observed that the abstinence percentages after 52 weeks were 33% and 34% for bupropion and placebo groups, respectively. The smoking cessation rate is also low in patients treated in specialized clinics (where patients have professional support and medication such as nicotine patches and bupropion when necessary). In an evaluation of 349 patients who completed a 1-year follow-up of a smoking cessation program it was detected that just 151 (43.26%) were successful in quitting (Akkaya et al., 2006). With the objective of reducing the negative impact of smoking on implant outcomes, without the problems related to smoking cessation, some authors have proposed the use of surface-treated titanium implants (which have properties that stimulate bone formation) for smokers. Kumar et al. (2002) retrospectively evaluated the effect of smoking on achieving initial osseointegration in 1,183 surface-modified dental implants placed in 461 patients. The group of smokers consisted of patients who smoked a half pack of cigarettes per day or more. The overall success rate for smokers and non-smokers in achieving osseointegration was 98.1%. Ninety-seven percent of the implants placed in smokers, and 98.4% of implants placed in non-smokers osseointegrated successfully. It appears from this short-term retrospective study that surface-modified dental implants may be an important alternative to improve success rates for osseointegrated implants placed in smokers. Bain et al. (2002) then examined the influence of smoking on the integration success and longevity of machined and acid-etched titanium implants. The study combined 3 prospective multicenter studies on machined implants (n= 2,614 implants) and six prospective multicenter studies on acid-etched implants (n=2,288 implants), all with standardized protocols. In all, 492 machined and 392 surface-treated implants were placed in smokers. Mean smoking consumption was 12.1 cigarettes each day in machined implants and 12.7 cigarettes each day in surface-treated implants. The overall cumulative success rates were 92.8% for the machined implants and 98.4% for the acid-etched implants. Although there was no significant difference between smokers and non-smokers in either type of surface, within the smoking sub-group cumulative success rates were 93.5% for the machined implants and 98.7 for the acid-etched implants. These results are in agreement with the ones of our pioneer study in rabbits that received nicotine injections (Stefani et al., 2002). In that study, thirty-two New Zealand rabbits received, in each tibia, either a machined or an AL_2O_3-blasted surface screw-shaped commercially available pure titanium implant, 7.0 mm in length and 3.75 mm. The animals were daily administered with subcutaneous injections of four different concentrations of nicotine. Forty-two days later, the degree of bone-to-implant contact and the bone area into the limits of the threads were obtained. It was concluded that modified implant surfaces may enhance osseointegration after nicotine administration. Although this result goes some way to explain clinical data, further clinical studies should be performed in order to investigate, on a long-term basis, whether the use of implants with special surface treatment is an alternative approach in order to offer a more predictable scenario for implants placed in smokers.

In summary, tobacco smoking represents a strong risk factor for implant failure and the poor bone quality promoted by cigarette smoke inhalation may be one of the causes of the increased failure rate observed in smokers. The mechanisms of the effect of smoking on bone metabolism are not clearly understood, but it seems to involve the regulation of genes important to bone formation and remodeling. The available evidence shows that smoking cessation is the best alternative to attenuate the negative influence of smoking on biological events. However, the great difficulty of smokers in quitting tobacco consumption must be considered. Preliminary studies have suggested that the use of surface-treated titanium implants seems to be a feasible alternative for smokers that are candidates for implant placement, but more studies are necessary to confirm such a hypothesis.

Conclusion

In the light of the existing evidence, it can be concluded that smoking is a strong risk factor for both periodontal diseases and implant failures. The mechanisms by which tobacco use favors periodontal destruction are not fully understood, but it seems that a down-regulation of anti-inflammatory/resorptive factors associated with an up-regulation of pro-inflammatory cytokines is involved. In addition, the higher rates of implant failures observed in smokers may be related with the decreased bone density around the implants. Smoking cessation is the main option to revert the harmful effect of tobacco on implant outcomes, periodontal risk and therapy; however, alternative approaches should also be investigated because of the low success obtained by smokers that attempt to quit cigarette consumption.

References

Adell, R; Eriksson, B; Lekholm, U; Branemark, PI; Jemt, T. Long-term follow-up study of osseointegrated implants in the treatment of totally edentulous jaws. *Int J Oral Maxillofac Implants.* 1990 Winter;5(4):347-59.

Akkaya, A; Ozturk, O; Cobanoglu, H; Bircan, HA; Simsek, S; Sahin, U. Evaluation of patients followed up in a cigarette cessation clinic. *Respirology*. 2006 May;11(3):311-6.

Bahat O. Branemark system implants in the posterior maxilla: clinical study of 660 implants followed for 5 to 12 years. *Int J Oral Maxillofac Implants*. 2000 Sep-Oct;15(5):646-53.

Bain, CA; Moy, PK. The association between the failure of dental implants and cigarette smoking. *Int J Oral Maxillofac Implants*. 1993;8(6):609-15.

Bain, CA; Weng, D; Meltzer, A; Kohles, SS; Stach, RM. A meta-analysis evaluating the risk for implant failure in patients who smoke. *Compend Contin Educ Dent*. 2002 Aug;23(8):695-706.

Bain, CA. Smoking and implant failure--benefits of a smoking cessation protocol. *Int J Oral Maxillofac Implants*. 1996 Nov-Dec;11(6):756-9.

Benatti, BB; Cesar-Neto, JB; Gonçalves, PF; Sallum, EA; Nociti, FH Jr. Smoking affects the self-healing capacity of periodontal tissues. A histological study in the rat. *Eur J Oral Sci*. 2005 Oct;113(5):400-3.

Bergstrom, J; Eliasson, S; Dock, J. A 10-year prospective study of tobacco smoking and periodontal health. *J Periodontol*. 2000 Aug;71(8):1338-47.

Bergstrom, J; Eliasson, S; Dock, J. Exposure to tobacco smoking and periodontal health. *J Clin Periodontol*. 2000 Jan;27(1):61-8.

Bergstrom, J; Eliasson, S. Noxious effect of cigarette smoking on periodontal health. *J Periodontal Res*. 1987 Nov;22(6):513-7.

Bergstrom, J; Persson, L; Preber, H. Influence of cigarette smoking on vascular reaction during experimental gingivitis. *Scand J Dent Res*. 1988 Feb;96(1):34-9.

Bergstrom, J; Preber, H. The influence of cigarette smoking on the development of experimental gingivitis. *J Periodontal Res*. 1986 Nov;21(6):668-76.

Bergstrom, J. Cigarette smoking as risk factor in chronic periodontal disease. *Community Dent Oral Epidemiol*. 1989 Oct;17(5):245-7.

Bergstrom, J; Preber, H. Tobacco use as a risk factor. *J Periodontol*. 1994 May;65(5 Suppl):545-50.

Bostrom, L; Linder, LE; Bergstrom, J. Smoking and cervicular fluid levels of IL-6 and TNF-alpha in periodontal disease. *J Clin Periodontol* 1999; 26:352-357.

Bostrom, L; Linder, LE; Bergstrom, J. Smoking and GCF levels of IL-1beta and IL-1ra in periodontal disease. *J Clin Periodontol* 2000; 27:250-255.

Bowers, GM; Schallhorn, RG; McClain, PK; Morrison, GM; Morgan, R; Reynolds, MA. Factors influencing the outcome of regenerative therapy in mandibular Class II furcations: Part I. *J Periodontol*. 2003 Sep;74(9):1255-68.

Calsina, G; Ramon, JM; Echeverria, JJ. Effects of smoking on periodontal tissues. *J Clin Periodontol*. 2002 Aug;29(8):771-6.

Carvalho, MD; Benatti, BB; Cesar-Neto, JB; Nociti, FH Jr; da Rocha Nogueira Filho, G; Casati, MZ; Sallum, EA. Effect of cigarette smoke inhalation and estrogen deficiency on bone healing around titanium implants: a histometric study in rats. *J Periodontol*. 2006 Apr;77(4):599-605.

Cendon, SP; Battlehner, C; Lorenzi Filho, G; Dohlnikoff, M; Pereira, PM; Conceicao, GM; Beppu, OS; Saldiva, PH. Pulmonary emphysema induced by passive smoking: an experimental study in rats. *Braz J Med Biol Res*. 1997 Oct;30(10):1241-7.

Cesar Neto, JB; de Souza, AP; Barbieri, D; Moreno, H Jr; Sallum, EA; Nociti, FH Jr. Matrix metalloproteinase-2 may be involved with increased bone loss associated with experimental periodontitis and smoking: a study in rats. *J Periodontol.* 2004 Jul;75(7):995-1000.

Cesar-Neto, JB; Duarte, PM; Casati, MZ; Oliveira, MCG; Tambeli, CH; Parada, CA; Sallum, E.A.; Nociti, F.H. Smoking modulates IL-6:IL-10 and RANKL:OPG ratios in the periodontal tissues. *J Periodontal Res*, 2006a (in press).

Cesar-Neto, JB; Duarte, PM; Casati, MZ; Oliveira, MCG; Tambeli, CH; Parada, CA; Sallum, EA; Nociti, FH Smoking modulates INF-γ expression in the gingival tissues of patients with chronic periodontitis. *Eur J Oral Sci* 2006b (in press).

Cesar-Neto, JB; Benatti, BB; Neto, FH; Sallum, AW; Sallum, EA; Nociti, FH. Smoking cessation may present a positive impact on mandibular bone quality and periodontitis-related bone loss: a study in rats. *J Periodontol.* 2005a Apr;76(4):520-5.

Cesar-Neto, JB; Benatti, BB; Sallum, EA; Casati, MZ; Nociti, FH Jr. The influence of cigarette smoke inhalation and its cessation on the tooth-supporting alveolar bone: a histometric study in rats. *J Periodontal Res.* 2006 Apr;41(2):118-23.

Cesar-Neto, JB; Benatti, BB; Sallum, EA; Nociti, FH Jr. Bone density around titanium implants may benefit from smoking cessation: a histologic study in rats. *Int J Oral Maxillofac Implants.* 2005b Sep-Oct;20(5):713-9.

Cesar-Neto, JB; Benatti, BB; Sallum, EA; Sallum, AW; Nociti, FH Jr. Bone filling around titanium implants may benefit from smoking cessation: a histologic study in rats. *J Periodontol.* 2005c Sep;76(9):1476-81.

Cesar-Neto, JB; Duarte, PM; Sallum, EA; Barbieri, D; Moreno, H Jr; Nociti, FH Jr. A comparative study on the effect of nicotine administration and cigarette smoke inhalation on bone healing around titanium implants. *J Periodontol.* 2003 Oct;74(10):1454-9.

Consensus report. Periodontal diseases: epidemiology and diagnosis. *Ann Periodontol.* 1996 Nov;1(1):216-22.

Dannewitz, B; Krieger, JK; Husing, J; Eickholz, P. Loss of molars in periodontally treated patients: a retrospective analysis five years or more after active periodontal treatment. *J Clin Periodontol.* 2006 Jan;33(1):53-61.

De Bruyn, H; Collaert, B. The effect of smoking on early implant failure. *Clin Oral Implants Res.* 1994 Dec;5(4):260-4.

Erdemir, EO; Duran, I; Haliloglu, S. Effects of smoking on clinical parameters and the gingival crevicular fluid levels of IL-6 and TNF-alpha in patients with chronic periodontitis. *J Clin Periodontol* 2004; 31:99-104.

Esposito, M; Hirch, J-M; Lekholm, U; Thomsen, P. Biological factors contributing to failures of osseointegrated oral implants (II). Etiopathogenesis. *Eur J Oral Sci* 1998; 106:721-764.

Fielding, JE. Smoking: health effects and control (1). *N Engl J Med.* 1985 Aug 22;313(8):491-8.

Fujiwara, S. Epidemiology of osteoporosis. *Clin Calcium.* 2005 Apr;15(4):577-82.

Fung, YK; Iwaniec, U; Cullen, DM; Akhter, MP; Haven, MC; Timmins, P. Long-term effects of nicotine on bone and calciotropic hormones in adult female rats. *Pharmacol Toxicol* 1999; 85: 181-7.

Gelskey, SC; Young, TK; Singer, DL. Factors associated with adult periodontitis in a dental teaching clinic population. *Community Dent Oral Epidemiol.* 1998 Aug;26(4):226-32.

Giannopoulou, C; Cappuyns, I; Mombelli, A. Effect of smoking on gingival crevicular fluid cytokine profile during experimental gingivitis. *J Clin Periodontol.* 2003 Nov;30(11):996-1002.

Giannopoulou, C; Geinoz, A; Cimasoni; G. Effects of nicotine on periodontal ligament fibroblasts in vitro. *J Clin Periodontol.* 1999 Jan;26(1):49-55.

Giannopoulou, C; Roehrich, N; Mombelli, A. Effect of nicotine-treated epithelial cells on the proliferation and collagen production of gingival fibroblasts. *J Clin Periodontol.* 2001 Aug;28(8):769-75.

Gonzalez, YM; De Nardin, A; Grossi, SG; Machtei, EE; Genco, RJ; De Nardin, E. Serum cotinine levels, smoking, and periodontal attachment loss. *J Dent Res.* 1996 Feb;75(2):796-802.

Gorman, LM; Lambert, PM; Morris, HF; Ochi, S; Winkler, S. The effect of smoking on implant survival at second-stage surgery. *Implant Dent.* 1994 Fall;3(3):165-8.

Goultschin, J; Cohen, HD; Donchin, M; Brayer, L; Soskolne, WA. Association of smoking with periodontal treatment needs. *J Periodontol.* 1990 Jun;61(6):364-7.

Gruica, B; Wang, HY; Lang, NP; Buser, D. Impact of IL-1 genotype and smoking status on the prognosis of osseointegrated implants. *Clin Oral Implants Res.* 2004 Aug;15(4):393-400.

Haas, R; Haimbock, W; Mailath, G; Watzek, G. The relationship of smoking on peri-implant tissue: a retrospective study. *Prosthet Dent.* 1996 Dec;76(6):592-6.

Haber, J; Wattles, J; Crowley, M; Mandell, R; Joshipura, K; Kent, RL. Evidence for cigarette smoking as a major risk factor for periodontitis. *J Periodontol.* 1993 Jan;64(1):16-23.

Heasman, L; Stacey, F; Preshaw, PM; McCracken, GI; Hepburn, S; Heasman, PA; The effect of smoking on periodontal treatment response: a review of clinical evidence. *J Clin Periodontol.* 2006 Apr;33(4):241-53.

Heitz-Mayfield, LJ. Disease progression: identification of high-risk groups and individuals for periodontitis. *J Clin Periodontol.* 2005;32 Suppl 6:196-209.

Henemyre, CL; Scales, DK; Hokett, SD; Cuenin, MF; Peacock, ME; Parker, MH; Brewer, PD; Chuang, AH. Nicotine stimulates osteoclast resorption in a porcine marrow cell model. *J Periodontol.* 2003 Oct;74(10):1440-6.

Hinode, D; Tanabe, S-I; Yokoyama, M; Fujisawa, K; Yamauchi, E; Miyamoto, Y. The influence of smoking on osseointegrated implant failure: a meta-analysis. *Clin. Oral Impl. Res.* doi: 10.1111/j.1600-0501.2005.01244. online early

Johnson, GK; Hill, M. Cigarette smoking and the periodontal patient. *J Periodontol* 2004; 75: 196–209.

Jones, JK; Triplett, RG. Relationship of cigarette smoking to impaired intraoral wound healing: a review of evidence and implications for patient care. *J Oral Maxillofac Surg.* 1992 Mar;50(3):237-40.

Kamma, JJ; Giannopoulou, C; Vasdekis, VG; Mombelli, A. Cytokine profile in gingival crevicular fluid of aggressive periodontitis: influence of smoking and stress. *J Clin Periodontol.* 2004 Oct;31(10):894-902.

Kan, JY; Rungcharassaeng, K; Lozada, JL; Goodacre, CJ. Effects of smoking on implant success in grafted maxillary sinuses. *J Prosthet Dent.* 1999 Sep;82(3):307-11.

Killen, JD; Fortmann, SP; Murphy, GM Jr; Hayward, C; Arredondo, C; Cromp, D; Celio, M; Abe, L; Wang, Y; Schatzberg, AF. Extended treatment with bupropion SR for cigarette smoking cessation. *J Consult Clin Psychol.* 2006 Apr;74(2):286-94.

Kourtis, SG; Sotiriadou, S; Voliotis, S; Challas, A. Private practice results of dental implants. Part I: survival and evaluation of risk factors--Part II: surgical and prosthetic complications. *Implant Dent.* 2004 Dec;13(4):373-85.

Krall, EA; Garvey, AJ; Garcia, RI. Alveolar bone loss and tooth loss in male cigar and pipe smokers. *J Am Dent Assoc.* 1999 Jan;130(1):57-64.

Kumar, A; Jaffin, RA; Berman, C. The effect of smoking on achieving osseointegration of surface-modified implants: a clinical report. *Int J Oral Maxillofac Implants.* 2002 Nov-Dec;17(6):816-9.

Kuri, M; Nakagawa, M; Tanaka, H; Hasuo, S; Kishi, Y. Determination of the duration of preoperative smoking cessation to improve wound healing after head and neck surgery. *Anesthesiology* 2005; 102: 892–896.

Lambert, PM; Morris, HF; Ochi, S. The influence of smoking on 3-year clinical success of osseointegrated dental implants. *Ann Periodontol.* 2000 Dec;5(1):79-89.

Lambrecht, JT; Filippi, A; Kunzel, AR; Schiel, HJ. Long-term evaluation of submerged and nonsubmerged ITI solid-screw titanium implants: a 10-year life table analysis of 468 implants. *Int J Oral Maxillofac Implants.* 2003 Nov-Dec;18(6):826-34.

Law, MR; Cheng, R; Hackshaw, AK; Allaway, S; Hale, AK. Cigarette smoking, sex hormones and bone density in women. *Eur J Epidemiol* 1997;13:553-558.

Lemmerman, KJ; Lemmerman, NE. Osseointegrated dental implants in private practice: a long-term case series study. *J Periodontol.* 2005 Feb;76(2):310-9.

Leung, WK; Ng, DK; Jin, L; Corbet, EF. Tooth loss in treated periodontitis patients responsible for their supportive care arrangements. *J Clin Periodontol.* 2006 Apr;33(4):265-75.

Levin, L; Schwartz-Arad, D. The effect of cigarette smoking on dental implants and related surgery. *Implant Dent.* 2005 Dec;14(4):357-61.

Lind, J; Kramhoft, M; Bodtker, S. The influence of smoking on complications after primary amputations of the lower extremity. *Clin Orthop Relat Res* 1991; 267: 211–217.

Linden, GJ; Mullally, BH. Cigarette smoking and periodontal destruction in young adults. *J Periodontol.* 1994 Jul;65(7):718-23.

Lindquist, LW; Carlsson, GE; Jemt, T. Association between marginal bone loss around osseointegrated mandibular implants and smoking habits: a 10-year follow-up study. *J Dent Res.* 1997 Oct;76(10):1667-74.

Liu, X; Kohyama, T; Kobayashi, T; Abe, S; Kim, HJ; Reed, EC; Rennard, SI. Cigarette smoke extract inhibits chemotaxis and collagen gel contractionmediated by human bone marrow osteoprogenitor cells and osteoblast-like cells. *Osteoporos Int.* 2003 Mar;14(3):235-42.

Liu, XD; Zhu, YK; Umino, T; Spurzem, JR; Romberger, DJ; Wang, H; Reed, E; Rennard, SI. Cigarette smoke inhibits osteogenic differentiation and proliferation of human osteoprogenitor cells in monolayer and three-dimensional collagen gel culture. *J Lab Clin Med.* 2001 Mar;137(3):208-19.

Machion, L; Andia, DC; Benatti, BB; Carvalho, MD; Nogueira-Filho, GR; Casati, MZ; Nociti, FH Jr; Sallum, EA. Locally delivered doxycycline as an adjunctive therapy to scaling and root planing in the treatment of smokers: a clinical study. *J Periodontol.* 2004 Mar;75(3):464-9.

Machion, L; Andia, DC; Lecio, G; Nociti, FH Jr; Casati, MZ; Sallum, AW; Sallum, EA. Locally delivered doxycycline as an adjunctive therapy to scaling and root planing in the treatment of smokers: a 2-year follow-up. *J Periodontol.* 2006 Apr;77(4):606-13.

Machion, L; Andia, DC; Saito, D; Klein, MI; Goncalves, RB; Casati, MZ; Nociti, FH Jr; Sallum, EA. Microbiological changes with the use of locally delivered doxycycline in the periodontal treatment of smokers. *J Periodontol.* 2004 Dec;75(12):1600-4.

Machtei, EE; Oettinger-Barak, O; Peled, M. Guided tissue regeneration in smokers: effect of aggressive anti-infective therapy in Class II furcation defects. *J Periodontol.* 2003 May;74(5):579-84.

Magnusson, I; Walker, CB. Refractory periodontitis or recurrence of disease. *J Clin Periodontol.* 1996 Mar;23(3 Pt 2):289-92.

Martins, AG; Andia, DC; Sallum, AW; Sallum, EA; Casati, MZ; Nociti Junior, FH. Smoking may affect root coverage outcome: a prospective clinical study in humans. *J Periodontol.* 2004 Apr;75(4):586-91.

Mascarenhas, P; Gapski, R; Al-Shammari, K; Hill, R; Soehren, S; Fenno, JC; Giannobile, WV; Wang, HL. Clinical response of azithromycin as an adjunct to non-surgical periodontal therapy in smokers. *J Periodontol.* 2005 Mar;76(3):426-36.

Moheng, P; Feryn, JM. Clinical and biologic factors related to oral implant failure: a 2-year follow-up study. *Implant Dent.* 2005 Sep;14(3):281-8.

Morozumi, T; Kubota, T; Sugita, N; Itagaki, M; Yoshie, H. Alterations of gene expression in human neutrophils induced by smoking cessation. *J Clin Periodontol* 2004; 31:1110-1116.

Motohashi, M; Shirota, T; Tokugawa, Y; Ohno, K; Michi, K; Yamagushi, A. Bone reactions around hydroxyapatite-coated implants in ovariectomized rats. *Oral Surg Oral Med Oral Pathol Oral Radiol Endod.* 1999 Feb;87(2):145-52.

Moy, PK; Medina, D; Shetty, V; Aghaloo, TL. Dental implant failure rates and associated risk factors. *Int J Oral Maxillofac Implants.* 2005 Jul-Aug;20(4):569-77.

Nitzan, D; Mamlider, A; Levin, L; Schwartz-Arad, D. Impact of smoking on marginal bone loss. *Int J Oral Maxillofac Implants.* 2005 Jul-Aug;20(4):605-9.

Nociti, FH Jr; Cesar Neto, JB; Carvalho, MD; Sallum, EA. Bone density around titanium implants may be influenced by intermittent cigarette smoke inhalation: a histometric study in rats. *Int J Oral Maxillofac Implants.* 2002 May-Jun;17(3):347-52.

Nociti, FH Jr; Nogueira-Filho, GR; Primo, MT; Machado, MA; Tramontina, VA; Barros, SP; Sallum, EA. The influence of nicotine on the bone loss rate in ligature-induced periodontitis. A histometric study in rats. *J Periodontol.* 2000 Sep;71(9):1460-4.

Nociti, FH Jr; Nogueira-Filho, GR; Tramontina, VA; Machado, MA; Barros, SP; Sallum, EA; Sallum, AW. Histometric evaluation of the effect of nicotine administration on periodontal breakdown: an in vivo study. *J Periodontal Res.* 2001 Dec;36(6):361-6.

Nociti, FH Jr; Stefani, CM; Sallum, EA; Duarte, PM; Sallum, AW. Nicotine and bone density around titanium implants: a histometric study in rabbits. *Implant Dent.* 2002;11(2):176-82.

Norderyd, O; Hugoson, A; Grusovin, G. Risk of severe periodontal disease in a Swedish adult population. A longitudinal study. *J Clin Periodontol.* 1999 Sep;26(9):608-15.

Ortorp, A; Jemt, T. Clinical experience of CNC-milled titanium frameworks supported by implants in the edentulous jaw: a 3-year interim report. *Clin Implant Dent Relat Res.* 2002;4(2):104-9.

Ouyang, Y; Virasch, N; Hao, P; Aubrey, MT; Mukerjee, N; Bierer, BE; Freed, BM. Suppression of human IL-1beta, IL-2, IFN-gamma, and TNF-alpha production by cigarette smoke extracts. *J Allergy Clin Immunol* 2000; 106:280-287.

Pan, J; Shirota, T; Ohno, K; Michi, K. Effect of ovariectomy on bone remodeling adjacent to hydroxyapatite-coated implants in the tibia of mature rats. *J Oral Maxillofac Surg.* 2000 Aug;58(8):877-82.

Payne, JB; Reinhardt, RA; Nummikoski, PV; Dunning, DG; Patil, KD. The association of cigarette smoking with alveolar bone loss in postmenopausal females. *J Clin Periodontol.* 2000 Sep;27(9):658-64.

Petropoulos, G; McKay, IJ; Hughes, FJ. The association between neutrophil numbers and interleukin-1alpha concentrations in gingival crevicular fluid of smokers and non-smokers with periodontal disease. *J Clin Periodontol* 2004; 31:390-395.

Pindborg, JJ. Tobacco and gingivitis. I. Statistical examination of the significance of tobacco in the development of ulceromembranous gingivitis and in the formation of calculus. *J Dent Res* 1947; 26:261-264.

Pindborg, JJ. Tobacco and gingivitis. II. Correlation between consumption of tobacco, ulceromembranous gingivitis and calculus. *J Dent Res* 1949; 28:460-463.

Preber, H; Bergstrom, J. Cigarette smoking in patients referred for periodontal treatment. *Scand J Dent Res.* 1986 Apr;94(2):102-8.

Preber, H; Bergstrom, J. Occurrence of gingival bleeding in smoker and non-smoker patients. *Acta Odontol Scand.* 1985 Oct;43(5):315-20.

Preshaw, PM; Hefti, AF; Bradshaw, MH. Adjunctive subantimicrobial dose doxycycline in smokers and non-smokers with chronic periodontitis. *J Clin Periodontol.* 2005 Jun;32(6):610-6.

Rawlinson, A; Grummitt, JM; Walsh, TF; Ian Douglas, CW. Interleukin 1 and receptor antagonist levels in gingival crevicular fluid in heavy smokers versus non-smokers. *J Clin Periodontol.* 2003 Jan;30(1):42-8.

Romeo, E; Chiapasco, M; Ghisolfi, M; Vogel, G. Long-term clinical effectiveness of oral implants in the treatment of partial edentulism. Seven-year life table analysis of a prospective study with ITI dental implants system used for single-tooth restorations. *Clin Oral Implants Res.* 2002 Apr;13(2):133-43.

Romeo, E; Lops, D; Margutti, E; Ghisolfi, M; Chiapasco, M; Vogel, G. Long-term survival and success of oral implants in the treatment of full and partial arches: a 7-year prospective study with the ITI dental implant system. *Int J Oral Maxillofac Implants.* 2004 Mar-Apr;19(2):247-59.

Roos-Jansaker, AM; Renvert, H; Lindahl, C; Renvert, S. Nine- to fourteen-year follow-up of implant treatment. Part III: factors associated with peri-implant lesions. *J Clin Periodontol.* 2006 Apr;33(4):296-301.

Ryder, MI; Hyun, W; Loomer, P; Haqq, C. Alteration of gene expression profiles of peripheral mononuclear blood cells by tobacco smoke: implications for periodontal diseases. *Oral Microbiol Immunol* 2004; 19:39-49.

Saldanha, JB; Pimentel, SP; Casati, MZ; Sallum, AW; Sallum, EA; Nociti, FH. Histologic evaluation of the effect of nicotine administration on bone regeneration. A study in dogs. *Pesqui Odontol Bras.* 2004 Oct-Dec;18(4):345-9.

Saldanha, JB; Pimentel, SP; Casati, MZ; Sallum, EA; Barbieri, D; Moreno, HJ; Nociti, FH. Guided bone regeneration may be negatively influenced by nicotine administration: a histologic study in dogs. *J Periodontol.* 2004 Apr;75(4):565-71.

Saldanha, JB; Casati, MZ; Haiter-Neto, F; Sallum, EA; Nociti, FH Jr. Smoking may affect the alveolar process dimensions and radiographic bone density in extraction sites. A prospective study in humans. *J. Oral Maxillofac.* Surg., 2006 (in press).

Schwartz-Arad, D; Samet, N; Samet, N; Mamlider, A. Smoking and complications of endosseous dental implants. *J Periodontol.* 2002 Feb;73(2):153-7.

Silva, CO; Sallum, AW; de Lima, AF; Tatakis, DN. Coronally positioned flap for root coverage: poorer outcomes in smokers. *J Periodontol.* 2006 Jan;77(1):81-7.

Slade, GD; Gansky, SA; Spencer, AJ. Two-year incidence of tooth loss among South Australians aged 60+ years. *Community Dent Oral Epidemiol.* 1997 Dec;25(6):429-37.

Smith, MR; Kinmonth, AL; Luben, RN; Bingham, S; Day, NE; Wareham, NJ; Welch, A; Khaw, KT. Smoking status and differential white cell count in men and women in the EPIC-Norfolk population. *Atherosclerosis* 2003 Aug;169(2):331-7.

Sorensen, LT; Horby, J; Friis, E; Pilsgaard, B; Jorgensen, T. Smoking as a risk factor for wound healing and infection in breast cancer surgery. *Eur J Surg Oncol* 2002; 28: 815–820.

Stefani, CM; Nogueira, F; Sallum, EA; de TS; Sallum, AW; Nociti, FH Jr. Influence of nicotine administration on different implant surfaces: a histometric study in rabbits. *J Periodontol.* 2002 Feb;73(2):206-12.

Sullivan, DY; Sherwood, RL; Porter, SS. Long-term performance of Osseotite implants: a 6-year clinical follow-up. *Compend Contin Educ Dent.* 2001 Apr;22(4):326-8, 330, 332-4.

Tanner, AC; Kent, R Jr; Van Dyke, T; Sonis, ST; Murray, LA. Clinical and other risk indicators for early periodontitis in adults. *J Periodontol.* 2005 Apr;76(4):573-81.

Theiss, SM; Boden, SD; Hair, G; Titus, L; Morone, MA; Ugbo, J. The effect of nicotine on gene expression during spine fusion. *Spine.* 2000 Oct 15;25(20):2588-94.

Tomar, SL; Asma, S. Smoking-attributable periodontitis in the United States: findings from NHANES III. National Health and Nutrition Examination Survey. *J Periodontol.* 2000 May;71(5):743-51.

Tonetti, MS. Cigarette smoking and periodontal diseases: etiology and management of disease. *Ann Periodontol.* 1998 Jul;3(1):88-101.

Trombelli, L; Cho, KS; Kim, CK; Scapoli, C; Scabbia, A. Impaired healing response of periodontal furcation defects following flap debridement surgery in smokers. A controlled clinical trial. *J Clin Periodontol.* 2003 Jan;30(1):81-7.

Walker, LM; Preston, MR; Magnay, JL; Thomas, PB; El Haj, AJ. Nicotinic regulation of c-fos and osteopontin expression in human-derived osteoblast-like cells and human trabecular bone organ culture. *Bone*. 2001 Jun;28(6):603-8.

Wallace, RH. The relationship between cigarette smoking and dental implant failure. *Eur J Prosthodont Restor Dent*. 2000 Sep;8(3):103-6.

Ward, KD; Klesges, RC. A meta-analysis of the effects of cigarette smoking on bone mineral density. *Calcif Tissue Int*. 2001; 68:259-70.

Wendell, KJ; Stein, SH. Regulation of cytokine production in human gingival fibroblasts following treatment with nicotine and lipopolysaccharide. *J Periodontol* 2001; 72:1038-1044.

WHO (World Health Organization) Tobacco Free Intiative. [on line] Url: *"http://www.who.int/tobacco/en/"*. 2005.

In: Smoking and Health Research Frontiers
Editor: Calvin B. Fong, pp. 213-230

ISBN 1-60021-480-0

Chapter IX

Passive Smoking in Oral Health Research

***Takashi Nanioka*[1] *and Miki Ojima*[2]**
[1]Department of Preventive and Public Health Dentistry, Fukuoka Dental College;
[2]Department of Preventive Dentistry, Osaka University Graduate School of Dentistry.

Abstract

ETS may deteriorate oral health as that has been demonstrated regarding with general health. The effects of ETS on oral health may be first noticed by practitioners who routinely see objective symptoms in oral cavity. Alternative pathway is epidemiological study where data-bases including information in large-scale survey on exposure to ETS and oral health are analyzed. Causal relationships must be discussed, further, based on evidences which could explain biological mechanisms. We address the possible effect of passive smoking on gingival pigmentation and dental diseases, pediatric caries and periodontal disease, in this chapter.

Oral symptoms could be addressed by both smokers and practitioners more easily relative to those of general diseases since the oral cavity is visible. Gingival pigmentation is strongly associated with active smoking. A dose-response relationship was exhibited in several epidemiological studies. Melanin pigmentation in the gingiva is common phenomena globally, however, current smokers are more likely exhibiting melanin pigmentation in the gingiva than non-smokers. Melanocytes were identified at the basal layer of the gingival epithelium. Tobacco smoking could stimulate production of melanin. Prevalence of pigmentation decreased in relation to the number of years following smoking cessation. These findings indicate a causal association.

An epidemiological study conducted in two workplace locations separately exhibited the association of active smoking with gingival pigmentation. Another finding of the study was a distinct difference in the prevalence of gingival pigmentation between groups of non-smokers in the workplaces, factory and office. We guess that smoking may have been prohibited in the factory and allowed in the office. This finding is indicative of the effect of passive smoking on gingival pigmentation. A dentist who works in the northern part of Japan suggested the effect of passive smoking on gingival pigmentation in children. We gathered digital images of gingiva in children and smoking status of their parents who visited a dental clinic where the weather is relatively cold. The investigation demonstrated an association of gingival pigmentation of children with parents who smoke. A possible mechanism will be discussed based on findings of the effect of active smoking on gingival pigmentation.

We review several studies on pediatric caries and a few studies on periodontal disease in terms of the effects of passive smoking. We discuss strength of evidence and the possible mechanisms.

INTRODUCTION

Effects of passive smoking in oral health research may be summarized by the following categories: gingival melanin pigmentation, dental caries, periodontal disease and tooth loss. Furthermore, effects in the oral region may function as a predictor of health consequences of passive smoking. Previous findings, which are summarized in Table 1, were derived from epidemiological investigation. Target populations consisted of children in those studies related to gingival melanin pigmentation and dental caries, and adults in those studies pertaining to periodontal disease and tooth loss.

Table 1. Epidemiologic studies regarding the association between passive smoking and oral diseases.

Diseases	Study	Population	Marker of ETS exposure	Findings
Gingival pigmentation	Hanioka et al 2005	59 children 6-16 years old Japan	Parental smoking (at least one parent smoked)	Existence of pigmentation adjusted for age and sex OR (95%CI) =5.6 (1.5-20.0) and 5.4 (1.4-21.2) for examiner A and B, respectively
Dental caries	Bolin et al. 1997	3,200 children 5 and 12 years old EU-countries (eight countries)	Parental smoking (maternal smoking)	Caries experience (dmfs/DMFS>0) adjusted for country, social class and number of siblings (5 years only) OR =3.2 (1.5-6.9) in Greek sample aged 5 years and 2.6 (1.4-4.8) in Swedish sample aged 12 years ORs in overall sample were not shown.
	Williams et al. 2000	749 children 3.0-4.5 years old UK	Parental smoking (maternal smoking)	Caries prevalence OR =1.96 (1.00-3.85) in social classes I, II and IIInm and 1.55 (1.02-2.35) in social classes IIIm, IV and V dmft =0.8 (Neither parent smoked), 1.5 (Only mother smoked) and 1.5 (Both parents smoked)
	Aligne et al. 2003	3,531 children 4-11 years old United States (NHANES III)	Serum cotinine level (0.2 to 10 ng/ml)	Deciduous caries experience adjusted for age, race/ethnicity, poverty status, region, education level of head of household, blood lead level and time since last dental visit OR =1.8 (1.2-2.7) for decayed surfaces and 1.4 (1.1-2.0) for filled surfaces and N.S. for permanent teeth PAR* = 27% for decayed surface and 14% for filled surface

Table 1. Epidemiologic studies regarding the association between passive smoking and oral diseases. (Continued)

Diseases	Study	Population	Marker of ETS exposure	Findings
	Shenkin et al. 2004	637 children 4-7 years old United States (Iowa)	Smoking in household (regular smoker at home)	Prevalence of caries adjusted for age, SES†, tooth brushing frequency, total ingested fluoride, and combined intake of soda pop and powdered drink beverages OR =3.38 (1.68-6.79); 44% for regular smokers and 25% for nonregular/non-smokers for over all subjects, and 52% and 24%, respectively, for subjects with middle SES
	Tanaka et al. in press	925 children 1-14 years old Japan	Smoking in household	Prevalence of DT‡ adjusted for age, gender, region of residence, tooth brushing frequency and experience of fluoride application; OR =1.34 (1.02-1.76), 33.6% for non-smoking and 40.6% for smoking in household Prevalence of FT§ ; OR =1.26 (0.93-1.69), 59.6% and 63.4%, respectively.
Periodontal disease	Arbes et al. 2001	6,611 persons 18+ years old United States (NHANES III)	Self-reported information Non-smokers having one or more persons smoked in their home, and/or one or more hours of smoke exposure at work	Prevalence of periodontal disease adjusted for age, sex, race/ethnicity, education, poverty index, history of diabetes and dental visits; Periodontal disease was defined as the presence of one or more sites with PPD¶ ≥ 4mm and CALⁿ ≥ 3mm OR =1.6 (1.1-2.2)
	Yamamoto et al. 2000	273 Japanese workers Aged 18-62 years Japan	Saliva cotinine level (1-7 ng/ml) Non smoking subjects including former smokers	Prevalence of periodontal disease adjusted for age, sex, alcohol consumption and body mass index; Periodontal disease was defined as the presence of two teeth with PPD¶ ≥3.5mm and CALⁿ ≥3.5mm OR =2.9(1.1-7.8)
Tooth loss	Tanaka et al. 2005	1,002 pregnant woman; mean age was 29.8 years and approximately 30% were between 29-31years of age	Self-reported information Non-smokers exposed to cigarette smoke at home or in workplace	Prevalence of tooth loss adjusted for age, gestation, parity, family income, education and body mass index; Prevalence of tooth loss was defined as extraction of one ore more teeth. OR = 0.77 (0.46–1.27) for subjects formerly exposed and 1.10 (0.67–1.82) for subjects currently exposed <10 cigarettes/day and 1.79 (1.08–2.94) for subjects currently exposed to 10+ cigarettes/day P for linear trend =0.03

*PAR = population attributable risk;
†SES = socioeconomic status;
‡DT = decayed deciduous and permanent teeth;
§FT= filled deciduous and permanent teeth;
¶PPD = probing pocket depth;
ⁿCAL = clinical attachment loss.

A brief explanation is provided regarding current etiology in order to describe the mechanism underlying the effects of passive smoking. Current information related to the relevant effect of active smoking may facilitate understanding of the mechanism of passive smoking: Many underlying mechanisms corresponding to increased risk of periodontal disease due to active smoking have been proposed. Effects of active smoking on gingival melanin pigmentation have also been demonstrated in epidemiological studies. Lack of data with respect to the effects of active smoking is evident in terms of dental caries and tooth loss.

In this chapter, we first present findings of black or brownish pigmentation in the gingiva of children as a predictor of the effect of passive smoking. Subsequently, we discuss several reports describing the effect of passive smoking on pediatric caries in epidemiological research and the possible mechanism. Finally, we review the literature in which the effect of passive smoking on periodontal disease and tooth loss as a consequence of periodontal disease was examined. We hope this chapter will enable researchers to address the issue in terms of the effects of passive smoking in the oral region.

1. Gingival Melanin Pigmentation

Epidemiology

Brownish or black discoloration in gingiva occurs as a solitary unit or as a continuous ribbon. Melanin pigmentation is distinguishable from other forms of oral pigmentation by macroscopic observation [1]. Melanin pigmentation in gingiva has been reported in many countries; however, prevalence rates are diverse, 5%-100%, according to race and country [2-10]. Gingival pigmentation is associated with that in the skin [2,3,11]. These characteristics are indicative of a hereditary connection. Intake of antimalarial drugs, including chloroquine [12] and quinidine [13], is associated with oral pigmentation; however, this phenomenon is rare.

Labial gingiva is the most evident localization of melanin pigmentation in Swedish [4] and Japanese [8]. Prevalence of pigmentation in labial gingiva of the anterior region is somewhat higher in mandible (53%) than in maxilla (43%) of Japanese. The prevalence rate decreased in buccal gingiva of posterior teeth (30%). In the palatal and lingual aspects of gingiva, the prevalence was less than 4%. However, melanin pigmentation was often observed in palatal gingiva of Malaysians [7].

Histopathology

Gingival melanin pigmentation derives from melanin granules in melanocytes, which are located at the basal layer of gingival epithelium [14]. Melanocytes were identified as dendritic cells, which are characterized by dendritic processes.

Melanin is synthesized from tyrosine and dihydroxyphenylalanine (DOPA) via dopaquinone by oxidation of tyrosinase [15]. Synthesis of melanin occurs in the melanosomes of melanocytes. Subsequently, melanin, which is transferred via specific processes to keratinocytes by phagocytic activity, is degraded as it ascends to the surface of the gingiva.

Effect of Active Smoking and Cessation

Active smoking enhances gingival pigmentation. This association has been reported in Israel [2], Great Britain and Sweden [5], Japan [6,8], Thailand and Malaysia [7], Turkey [9] and India [10]. Among 214 Swedish subjects, in particular, all individuals who displayed melanin pigmentation of the gingiva were smokers; the phenomenon was referred to as "smoker's melanosis" [7]. Tobacco smoking may stimulate melanin production in gingival tissue. Melanin pigmentation in smokers begins as a solitary unit in attached gingiva between the lateral incisor and the canine. Then, the number of solitary units increases in the labial gingiva such that the pigmentation appears as a continuous ribbon [4]. In the case of reverse smoking, excessive pigmentation due to tobacco smoke was observed in palatal mucosa [16]; however, this phenomenon is rare.

In addition to the fact that smokers exhibited a greater propensity toward pigmentation than did non-smokers, some evidence suggests the presence of a causal association between active smoking and gingival melanin pigmentation. Firstly, a dose-response relationship was observed [5-8]. Second, prevalence of pigmentation decreased in relation to the number of years following smoking cessation [17]. Rate of pigmentation decreased two years after cessation by approximately one half; moreover, the level of pigmentation was identical to that of never smokers more than three years after smoking cessation. Third, the biological mechanism of the association may be explained. Nicotine in tobacco smoke may enhance synthesis of DOPA, which produces melanin from tyrosine [15]. The stimulatory effect could occur as a result of the high affinity function of nicotine [18] and benzpyrene [19] in tobacco smoke relative to melanin.

The aforementioned mechanism is controversial. Exposure to ultraviolet light may contribute to melanin pigmentation in the gingiva since pigmentation often occurs in labial gingiva. This phenomenon is suggestive of a protective function of melanin pigmentation in terms of external attack. However, the wavelength of ultraviolet light is insufficiently short to penetrate lip and labial tissue. The protective function may be negligible with respect to tobacco smoke since exposure to tobacco smoke often occurs in palatal gingiva where melanin pigmentation is rarely observed. A scavenger function may be significant as the affinity of melanin to nicotine and benzpyrene is high. A predictor function, which indicates exposure to toxic substances, may be considered.

Production of melanin might be enhanced in the presence of gingival inflammation. A variety of inflammatory substances is produced in lesions of gingival tissue. A positive correlation was observed between density of melanophores in the vestibular epithelium and numbers of inflammatory cells in the attached gingiva [20]. However, correlation between the number of melanocytes in gingival tissue and visible pigmentation was not significant [21]. Inflammatory response in gingiva was suppressed in smokers in comparison with non-smokers [22]. Contrarily, gingival melanin pigmentation exhibits higher prevalence in smokers than in non-smokers. Therefore, the relationship between gingival pigmentation and inflammation should be addressed with caution. This relationship may be examined in the gingiva of smokers and non-smokers separately.

Gingival pigmentation is a normal symptom given that melanocytes were identified in the basal layer of gingival tissue in all subjects. However, some individuals desired removal of excessive gingival pigmentation for aesthetic reasons. Surgical and non-surgical methods, for example, Laser surgery and application of hydrogen peroxide to the gingiva, respectively, could evacuate melanin pigmentation from gingival tissue; however, in smokers, recurrence of pigmentation occurred following surgery [23].

Direct and indirect pathways may provide a mechanism with respect to how stimulatory substances in tobacco smoke reach melanocytes in gingiva. The most direct route is the penetration of substances through oral mucosa. Stimulatory substances can be dissolved in saliva and might reach melanocytes through gingival epithelium. Melanin pigmentation was often observed in the labial aspect of attached gingiva [4,7,8,10] where tobacco smoke may not overlap directly, although the majority of smoke is aspirated through the mouth. The palatal and lingual aspects of gingiva were exposed to the majority of tobacco smoke. Therefore, indirect stimulation of gingival pigmentation by nicotine and benzpyrene in tobacco smoke via the bloodstream may afford a more plausible mechanism.

Background Pertaining to the Effects of Passive Smoking

Melanin pigmentation production may be sensitive to tobacco smoke. Gingival melanin pigmentation in 317 Japanese men was surveyed in relation to active smoking at two workplace locations. Smoking rate by age group was similar between the locations. Prevalence of gingival pigmentation in smokers increased and approached maximum levels upon slight exposure to smoking in minimal categories of duration of smoking and number of cigarettes smoked (Figure 1). Melanin index was employed as an indicator of severity of pigmentation. Extent of pigmentation was evaluated according to type of formation of pigmentation, e.g., solitary unit or continuous ribbon. Severity of pigmentation exhibited a similar trend. These findings suggest that gingival melanocytes are sensitive to tobacco smoke with respect to production of melanin.

Subsequently, prevalence of melanin pigmentation was compared according to smoking status in two workplace locations. Prevalence of pigmentation in current smokers was similar, 81% and 85%, at the two locations. However, prevalence differed at the two locations among former and never smokers. Office workers displayed a higher prevalence rate relative to chemical plant workers, 70% versus 27% in former smokers and 37% versus 15% in never smokers, respectively (Figure 2). Odds ratios (OR) were 9.3 (95% confidence interval (CI) =2.2-38.9) in office workers and 21.1 (4.8-92.7) in chemical plant workers. This survey was performed in 1994. A national law prohibiting smoking in public space has been in effect since 2004; however, restriction of smoking in offices was a scarcely enforced regulation at that time. Regulation of smoking in the chemical plant was common due to fire prevention measures. Therefore, the apparent distinction in the prevalence rates of non-smoking workers may be attributable to differences in environmental tobacco smoke (ETS) between workplace locations.

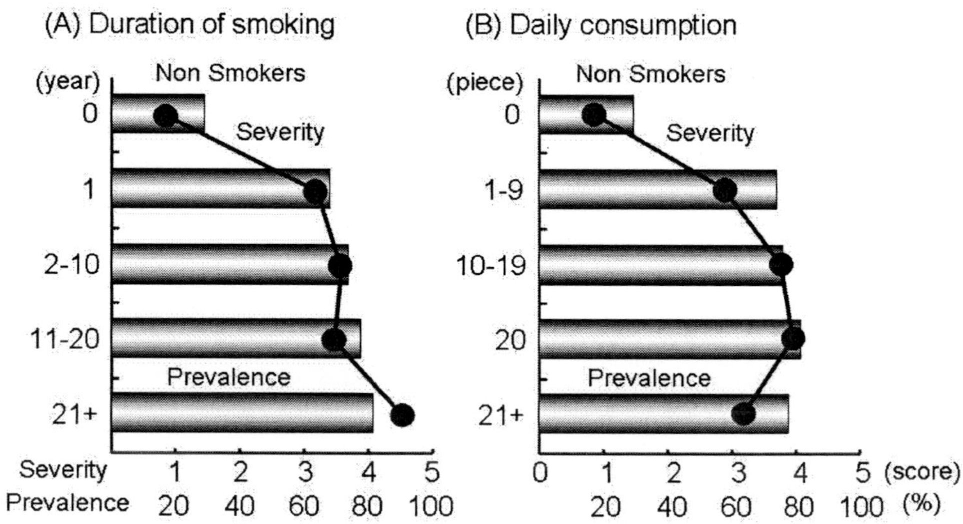

Figure 1. Prevalence and severity (Melanin Index) of gingival melanin pigmentation by duration of smoking (A) and daily consumption (B) indicating sensitivity of melanin production to tobacco smoke.

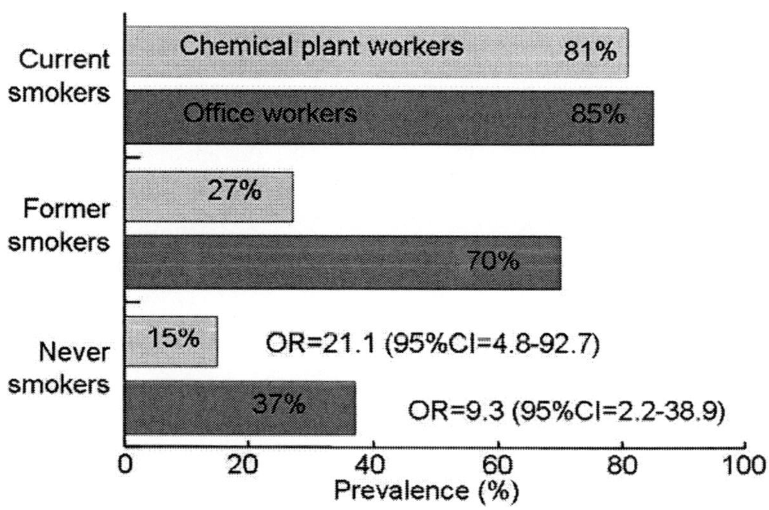

Figure 2. Differences in the prevalence of gingival melanin pigmentation between two workplace locations.

Effect of Passive Smoking on Gingival Melanin Pigmentation

Oral photographs of children were selected randomly from patient records of a private dental clinic in the northern region of Japan. Subjects consisted of 59 children (22 males and 37 females) aged 6 to 16 years (11.3 ± 2.5). Smoking status of children and parents was established via interview. Oral images of the frontal mouth were acquired with a digital camera (EOS D30, Canon Inc., Tokyo) equipped with wide-angle conversion lens (C-AF1 2X TELEPLUS MC7, Kenko Co., Tokyo).

No objective methodology has been developed for evaluation of gingival melanin pigmentation. Degree of gingival pigmentation was first introduced as scores of the Melanin Index [4]. Classification in terms of the assessment is subjective. The Melanin Index classifies gingival pigmentation in the labial aspect of anterior teeth utilizing the following criteria for each jaw: a score of 0 indicates no visible pigmentation; a score of 1 indicates one or two solitary unit(s) of pigmentation in attached gingiva without formation of a continuous ribbon of pigmentation between solitary units; a score of 2 indicates more than three units of pigmentation in papillary gingiva without formation of a continuous ribbon; a score of 3 indicates one or more short continuous ribbons of pigmentation; a score of 4 indicates one continuous ribbon including the entire area between canines. Total scores of the upper and lower jaws served as the Melanin Index score of each subject.

Gingival pigmentation in children is distinct from that in adults. Since keratinization of gingival tissue in children is often premature, gingival melanin may not be masked even in instances of slight pigmentation. We employed modifications of the Melanin Index categories in the assessment of gingival pigmentation of children. Each jaw was classified according to three categories (Figure 3): a score of 0 indicates no visible pigmentation; a score of 1 indicates solitary unit(s) of pigmentation in attached gingiva without formation of a continuous ribbon of pigmentation between solitary units; a score of 2 indicates at least one unit of continuous ribbon formation extending from two neighboring solitary units. Scores of 1 and 2 with respect to gingiva of children correspond to scores of 1 and 2 and scores of 3 and 4 of the Melanin Index, respectively.

These assessments were subjective; consequently, evaluation of the accuracy of the assessment is necessary in order to ensure proper methodology. The protocol of this retrospective study involved assessment of gingival pigmentation of children in oral photos, which were reproduced in a computer display. Melanin pigmentation was not masked in the gingiva of children; therefore, these reproductions exhibited size similar to that of the actual mouth. Two examiners were trained and calibrated using photographs which depicted typical examples of pigmentation. Subsequently, the examiners reviewed identical photos and inter-examiner agreement for the existence and extent of melanin pigmentation was evaluated with the K (kappa) statistic. Status of parental smoking, which was assessed via questionnaire, was withheld from the examiners. The K statistic for existence and extent of pigmentation was 0.73 and 0.68, respectively; these results indicated satisfactory inter-examiner agreement

No child reported active smoking. At least one parent of 36 children (61%) smoked. Mean duration of smoking was 19.8 (±4.2) years and mean number of daily consumption was 19.3 (±9.0) cigarettes. Two thirds of these parents smoked heavily (more than 20 cigarettes per day). Distribution of sex was similar between the non-smoking (39% in males) and smoking (36% in males) groups. Age was also similar, 11.4 ± 2.5 years in the non-smoking group and 11.4 ± 2.5 years in the smoking group.

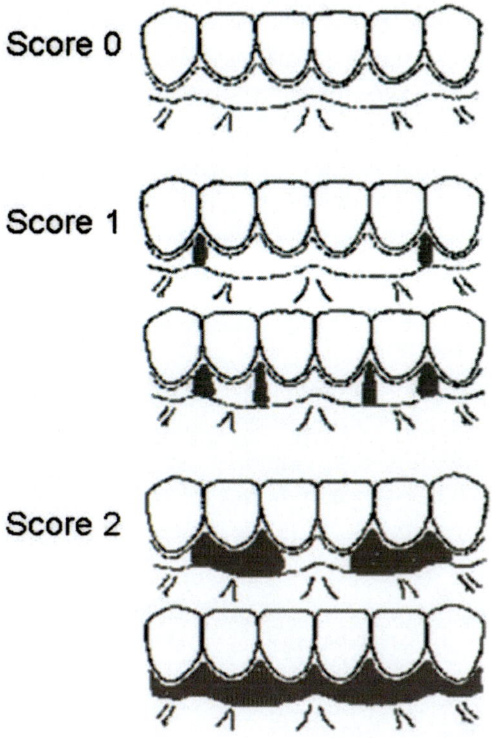

Figure 3. Modifications of the Melanin Index categories in the assessment of gingival pigmentation of children.

Typical photographs in which visible pigmentation in the gingiva of children is apparent or lacking are presented in Figure 4. Gingival pigmentation was assessed in the oral photos, which were reproduced in a computer display; furthermore, these reproductions exhibited size similar to that of the actual mouth.

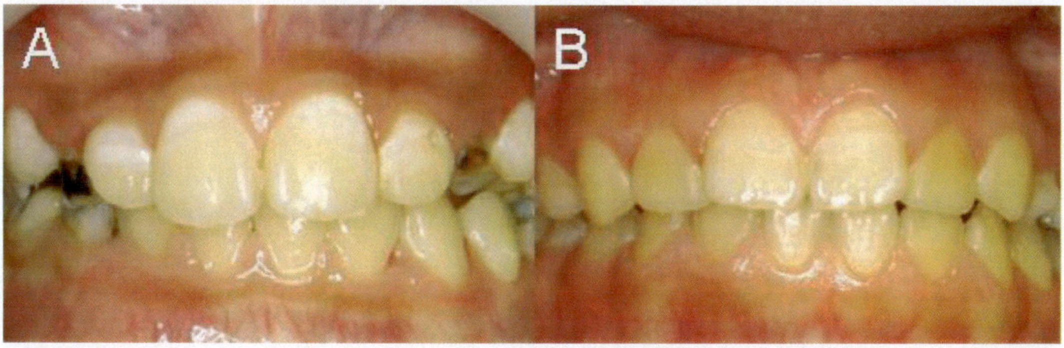

Figure 4. Typical photographs with (A) and without (B) visible pigmentation in the gingiva of children: the assessment of pigmentation was based on the oral photos, which were reproduced in a computer display with magnification of x 1.

Examiners A and B detected gingival pigmentation in 71% and 78% of children, respectively. Prevalence of pigmentation was similar in males and females. The percentage of children whose parents did not smoke was lower in subjects lacking visible pigmentation (35%) than in subjects displaying gingival pigmentation (70-71%, Figure 5). Continuous pigmentation (score 2), a form more distinct than solitary pigmentation, was noted in 42-46% of the children. Results of the assessment by examiner A revealed a higher percentage of smoking parents among children exhibiting solitary pigmentation (82%) in comparison to those characterized by continuous pigmentation (64%). The percentage was consistent with that of the assessment by examiner B. When children were grouped according to parental smoking status, prevalence of gingival pigmentation in children with at least one smoking parent was 83-89%. Gingival pigmentation in children whose parents did not smoke was less prevalent (52-60%).

Prevalence of gingival pigmentation in children demonstrated significant correlation with parental smoking status (Table 2). Crude Ors of parental smoking were 4.6 (1.4-15.2) and 5.1 (1.4-20.0) based on the assessments of examiners A and B, respectively. Adjusted ORs by sex and age were 5.6 (1.5-20.0) and 5.4 (1.4-21.2), respectively.

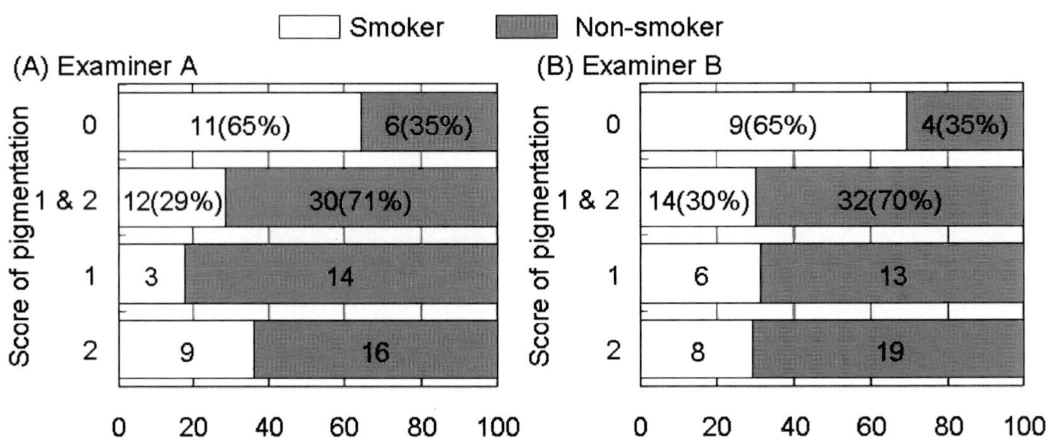

Figure 5. Distribution of smoking parents by melanin pigmentation score in the gingiva of their children according to observations of two examiners.

Table 2. Odds ratios (OR) and 95% confidence intervals (CI) of gingival pigmentation to parental smoking status based on the assessment of two examiners.

		Crude*		Adjusted	
Examiner	Parents	OR(95% CI)	P	OR(95% CI)	P
A	Non-smoker	1.0 (Reference)		1.0 (Reference)	
	Smoker	4.6 (1.4-15.2)	0.013	5.6 (1.5-20.0)	0.010
B	Non-smoker	1.0 (Reference)		1.0 (Reference)	
	Smoker	5.1 (1.4-20.0)	0.016	5.4 (1.4-21.2)	0.015

*Adjusted by sex and age.

In this study, accuracy of subjective assessment with respect to detection of gingival pigmentation was essential. Examiners detected pigmentation in 71-78% of children; additionally, percentages of parental smoking on the basis of the Melanin Index score and

ORs were similar between examiners. Furthermore, the K statistic was satisfactory with respect to inter-examiner reliability. The relationship between parental smoking status and degree of pigmentation was not clear. Development of objective measures to evaluate gingival melanin pigmentation may provide a suitable topic for a future investigation.

Chemical validation of exposure to ETS, for example, determination of cotinine level in serum and urine by gas chromatography, should be included in a future investigation. No data corresponding to the exact amount of time that smoking parents and their children spent together were available. Subjects in the present study resided in the northern region of Japan, where the climate is cold throughout the year. Most parents smoked moderately or heavily. Therefore, their children may be exposed to ETS for certain hours each day consequent to parental smoking. The meaningful relationship between parental smoking and gingival pigmentation in their children suggests the presence of an ETS effect.

Active smoking of participants was verified via an interview. In Japan, the smoking rate of adult males at ages corresponding to participating parents was approximately 60%. The smoking rate of adult females, which was less than 15%, was substantially lower than that of males. Therefore, a smoking rate among parents of 61% is a reasonable figure. In children, data from a national survey may also be suggestive with respect to estimation of the accuracy of the interview. Data of a national survey conducted in 1996 revealed that the smoking rate at the age of approximately 13 years was 0.7% in males and 0.4% in females. We believe that the influence of smoking parents and children who failed to report is minimal. The present study suggested an indirect association between passive smoking and gingival pigmentation.

The effect of ETS of parental origin may be underestimated due to the impact of ETS from additional sources. Passive smoking, other than that of parental origin, potentially may be similar or slightly higher in the smoking parental group than in the non-smoking parental group. National law restricting smoking in public areas was recently introduced in Japan.

Gingival pigmentation is not a predictor of parental smoking. Gingival pigmentation was frequently observed in children. In the present study, examiners observed photographs, which were similar in terms of actual mouth size; moreover, the prevalence of gingival pigmentation was 71-78% as a total. Melanocytes normally occur in the gingiva of all humans [1]. The results of the current study were suggestive of a relationship between excessive pigmentation in the gingiva of children and passive smoking [24].

2. Dental Caries

Etiology of Dental Caries

Dental caries are an infectious and communicable disease [25]. Dental caries, which are a multifactorial condition, are caused by the interaction of three major factors: tooth surface, cariogenic bacteria and fermentable carbohydrates. Cariogenic bacteria, in particular, *Streptococcus mutans* and *S. lactobacill*, convert carbohydrates into acids, e.g., lactic acid, via fermentation processes. Dental plaque consists of bacteria and bacterial metabolic products such as water-insoluble glucan, which adheres to the tooth surface. When plaque remains in contact with the tooth surface, acid produced in the plaque induces demineralization, i.e., dissolution of the mineral content of the tooth enamel.

Dental caries, if untreated, generally progress to incapacitating pain and bacterial infection, which leads to pulpal necrosis, tooth extraction and loss of dental function. Furthermore, untreated dental caries may result in an acute systemic infection.

Epidemiological Findings of Passive Smoking

To identify those epidemiologic studies pertaining to the association between ETS exposure and dental caries, a search of the PubMed databases of the National Library of Medicine was conducted for English language publications from 1965-2005. The following MeSH keywords were used: "passive smoking", "environmental tobacco smoke", "second-hand smoke" and "dental caries". These keywords were entered in the title/abstract field. Four studies that addressed the association between ETS exposure and dental caries were published between 1997 and 2004. One on-going investigation was also included (Table 1).

Relationships between socioeconomic and sociodemographic factors as well as caries experience in 5- and 12-year-old children were represented by samples from eight countries of the European Union [26]. In both age groups, risk indicators for dental caries were social class of the family, the mother's smoking habits, and, in the 5-year-olds, the number of siblings.

The relationship between parental smoking practices and caries prevalence among pre-school children was examined using data derived from the UK National Diet and Nutrition Survey in 1995 [27]. Social class, which was a confounding factor with smoking practices, was categorized into non-manual and manual occupation groups. Maternal smoking practices were correlated with prevalence of caries in each social class. ORs in manual and non-manual social classes were 1.55 and 1.96, respectively.

The association between exposure to ETS and risk of dental caries was tested in databases of a nationally representative population of the NHANES III [28]. Serum cotinine level served as a measure of ETS exposure; the cutoff value was 0.2 ng/ml. In deciduous teeth, elevated cotinine levels displayed significant correlation with dental caries. Adjusted ORs were 1.8 (1.2-2.7) for risk of decayed surfaces and 1.4 (1.1-2.0) for filled surfaces. In permanent teeth, the relationship between cotinine level and dental caries was not meaningful. These data also suggested a dose-response relationship between cotinine level and risk of decayed surfaces in deciduous teeth.

The association between exposure to ETS and primary dental caries among a birth cohort in the Iowa Fluoride Study was examined [29]. Children residing with individuals who smoked were at increased risk for developing dental caries. Overall, children residing with individuals who regularly smoked displayed a higher prevalence of dental caries. For the middle socio-economic status (SES) group and overall, children from smoking homes demonstrated a markedly higher prevalence of caries in comparison to children from non-regular/non-smoking homes (52% vs 24%, P=0.05 and 44% vs 25%, P=0.002, respectively). Following adjustment for age, SES, toothbrushing frequency, total ingested fluoride and combined intake of soda pop and powdered beverages, the relationship between smoking and dental caries remained significant (OR=3.38, P=0.001).

Smoking in the household was independently associated with increased prevalence of decayed teeth in Japanese children [30]. The adjusted mean of filled teeth among children exposed to household smoking was higher than that among non-exposed subjects. However, no statistically significant relationship was observed between household smoking and caries experience.

Possible Mechanism

Several key components may underlie the association between active smoking and dental caries: bacterial profile, formation of dental plaque, pH of dental plaque and buffering capacity as well as the protective function of saliva with respect to enamel demineralization. Most epidemiological studies that addressed the relationship between active smoking and dental caries did not include potential confounders [31]. Furthermore, exposure to ETS may be correlated with SES, poor dietary habits, low fluoride exposure or other unknown factors that may influence the oral health of children.

Health consequences of active smoking were examined in adolescents and adults; children were the focal point in terms of the effects of passive smoking. Those effects of passive and active smoking on dental caries that may operate via common mechanisms are unclear. Evidence is inconsistent with respect to effects of active smoking on increased risk of dental caries. In the chapter of dental diseases of the Surgeon General's Reports in 2004 [31], a conclusion indicated that the evidence was inadequate to infer the presence or absence of a causal relationship between active smoking and coronal dental caries.

Substances in tobacco products may influence the growth of oral cariogenic streptococci. However, this *in vitro* study involved only smokeless tobacco products. Sugar in smokeless tobacco, which may be added to the product, enhances oral cariogenic streptococci growth. The potential relationship between tobacco smoke and growth of cariogenic oral flora has not been examined.

Biological evidence in terms of causal role of ETS with dental caries are scarce: Mothers who smoke may be more likely than nonsmokers to transmit *S. mutans*. to their children since nicotine may promote the growth of this microorganism [32]. ETS possesses immunosuppressive properties and may cause infections in children [33].

3. Periodontal Disease

Etiology of Periodontal Disease and Measures of the Disease

The periodontium includes hard and soft tissue structures that support the teeth, namely, gingiva, cementum, periodontal ligament and alveolar bone. The cementum covers the root surfaces of the teeth and the periodontal ligament attaches the tooth root surfaces to the adjacent alveolar bone, which supports each tooth. The most common categories of periodontal diseases and conditions are gingivitis and chronic periodontitis. Gingivitis is defined as an inflammation of the gingiva. Clinically, gingivitis is characterized by redness, gingival bleeding, edema or enlargement. Gingival sensitivity and tenderness are occasionally observed. Chronic periodontitis is an inflammation of the gingiva and the adjacent attachment apparatus. This inflammatory disease is characterized by loss of clinical attachment due to destruction of the periodontal ligament and loss of the adjacent supporting bone. Clinical features include edema, erythema, gingival bleeding upon periodontal probing, periodontal pocket formation or suppuration. The most common forms of both diseases involve bacterial infection. Destruction of periodontal tissue is attributable to bacterial toxins and proteases, and hyperresponsiveness and reactivity of various components of the immune system, for example, cytokines and prostaglandins.

Periodontal destruction may be estimated by dental professionals utilizing a periodontal probe. Probing pocket depth (PPD) is the most frequent measure of periodontal destruction. A calibrated probe is inserted into the gingival pocket and the distance from the gingival margin to the bottom of the gingival pocket is measured in millimeters. PPD greater than 4 mm indicates the presence of disease at the specific site. The pathogenesis of periodontitis involves destruction of the junctional epithelium at the base of the sulcus; consequently, clinical attachment level (CAL) is the second common measure of periodontitis. CAL is measured as the distance from the cement-enamel junction to the base of the gingival pocket in millimeters. Currently, change in CAL is considered the superior indicator of periodontal destruction.

Epidemiological Findings of Active Smoking

The epidemiologic literature is highly consistent in terms of the existence of a moderate to strong correlation between cigarette smoking and periodontal destruction [31]. The association is consistent throughout case definitions, populations and study designs, which display a wide range of variability. Findings of case-control and cross-sectional studies were consistent; furthermore, cohort studies documented risk ratios of 1.4 to more than 10 with respect to the relationship between active smoking and onset or progression of periodontitis. These investigations also employed a wide range of outcome measures. Cross-sectional studies reported that current smokers were more likely to exhibit periodontitis than former smokers. A dose-response relationship was evident between the amount of smoking and risk and severity of periodontitis.

The risk of periodontitis diminished following smoking cessation. The risk of periodontitis decreased as the duration of successful cessation increased. A few prospective cohort studies consistently found that smokers were more likely than nonsmokers to experience onset or progression of disease. The Surgeon General's Reports in 2004 concluded that evidence is sufficient to infer a causal relationship between smoking and periodontitis [31].

Epidemiological Findings of Passive Smoking

The association between ETS and periodontal disease was initially reported based on analysis of the national database of NHANES III [34]. Adjusted odds for periodontal disease were 1.6 times greater for individuals exposed to passive smoke than for those not exposed via evaluation of self-reported ETS exposure in the home and in the workplace.

Non-smokers, passive smokers and active smokers were defined according to the level of cotinine in saliva [35]. Odds ratios in passive and active smokers relative to non-smokers following adjustment for other lifestyle factors were 2.87 (1.05–7.82) and 4.91 (1.80–13.35), respectively.

The relationship between passive smoking and tooth loss was examined in pregnant Japanese woman [36]. A significant positive correlation was observed between current heavy passive smoking (more than 10 cigarettes / day) at home and tooth loss. In Japan, periodontal disease is a major factor in tooth loss.

The design of these epidemiological studies was cross-sectional; as a result, current or recent exposure to ETS was evaluated. To characterize the relationship between passive smoking and periodontal disease in greater detail, future investigations might employ the cohort design; however, this type of study may not be permissible due to ethical concerns.

Possible Mechanism

In a manner similar to the mechanisms governing the relationship between passive smoking and dental caries, exposure to ETS and active cigarette smoking likely affect periodontal disease via common mechanisms. The mechanisms involved in smoking-associated periodontal destruction have not been fully elucidated [31].

An immune mechanism is plausible as smoking affects various components of the immune system. Decreases in local and systemic immune function in smokers may elevate susceptibility to bacterial infection. Local effects of smoking on vasoconstriction and reduction in oxygen tension in periodontal tissue may create a favorable subgingival environment for colonization by anaerobic bacteria. Systemic effects include impairment of chemotaxis and of both oral and peripheral neutrophil phagocytosis and chemotaxis, suppression of osteoblast proliferation and stimulation of alkaline phosphatase activity.

ETS may be inhaled via the nose rather than via the mouth. Thus, ETS is likely to affect periodontal disease based on systemic mechanisms. Substantially, smoking impairs regeneration and repair of periodontal tissues. Qualitative as well as quantitative evidence is inconsistent regarding alteration by smoking of microflora of subgingival plaque.

Conclusion

Oral health research in terms of passive smoking has been initiated only recently. The evidence is suggestive with respect to gingival melanin pigmentation, dental caries, periodontal disease and tooth loss. Additional research may involve epidemiologic studies.

Although results of biological investigations related to active smoking may support a relevant association regarding passive smoking, a more accurate explanation than that afforded by current findings is required.

References

[1] Çiçek, Y. & Ertas, Ü. (2003). The normal and pathological pigmentation of oral mucous membrane: a review. *J Contemp Dent Pract, 15*, 76-86.

[2] Steigmann, S. (1965). The relation between physiologic pigmentation of the skin and the oral mucosa in Yemenite Jews. *Oral Surg, 19*, 32-8.

[3] Fry, L. & Almeyda, J. R. (1968). The incidence of buccal pigmentation in Caucasoids and Negroids in Britain. *Br J Dermatol, 80*, 244-7.

[4] Hedin, C. A. (1977). Smoker's melanosis. Occurence and localization in the attached gingiva. *Arch Dermatol*, 1977;113:1533-1538

[5] Axell, T. & Hedin, C. A. (1982). Epidemiologic study of excessive oral melanin pigmentation with special reference to the influence of tobacco habits. *Scand J Dent Res, 90*, 434-42.

[6] Araki, S., Murata, K., Ushio, K., Sakai, R. (1983). Dose-response relationship between tobacco consumption and melanin pigmentation in the attached gingiva. *Arch Environ Health, 138*, 375-8.

[7] Hedin, C. A. & Axell, T. (1991). Oral melanin pigmentation in 467 Thai and Malaysian people with special emphasis on smoker's melanosis. *J Oral Pathol Med, 20*, 8-12.

[8] Hanioka, T., Tanaka, M., Tamagawa, H., Shizukuishi, S. (1993). Epidemiologic study of melanin pigmentation in the attached gingiva in relation to cigarette smoking. *J Dent Health, 43*, 40-7 (in Japanese).

[9] Ünsal, E., Paksoy, C., Soykan, E., Elhan, A. H., Şahin, M. (2001). Oral melanin pigmentation related to smoking in a Turkish population. *Community Dent Oral Epidemiol, 29*, 272-7.

[10] Sarswathi, T. R., Kumar, S. N., Kavitha, K. M. (2003). Oral melanin pigmentation in smoked and smokeless tobacco users in India. Clinico-pathological study. *Indian J Dent Res, 14*, 101-6.

[11] Dummett, C. O. (1959). Oral pigmentation –physiologie and pathologie. *NY State Dent J, 25*, 188-90.

[12] Dencker, L., Lindquist, N. G., Tjalve, H. (1976). Uptake of ^{14}C-labelled chloroquine and an ^{125}I-labelled chloroquine analogue in some polypeptide hormone producing cell systems. *Med Biol, 54*, 62-8.

[13] Main, J. H. P. (1988). Two cases of oral pigmentation associated with quinidine therapy. *Oral Surg, 66*, 59-61.

[14] Hedin, C. A. &, Larsson, A. (1984). The ultrastructure of the gingival epithelium in smoker's melanosis. *J Periodont Res, 19*, 177-190.

[15] Halaban, R., Cheng, E., Svedine, S., Aron, R., Hebert, D. N. (2001). Proper folding and endoplasmic reticulum to golgi transport of tyrosinase are induced by its substrates, DOPA and tyrosine. *J Biol Chem, 276*, 11933-8.

[16] Hedin, C. A., Pidborg, J. J., Daftary, D. K., Mehta, F. S. (1992). Melanin pigmentation of the palatal mucosa in reverse smokers: a preliminary study. *J Oral Pathol Med, 21*, 440-4.

[17] Hedin, C. A., Pindborg, J. J., Axell, T. (1993). Disappearance of smoker's melanosis after reducing smoking. *J Oral Pathol Med, 22*, 228-30.

[18] Claffey, D. J., Stout, P. R., Ruth, J. A. (2001). ^{3}H-nicotine, ^{3}H-flunitrazepam, and ^{3}H-cocaine incorporation into melanin: a model for the examination of drug-melanin interactions. *J Anal Toxicol, 25*, 607-11.

[19] Roberto, A., Larsson, B. S., Tjarve, H. (1996). Uptake of 7,12-dimethylbenz(a)anthracene and benzo(a)pyrene in melanin-containing tissues, *Pharmacol Toxicol, 79*, 92-9.

[20] Patsakas A, Demetriou N, Angelopoulos A (1981). Melanin pigmentation and inflammation in human gingiva, *J Periodontol, 52*, 701-4.

[21] Schreoder, H. E. (1969). Melanin containing organelles in cells of the human gingiva. II. Keratinocytes. *J Periodont Res, 4*, 235-47.

[22] Lie, M. A., Timmerman, M. F., van der Velden, U., van der Weijden, G. A. (1998). Evaluation of 2 methods to assess gingival bleeding in smokers and non-smokers in natural and experimental gingivitis. *J Clin Periodontol 25*: 695-700.

[23] Tamizi, M. & Taheri M. (1996). Treatment of severe physiologic pigmentation with free gingival autograft. *Quintessence Int, 27*, 555-8.

[24] Hanioka, T., Tanaka, K., Ojima, M., Yuuki, K. (2005). Association of melanin pigmentation in the gingiva of children with parents who smoke, Pediatrics, 116, 186-90.

[25] Featherstone, J. D. B. (1999) Prevention and reversal of dental caries: role of low level fluoride. *Community Dent Oral Epidemiol, 27*, 31-40.

[26] Bolin, A. K., Bolin, A., Jansson, L., Calltorp, J. (1997). Children's dental health in Europe. *Swed Dent J, 21*, 25-40.

[27] Williams, S. A., Kwan, S. Y. L., Parsons, S. (2000). Parental smoking practices and caries experience in pre-school children. *Caries Res, 34*, 117-22.

[28] Aligne, C. A., Moss, M. E., Auinger, P., Weitzman, M. (2003). Association of pediatric dental caries with passive smoking. *JAMA, 12*, 1258-64.

[29] Shekin, J. D., Broffitt, B., Levy, S. M., Warren, J. J. (2004). The association between environmental tobacco smoke and primary tooth caries. *J Public Health Dent 64*, 184-6.

[30] Tanaka, K., Hanioka, T., Miyake, Y., Ojima, M., Aoyama, H. Association of smoking in household and dental caries in Japan, *J Public Health Dent*, in press.

[31] USDHHS. Dental diseases, In: *The health consequences of smoking: a report of the Surgeon General*, Washington DC, USDHHS, 2004; 732-66.

[32] Lindemeyer, R. G.., Baum, R. H., Hsu, S. C., Going, R. E. (1981), In vitro effect of tobacco on the growth of oral cariogenic streptococci. *J Am Dent Assoc, 103*, 719-22.

[33] Kum-Nji, P., Meloy, L., Herrod, H. G. (2006). Environmental tobacco smoke exposure: prevalence and mechanisms of causation of infections in children. *Pediatrics, 117*, 1745-54.

[34] Arbes, S. J. Jr, Ágústsdósttir, H., Slade, G. D. (2001) Environmental tobacco smoke and periodontal disease in the United States. *Am J Public Health, 91*, 253-7.

[35] Yamamoto, Y., Nishida, N., Tanaka, M., Hayashi, N., Matsuse, R., Nakayama, K., Morimoto, K., Shizukuishi, S. (2005) Association between passive and active smoking evaluated by salivary cotinine and periodontitis. *J Clin Periodontol, 32*, 1041-6.

[36] Tanaka, K., Miyake, Y., Sasaki, S., Ohya, Y., Miyamoto, S., Matsunaga, I., Yoshida, T., Hirota, Y., Oda, H., The Osaka Maternal and Child Health Study Group. (2005). Active and passive smoking and tooth Loss in Japanese women: baseline data from the Osaka Maternal and Child Health Study. *Ann Epidemiol, 15*, 358–64.

INDEX

A

B

C

D

E

F

G

H

I

J

K

N

O

P

Q

R

S

T

U

V

W

Y

Z